Values and Vaccine Refusal

In this first book-length philosophical treatment of vaccine refusal, Mark Navin argues that we can best understand current debates by placing them in a broader narrative about medical expertise and civic engagement. *Values and Vaccine Refusal* focuses on the shifting epistemic and moral terrain surrounding an educated public's relationship with health care and society – a relationship characterized by wariness of experts and elites, withdrawal from participation in public projects, and do-it-yourself models of reasoning and practice. This is a must-read for students and researchers interested in public health, social epistemology, and the ethical dimensions of both.

Mark Navin is Associate Professor of Philosophy at Oakland University (Rochester, MI). His research focuses on ethical issues in law and public policy. In addition to his work on vaccine refusal, he has published on topics including human rights, inequality, conscientious objection, international development assistance, social segregation, and food justice.

Values and Vaccine Refusal

Hard Questions in Ethics, Epistemology, and Health Care

Mark Navin

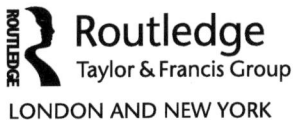

LONDON AND NEW YORK

First published 2016
by Routledge

2 Park Square, Milton Park, Abingdon, Oxfordshire OX14 4RN
711 Third Avenue, New York, NY 10017

Routledge is an imprint of the Taylor & Francis Group, an informa business

First issued in paperback 2017

Library of Congress Cataloging in Publication Data
Navin, Mark.
Values and vaccine refusal : hard questions in ethics, epistemology,
and health care / Mark Navin.
pages cm
Includes bibliographical references and index.
1. Vaccines. 2. Vaccination. 3. Knowledge, Theory of. I. Title.
QR189.N38 2015
615.3'72--dc23
2015012693

ISBN: 978-1-138-79065-0 (hbk)
ISBN: 978-1-138-47821-3 (pbk)

Typeset in Goudy
by Taylor & Francis Books

For my parents

Contents

Preface

Some books about vaccine refusal begin with stories of small children fighting vaccine-preventable diseases, including rotavirus (Largent 2012), *Haemophilus influenzae* type b (Hib) (Mnookin 2011), and measles (Offit 2010). I am moved by the suffering of infants, but compassion did not drive me to write this book. I wrote out of anger.

I started thinking about vaccine refusal in 2011, when I realized that some of my friends and acquaintances were choosing not to vaccinate their children. I discovered through casual conversations what recent research (e.g. Nyhan et al. 2014) has confirmed: People who believe vaccines are harmful or ineffective usually cannot be convinced otherwise, even though there is overwhelming scientific evidence they are wrong. In the summer of 2011, my son was only a few months old. He was too young to have received more than a handful of vaccines. Yet people around me had chosen to put him at risk of vaccine-preventable diseases, even though they could have easily avoided doing so. I thought these people were ignorant, irrational, and wicked. I seethed just to think of them.

Philosophy can be therapeutic for people who are plagued by anger or resignation. In ancient Athens, Epicurus taught that rational reflection about our world cultivates tranquility of mind. In 19th-century Germany, Hegel wrote that philosophy reconciles us to an otherwise alienating world, by revealing that there are reasons for what may seem to be irrational. I confess I have not yet achieved tranquility in my thinking about vaccine refusal, and I continue to believe there are overwhelming reasons to vaccinate one's children. But I have gone a long way towards making sense of the apparent nonsense of refusing vaccines. This book is the evidence of my progress, such as it is. In the following chapters, I argue that a decision to refuse vaccines is often an understandable consequence of psychological, social, and political forces beyond an individual parent's control. I no longer think vaccine refusal is a sign of unusual cognitive or moral deficiencies. Instead, the vices that lead to vaccine refusal are all too common, including among people who vaccinate.

Vaccine refusal matters. Vaccines have saved millions of lives and have prevented disease and serious complications for countless more. For many decades, parents in the developed world have lived without much fear of their young children suffering and dying in disease outbreaks. The public health benefits of mass vaccination should be obvious, but significant (though less visible) benefits have also accrued to education, public trust, national security, and the economy. Parents who refuse routine vaccines may place all these goods at risk. We must understand and evaluate vaccine refusal, to ensure that our responses to it will be justified and effective.

Many good books have been written about historical and contemporary vaccine refusal, but I have tried to do something new. In this book I evaluate and explain vaccine refusal by reflecting on complex relationships between knowledge, gender, science communication, democracy, the moral and political status of children, and the rights and duties of parents. I have drawn on work in bioethics, social and political philosophy, social epistemology, and socially relevant philosophy of science. One of my main goals is to show that vaccine refusal often results from (or manifests) disagreements about non-epistemic values. Vaccine refusal is, therefore, a case study of how disputes about science-informed policy are (also) often disagreements about what matters in our social and political worlds.

Bibliography

Largent, M. A. 2012. *Vaccine: The Debate in Modern America.* Johns Hopkins University Press.

Mnookin, Seth. 2011. *The Panic Virus: A True Story of Medicine, Science, and Fear.* Simon & Schuster.

Nyhan, Brendan, Jason Reifler, Sean Richey, and Gary L. Freed. 2014. "Effective Messages in Vaccine Promotion: A Randomized Trial." *Pediatrics* 133(4): e835–e842. doi: 10.1542/peds.2013-2365.

Offit, Paul A. 2010. *Deadly Choices: How the Anti-Vaccine Movement Threatens Us All.* Basic Books.

Acknowledgments

I thank Phyllis Rooney for encouraging me to consider how epistemology and the philosophy of science could inform my work on ethical and political questions. Phyllis and Ami Harbin read and commented on drafts of each chapter, and they were the first to encourage me to develop this project into a book. I have been fortunate to have such supportive colleagues. Indeed, I am grateful for the support I received from so many of my colleagues at Oakland University – in the Philosophy Department and beyond.

I thank the many people who read and commented on individual chapters, and whose conversations forced me to reconsider and refocus my views. These include Jacob Affolter, Michael Doan, Jessica Flanigan, Leslie Francis, Maya Goldenberg, Melinda Hall, Peter Higgins, Mark Huston, Kristen Intemann, Dan Kahan, Anna Kirkland, Ashley Kennedy, Mark Kuczewski, Mark Largent, Heidi Malm, Adrienne Martin, Michael Merry, Nicolae Morar, Dan Moseley, Tatiana Patrone, Roland Pierik, Susan Purviance, Abraham Schwab, Jonathan Simmons, and Sarah Wieten. I am also grateful to participants at Western Michigan University's Medical Humanities Conference (2012, 2013, and 2014), the Values in Medicine, Science, and Technology Conference at the University of Texas at Dallas (2013), the North American Society for Social Philosophy's International Social Philosophy Conference (2014), the Michigan Academy of Science, Arts and Letters (2014), AMINTAPHIL (2014), the Central Division Meeting of the APA (2015), and colloquia at both Eastern Michigan University and Oakland University. I also thank the students in my winter 2015 course on "Science Denialism and Democracy," and especially those who offered comments on my manuscript: Jenna Duronio, Katherine Eckenwiler, Olivia Hardin, Megan Luther, and Brooke Shepard.

During the past four summers, Oakland University funded undergraduate research assistants. Chief among these was Karl Martin Adam, whose comments and research inform every page of this book. I am also grateful for the research support of Nikole Fisher, Brooke Shepard, Caroline Fienberg, Paul Albarran, Brett Ammon, Jennifer Cepnick, and Lisa Vecchio.

I appreciate the guidance of Andrew Beck at Routledge. Andy and his assistants, John Downes-Angus and Laura Briskman, helped me along at every stage. I also thank the three anonymous reviewers for their many helpful comments and suggestions.

Finally, thank you to my family. Lillian, Phoebe, and Ezra often played quietly while I wrote a bit on weekend mornings. This project began in late-night conversations I had with Debra, as we puzzled over the fact that some of our friends had not vaccinated their children. Like many of the best things in my life, my work on this project has been sustained by Debra's love for me.

Chapter one includes material that was previously published in "Competing Epistemic Spaces: How Social Epistemology Helps Explain and Evaluate Vaccine Denialism," *Social Theory and Practice* 39/2 (April 2013), 241–64. (Copyright 2013 by *Social Theory and Practice*.) Chapter four includes material that was previously published in "Resisting Moral Permissiveness about Vaccine Refusal," *Public Affairs Quarterly* 27/1 (January 2013), 69–85. (Copyright 2013 by the Board of Trustees of the University of Illinois Press.) I thank the publishers of both journals for allowing this material to be reprinted here.

Introduction

We live in a hopeful age for vaccines. In most societies, vaccination rates are at historical highs. Many societies possess *herd immunity* against diseases that previously ravaged their populations: It is unlikely that unvaccinated members of these societies will be exposed to the diseases against which vaccines offer protection. We have new vaccines against deadly pathogens, including human papillomavirus (HPV), which causes most of the cancers of the cervix, vagina, and anus. Public and private actors, such as the Bill and Melinda Gates Foundation, have dedicated billions of dollars to vaccination efforts in the developing world, and we may eradicate polio within a generation.

But all is not well. Many parents in the United States are hesitant to vaccinate their children. Increasing numbers are rejecting some vaccines, or are slowing down the vaccine schedule, or are choosing not to vaccinate at all. In absolute terms, rates of vaccination remain high enough not to place the country at significant risk of massive disease outbreaks. But there are more vaccine refusers every year. Also, parents who refuse vaccines are often geographically clustered, which makes smaller outbreaks more likely. Recent outbreaks of mumps in Ohio, pertussis in Michigan, and measles in California are evidence of the magnifying effects of geographic clustering.

In this book, I argue that vaccine refusal is a symptom of changes in the educated public's relationship with both health care and the political community. We are less trusting of experts and elites, less engaged in public projects, and more attracted to do-it-yourself models of reasoning and practice. On my view, vaccine refusers are often committed to ways of reasoning – both about what to believe and what to do – that are understandable (and sometimes commendable) given the conditions under which they are making up their minds. So, if we are committed to protecting vaccination programs, we ought to focus our attention on the deeper social and political causes of contemporary vaccine refusal.

In this Introduction, I provide background information about the science and history of vaccines (and vaccine refusal) to inform the epistemological and ethical arguments I develop throughout the rest of the book. I begin by defining some key terms. Then, I review the history of vaccination (especially in English-speaking countries), with a special focus on early vaccine refusers. I follow with an outline of the ways in which contemporary vaccines work and the manner in which contemporary vaccination policies proceed. Then, I review the main complaints of today's vaccine refusers, and I conclude with an outline of the six chapters of the book.

Key terms

There is a contentious debate about what to call people who reject mainstream beliefs and practices surrounding vaccination. Some say that these people are *anti-vaccine* (Jacobson, Targonski, and Poland 2007; Ołpiński 2012; Wolfe and Sharp 2002). But many people who have been labeled this way describe themselves as advocates of *vaccine safety* (National Vaccine Information Center 2015; Wakefield 2011).

In an attempt to sidestep terminological disputes, I will use the term *vaccine denialist* to name people who deny significant aspects of the mainstream medical consensus regarding the risks and benefits of vaccines. This term is common in the literature (MacKenzie 2010). Vaccine denialism exists along a spectrum: An extreme vaccine denialist believes that vaccines are entirely ineffective and always cause at least some harms. A more moderate vaccine denialist may believe that a child's immune system can be overwhelmed if a child receives more than one vaccine at a time (Sears 2007). This form of vaccine denialism is consistent with the belief that individual vaccines are safe and effective, but is nonetheless false and, therefore, an instance of vaccine denialism (Centers for Disease Control and Prevention 2012b; DeStefano, Price, and Weintraub 2013; M. J. Smith and Woods 2010).

I will use the term *vaccine refuser* to identify people who have actively refused (or who intend to refuse) routine childhood vaccines for non-medical reasons.[1] This is also a standard term (Glanz et al. 2009; Omer et al. 2009; Wei et al. 2009). There is a great deal of overlap between vaccine denialists and vaccine refusers, but the memberships of these groups are not perfectly coextensive: Some vaccine refusers do not reject the scientific consensus about vaccine risks, and some vaccine denialists choose to vaccinate their children. Like vaccine denialism, vaccine refusal also exists along a spectrum. On one extreme are people who never vaccinate their children against any diseases. On the other extreme are people who may delay some routine vaccines, but who intend for their children to become fully vaccinated. It is also important to distinguish vaccine refusers from the *undervaccinated*. The parents of undervaccinated children are often socially and economically disadvantaged and are not usually vaccine denialists. Their failure to be up-to-date on their children's vaccinations is caused by their inability to access medical care; it is not a goal they have purposefully pursued (Healy and Pickering 2011; Omer et al. 2009).

I will sometimes speak of *vaccine hesitancy*, by which I mean a hesitation to defer to medical experts and public health advocates about either *what to believe* about vaccines or *what to do* in the face of vaccine choices. Vaccine hesitancy is also a standard term (Dubé et al. 2013; M. J. Smith and Marshall 2010). It is a common gateway to both vaccine denialism and vaccine refusal.

Finally, I will often talk about vaccine denialism and vaccine refusal as organizing ideas for collective activities. Here, I include everything from group discussion of key literature (books, websites), to participation in advocacy groups, to membership in online parenting communities. The social groups which promote vaccine denialism and vaccine refusal differ according to the additional social causes they often advocate. For example, vaccine denialism and refusal may be complementary practices for groups focused on early childhood issues (alternative birthing practices, breast-feeding, autism 'prevention' and 'treatment'), broader social issues (food politics, environmental sustainability), and explicitly political concerns (libertarianism, 'parents' rights').

Vaccines

Immunity is an old idea. Many people in the ancient world knew they could be resistant to diseases from which they had recovered. For example, the ancient Greek historian Thucydides wrote in the 5th century BCE that Athenians who had recovered from a disease were able to safely tend to those who were still suffering from it (Thucydides 1972, bk. 2.51).

The active cultivation of immunity is an old practice. We have evidence that the Chinese were deliberately immunizing themselves against smallpox a thousand years ago, by inhaling powders made from the dried blisters of smallpox sores (Behbehani 1983; Leung 2011). By the 16th century, active cultivation of smallpox immunity through hypodermic exposure to antigenic material was common in India and Turkey. Here, the idea was to introduce material from the blister of a person with a mild case of smallpox (*Variola minor*) into a wound on a healthy person's body. These people would contract a mild form of smallpox and would thereafter be immune to subsequent (and more severe) infections (of *Variola major*). This process was called *variolation* (after the name of the smallpox pathogen, *variola*).

Lady Mary Wortley Montagu learned of variolation in the late 1710s while living in Istanbul as the wife of the British ambassador to the Ottoman Empire, where the practice had long been common (Fenner et al. 1988). She introduced smallpox variolation to British high society in the 1720s. Variolation was introduced in the American colonies at around the same time. Cotton Mather, a famous early American religious leader, learned of the method from one of his slaves, Onesimus, and Mather worked to spread variolation in the American colonies (Henderson 2009; Silverman 2001).

The age of vaccination began in 1796, when Edward Jenner first successfully immunized people against smallpox (Jenner 1798). What made Jenner's active cultivation of smallpox immunity unique is that it used material from cowpox sores. (Hence *vaccination*, which derives from the Latin word for cow.) When Jenner's method was successful, a vaccinated person would receive lifelong immunity against smallpox, but would never have suffered from that disease. As the 19th century progressed, there was a gradual transition away from smallpox variolation towards (the much safer) smallpox vaccination.

For most of the 19th century, the smallpox vaccine was the only vaccine. However, by the beginning of the 20th century, researchers had developed vaccines against cholera, rabies, tetanus, typhoid fever, and the bubonic plague (College of Physicians of Philadelphia 2014). And by the beginning of the 21st century, two dozen additional major vaccines had been developed, including vaccines against polio and measles. Today, there are new vaccines in various stages of research and regulatory approval.

It may be helpful to say something about the different types of vaccines that are now in use.[2] The initial vaccines cultivated immunity by introducing a weaker (or weakened) version of an antigen. For example, Jenner's vaccine cultivated immunity against smallpox by exposing the immune system to the weaker cowpox virus. In contrast, the rabies vaccine uses the actual rabies virus, but it is a weakened (attenuated) version of that antigen. The use of live attenuated viruses is still common. Vaccines against measles, mumps, rubella, varicella, and rotavirus are all of this type, as is the oral polio vaccine. Vaccines against other diseases include an antigen that has been inactivated. The vaccine for hepatitis A and the injected form of the polio vaccine are of this type. Still other vaccines use inactivated toxins (toxoids), to cultivate immunity against bacterial infections that cause illness by generating toxins. These include vaccines for diphtheria and tetanus. Finally, some vaccines use only part of an antigen, or they use genetic engineering to attach an antigen (or a part of one) to another protein. These include vaccines against hepatitis B and pertussis.

The immediate goal of vaccination is the development of individual immunity. Individuals who become immune from a vaccine are not susceptible to the infection they have been vaccinated against, at least for some time after they have been vaccinated. Vaccines are very effective at cultivating individual immunity, though they are not perfect. For example, more than 96% of children develop immunity against measles, mumps, and rubella after their second dose of the measles, mumps, and rubella (MMR) vaccine (Pebody et al. 2002). And after three doses of the Diphtheria, Tetanus, and acellular Pertussis (DTaP) vaccine, more than 97% develop immunity against diphtheria, more than 99% develop immunity against tetanus, and more than 95% develop immunity against pertussis (Capeding et al. 2008).

Individual immunity is not the only goal of vaccination. If a sufficiently large percentage of the population develops individual immunity, then that population will possess 'herd immunity': It will be extremely unlikely for members of the community to be exposed to the diseases against which most members of the community are individually immune (Anderson and May 1985; Fine 1993). Even people who lack individual immunity are relatively safe when a community has herd immunity. This is important because there will always be members of the community who do not possess individual immunity, because they are too young or too immunocompromised to be vaccinated, or because their vaccines failed to develop individual immunity. Herd immunity keeps these people safe. Fortunately, herd immunity does not require 100% vaccination rates, but it often requires something close. For example, herd immunity against measles requires 92–95% of the population to be immunized, while herd immunity against rubella requires 83–90% (Fine 1993; Meissner, Strebel, and Orenstein 2004; Wright and Polack 2006).[3]

For the purposes of this book, I focus on *routine childhood vaccines*. But the word 'vaccine' is also sometimes used to name immunotherapies that treat ongoing diseases and disorders. For example, various cancer vaccines improve a person's ability to fight against the cancer she already has (Finn 2008; Sioud 2007). Also, some vaccines are used in treatments for allergies. In these treatments, patients are injected with progressively larger doses of an allergen to hyposensitize them to that allergen (Bousquet, Lockey, and Malling 1998; Till et al. 2004).

I am not committed to the existence of a clear demarcation between routine childhood vaccines and other immunotherapies. Nevertheless, two main differences between vaccines for cancer/allergies and vaccines to prevent childhood diseases may help to justify my decision to focus upon the latter kind of vaccines. First, if a vaccine is used only to treat a disease, then questions about risk assessment are likely to be more straightforward. The patient needs only to weigh the risks and benefits of the treatment against the undesirability of the disease from which she currently suffers. In contrast, risk assessment in the case of childhood vaccination is more difficult, since we vaccinate only healthy children, and since their risk of becoming infected with vaccine-preventable diseases depends upon the rates at which others vaccinate. Second, most immunotherapies for ongoing diseases and disorders aim at treating non-communicable diseases and disorders. Allergies are not generally contagious, nor are most cancers.[4] In contrast, routine childhood vaccines often protect against infectious diseases. Much of the ethical and political significance of routine childhood vaccination arises from the fact that vaccinated persons contribute to the formation of herd immunity and are much less likely to infect others.

Safety and success

Vaccines have been a huge success. In the United States, vaccines have prevented over 100 million cases of previously routine childhood diseases, such as polio and measles (Van Panhuis et al. 2013). Another study found that US domestic vaccination efforts annually prevent about 42,000 early deaths, save $13.5 billion in direct medical expenses, and save $68.8 billion in broader social costs (Zhou et al. 2014). For all of these reasons, the Centers for Disease Control and Prevention conclude that "[p]erhaps the greatest success story in public health is the reduction of infectious diseases resulting from the use of vaccines" (Centers for Disease Control and Prevention 2011).

Vaccines have achieved such great successes with very low rates of adverse complications.[5] The most common vaccine complications are mild. For example, of the children who receive the DTaP vaccine, 1 in 4 will have redness or tenderness where the shot was given (Centers for Disease Control and Prevention 2007). Of the children who receive the MMR vaccine, 1 out of 20 will develop a mild rash (Centers for Disease Control and Prevention 2012a). More serious complications are very rare. For example, only 1 child out of 16,000 will develop a fever greater than 105 degrees after receiving the DTaP vaccine (Centers for Disease Control and Prevention 2007). And about 1 out of every 50,000 children who are vaccinated against rotavirus develop an intussusception (a bowel blockage that may require hospital treatment) (Centers for Disease Control and Prevention 2013a). The most severe complications are extremely rare; they are often so rare that we do not have accurate data on the risks. For example, less than one child out of 1,000,000 will develop long-term seizures or brain damage after receiving the DTaP vaccine (Centers for Disease Control and Prevention 2007). Children face a similarly low risk of becoming deaf after the MMR vaccine (Centers for Disease Control and Prevention 2012a).

Some parents today are concerned that vaccination may contribute to autism spectrum disorders. Among other reasons, this is because of a (now-retracted) paper by Andrew Wakefield et al. that claimed the MMR vaccine was linked to inflammatory bowel disease and behavioral regression (Wakefield et al. 1998).[6] But these claims are not supported by the evidence (Baird et al. 2008; Davis et al. 2001; Farrington, Miller, and Taylor 2001; Kaye, del Mar Melero-Montes, and Jick 2001; Peltola et al. 1998; Taylor et al. 1999). Furthermore, the MMR vaccine does not increase the risk of encephalitis, meningitis, or developmental disorders (Fombonne et al. 2006; Mäkelä, Nuorti, and Peltola 2002; Smeeth et al. 2004). Also, there is no evidence of a connection between vaccination with vaccines that contain thimerosal/thiomersal and autism spectrum disorders (Heron, Golding, and the ALSPAC Study Team 2004; Hviid et al. 2003; Price et al. 2010; Schechter and Grether 2008). Finally, following the regular vaccine schedule (as opposed to a delayed schedule of the sort recommended by Dr. Bob Sears (2007)) does not increase the risks of vaccine complications (DeStefano, Price, and Weintraub 2013; Klein et al. 2011; Klein et al. 2012; M. J. Smith and Woods 2010).

Vaccine policy

Vaccines are not merely private medical treatments. They prevent people from harming each other, and they offer a means for generating and maintaining herd immunity, a valuable public good. Among the core purposes of government is to prevent people from harming each other and to ensure people contribute to public goods. Therefore, it makes sense that government has long been involved in vaccine policy.

Beginning in the middle of the 19th century, the government of the United Kingdom sought to increase smallpox vaccination rates through legal measures.[7] An 1840 law prohibited the older (and more dangerous) practice of variolation and provided public funds to make smallpox vaccination freely available. In 1853, smallpox vaccination was made compulsory for infants. Later laws (in 1867, 1871, and 1873) expanded this requirement to include older children and introduced penalties for non-compliance. In the United States, coercive vaccination proceeded more sporadically, since public health law was largely left up to individual states. But some states (including Massachusetts and New York) followed the model of the United Kingdom and made vaccines mandatory for children, especially for children who wished to enter school.

The first vaccine refusal mass movements emerged in response to compulsory vaccine laws. These protest movements focused their attention on the penalties that could be imposed on parents who refused to comply with the law. (For example, people who refused to pay the United Kingdom's £1 fine for refusing to vaccinate could have their property seized and sold to pay the fine.) Many anti-vaccine groups sprung up in the United Kingdom, including the Anti-Compulsory Vaccination League and the National Anti-Vaccination League. They had an array of complaints about vaccination: vaccines violated biblical prohibitions on bodily mutilation, vaccines were more dangerous than the diseases against which they were supposed to protect, and the state had no right to compel vaccination. Similar organizations emerged in the United States, including the Anti-Vaccination Society of America, the New England Anti-Compulsory Vaccination League, and the Anti-Vaccination League of New York City. These groups often echoed the concerns raised by the anti-vaccine societies of the United Kingdom.

The anti-vaccine movements of the late 19th century led to changes in vaccine policies. The United Kingdom passed a set of laws in 1889, 1898, and 1907 that provided a means for 'conscientious objectors' to be exempted from compulsory vaccination. (It is notable that the first legally protected exemption rights for conscientious objectors were established for *vaccine refusers*, and were only later offered to *war resisters*.) The new laws also lessened or eliminated penalties for vaccine refusal. In the United States, some states began providing exemptions to vaccine refusers, too. However, even in the light of expanding exemption practices, the US Supreme Court held in Jacobson v. Massachusetts, 197 U.S. 11 (1905), that it was not unconstitutional for a state to compel vaccination for the sake of public health. But this decision did not defend as much state coercion as people who invoke this court case sometimes suggest. *Jacobson* upheld only the right of the state of Massachusetts to impose a fine on people who refused to vaccinate; it did not uphold the con-stitutionality of forcible vaccination. And with rare exceptions, vaccina-tion policies have never involved the forcible physical imposition of vaccination on unwilling citizens. Instead, states have usually resorted only to imposing economic or social burdens on vaccine refusers, for example, making them pay fines or excluding them from schools and (some) workplaces.

World War I ushered in a new set of efforts aimed at mass vaccination. Military mobilization for the Great War required a massive expansion of government and included efforts to cultivate (what Christopher Capozzola has called) 'coerced voluntarism' among previously disengaged citizens (Capozzola 2008). State propaganda machines used their new powers to drive young men to enlist, but these powers were also used to encourage other members of society to offer material and psychological support to the war, e.g. through buying war bonds and reporting on neighbors who they believed to be disloyal to the war effort. Public health officials made effective use of the new physical and psychological powers of the state in their efforts to encourage vaccination and to discourage participation in anti-vaccine movements. For example, they portrayed vaccine refusal as an unpatriotic form of domestic sabotage (Willrich 2008). (In the light of this history, it is odd for contemporary vaccine refusers to complain that the use of state power to promote vaccination is a new phenomenon (see e.g. Wagner 2011).) The state's efforts to harness patriotism in sup-port of vaccination programs continued through the interwar period and only expanded through World War II. As the 1950s began, widespread patriotism and public feeling – combined with a new public reverence for the 'miracles of science' – lent even more support to mass vaccination policies. A high point for this public commitment to vaccination was the success of Jonas Salk's polio field trials – a process in which millions of American parents agreed to have their children participate. These trials involved the cooperation of countless teachers, school nurses, and public officials of all stripes.

Children today have access to vaccines against many diseases to which they would have been vulnerable in previous generations. While there is some diversity between countries, there are more or less standard vaccination schedules in the developed world (Australian Government – Department of Health 2013; Centers for Disease Control and Prevention 2014a; National Health Service 2014). Children are generally vaccinated against hepatitis B, rotavirus, diphtheria, tetanus, pertussis, *Haemophilus influenzae* type b (Hib), pneumococcal infections, polio, measles, mumps, rubella, and hepatitis A. Vaccination against varicella and meningitis has become standard more recently; vaccination against human papilloma-virus is becoming normalized only now. Clearly we have come a long way from the days in which smallpox vaccine was the only show in town. Even in the past sixty years change has happened quickly. As late as the 1950s, children were routinely vaccinated against only a handful of diseases, including smallpox, diphtheria, tetanus, pertussis, and polio (Children's Hospital of Philadelphia 2013).

Contemporary vaccine refusal and denialism

Parents in the United States, Australia, and the United Kingdom (among other countries) are increasingly refusing (some) routine childhood vaccines (Glanz et al. 2013; Konner 2011; Nicholson and Ramet 2013; Omer et al. 2009; Omer et al. 2012; Tafuri et al. 2014; Williams and Swan 2014). While less than 2% of parents in the United Kingdom and about 1% of parents in the United States refuse *all vaccines*, 5–10% refuse some vac-cines and a significantly larger percentage practice a 'slowed-down' vaccine schedule (Brown et al. 2010; Diekema 2005; Dubé et al. 2013; Healy and Pickering 2011; Leask et al. 2012).

The MMR vaccine is one of the most commonly refused vaccines. As of 2011, over 15% of five-year-old children in the United Kingdom had not received the recommended two doses of the MMR vaccine, and 75% of those were vaccine refusers (rather than the merely undervaccinated) (Brown et al. 2012; Diekema 2005). Some of the decline in MMR vaccination rates seems tied to the publicity surrounding the Wakefield paper, but rates have not much recovered even after the paper has been retracted and after Wakefield has been barred from practicing medicine (Brown et al. 2012; Einsiedel 2011). In contrast, Gust et al. have found that parents in the United States most frequently *refuse* varicella (chicken pox) vaccine, but they most commonly *delay* MMR (Gust et al. 2008). Freed et al. arrived at a similar result: Varicella was the most commonly refused routine early childhood vaccine, followed by meningococcal conjugate and MMR (Freed at al. 2010).[8]

Dan Kahan advises that we should not become overly alarmed by vac-cine refusal since, in the United States, "the proportion of children receiving no vaccinations has remained below 1%" (Kahan 2013, 54; Kahan is citing Centers for Disease Control and Prevention 2013b). Kahan is right; we do not have a large population of parents who refuse *all* vaccines. In many communities, vaccination rates for some vaccines are at or near record highs, though this is often due to effective efforts at vaccinating those who would otherwise remain undervaccinated (Healy and Pickering 2011; Omer et al. 2009). However, we should be careful not to let the '1%' number contribute to complacency about vaccine refusal. First, as I mention above, many parents are selectively vaccinating and the rates of vaccine refusal for some vaccines are quite high. Second, delayed vaccination is also a problem since it leaves infants and young children unnecessarily vulnerable to dangerous infections (Dempsey et al. 2011; Robison, Groom, and Young 2012).[9] Finally, vaccine refusers are often geographically clustered. So, even when overall vaccination rates are relatively high, they can be low enough to lead to outbreaks in some areas (May and Silverman 2003; Omer et al. 2008; Sadaf et al. 2013; Salathé and Bonhoeffer 2008).[10]

There have been numerous recent disease outbreaks tied to vaccine refusal. For example, various outbreaks of measles, mumps, and rubella in the United Kingdom have occurred over the past fifteen years (Einsiedel 2011). In communities where rates of pertussis vaccination have fallen, pertussis infection rates have increased 100 times faster than in communities that have maintained their pertussis vaccination rates (Dubé et al. 2013). The rate of measles infection in California is the highest it has been in twenty years (Centers for Disease Control and Prevention 2014c). As I complete the revisions on this book in the winter of 2015, a measles outbreak is still spreading across the western states of the United States.

Who are the vaccine refusers?

Vaccine refusers tend to be more educated and higher paid than either parents who vaccinate their children or parents whose children are undervaccinated because of difficulties accessing medical care (Gust et al. 2008; Healy and Pickering 2011; Mnookin 2011; Omer et al. 2009; Salmon et al. 2005; P. J. Smith, Chu, and Barker 2004; Wei et al. 2009). Vaccine refusers are disproportionately white and they tend to be married (Healy and Pickering 2011; Omer et al. 2009).

Vaccine refusers are not only more educated, but they also often have more knowledge about vaccines than parents who vaccinate. This is especially true of parents who selectively vaccinate. Vaccine refusers who delay vaccination or selectively vaccinate have more correct beliefs about vaccines than parents who follow the vaccination schedule or parents who refuse all vaccines (Benin et al. 2006; Leask et al. 2012).

Some writers and entertainers for popular audiences have claimed that vaccine denialism and vaccine refusal are correlated with a commitment to liberal political ideology (see e.g. Abrams 2014). But there is little evidence to support this conclusion. If anything, there is better evidence that vaccine refusal and denialism correlate with conservative political ideology. For example, a 2013 Public Policy Polling survey found that 16% of Democrats believe vaccines cause autism, but 26% of Republicans endorse this belief (Public Policy Polling 2013, 21). A 2012 YouGov poll was more mixed. It showed that 31% of Republicans thought that vaccines are linked to autism versus 27% for Democrats; but it also found that 8% of Democrats thought vaccines were linked to diabetes, versus only 5% for Republicans (Berinksy 2012). A more recent study by Dan Kahan shows that there is almost no correlation between vaccine denialism and political ideology (Kahan 2014).[11] So, vaccine denialism is unlike other contemporary forms of mass science refusal, which are strongly correlated with political ideology (e.g. denial of evolution and climate change among conservatives; denial of GMO safety among liberals) (Kahan and Braman 2006).

The most common concerns that vaccine refusers have are about the potential for adverse effects of vaccination. For example, Omer et al. (2009) reported that 69% of refusers stated that they were afraid that a vaccine might cause harm. The most common adverse effect that vaccine refusers worry about is autism, specifically with regards to the MMR vaccine (Brown et al. 2010; Dubé et al. 2013; Healy and Pickering 2011). Parents are also worried about Guillain–Barré syndrome, asthma, and allergies (Brown et al. 2010; Brown et al. 2012). Many parents have less specific worries and they focus on unnamed short- and long-term possible harms (Brown et al. 2010; Dempsey et al. 2009).

While most vaccine refusers focus primarily on concerns about safety, many vaccine refusers also believe that vaccines are not effective. Omer et al. (2009) notes that 54% of vaccine refusers rate the efficacy of vaccines as low.

Many parents identify worries about health considerations, but a smaller number of parents refuse vaccines for religious or philosophical reasons (Downs, Bruine de Bruin, and Fischhoff 2008; Leask et al. 2012; Sadaf et al. 2013; Tafuri et al. 2014). Other parents have political reasons for refusing: they embrace libertarian politics and they resist participation in collective projects, such as efforts to promote herd immunity (Luyten et al. 2013). Some parents are just happy to free-ride on the herd immunity others have generated (Benin et al. 2006). That is, parents whose decisions about childhood vaccination are based exclusively on considerations of their own children's well-being may choose not to vaccinate, because they know that the high rates of vaccination in their communities mean that their child is unlikely to be exposed to the diseases she is not vaccinated against (May and Silverman 2005; Spier 1998; Viens, Bensimon, and Upshur 2009).

Finally, some parents who refuse routine childhood vaccines think the diseases vaccines protect against are not very severe. And if their children are going to develop immunity, they would rather it happened as a result of their child recovering from a disease than from a vaccine (Benin et al. 2006; Brown et al. 2010; Downs, Bruine de Bruin, and

Fischhoff 2008; Omer et al. 2009; Sadaf et al. 2013; Tafuri et al. 2014; Wei et al. 2009).

Outline of chapters

In chapter one, I argue that vaccine denialists sometimes disagree with mainstream medical authorities about the sorts of practices and communities that are conducive to good reasoning about health care choices. Of particular interest to me is the fact that vaccine-hesitant parents – usually mothers – have sometimes created resistant epistemological communities. These communities practice democratic epistemic norms, but they are also often committed to poor epistemic practices. In chapter two, I argue that vaccine denialism may result from parental epistemic self-reliance and from parents' isolation from communities of inquiry whose practices could check their overconfidence. Vaccine denialists feel entitled to do their own research about vaccines, but this tendency leaves them especially vulnerable to a host of cognitive biases. In chapter three, I argue that the concerns vaccine refusers express about 'safety' are sometimes not examples of vaccine denialism. Instead, vaccine refusers may be motivated by a commitment to 'natural' forms of bodily purity (including the avoidance of 'unnatural' contaminants). Such a commitment is often fueled by both moralized and non-moralized forms of disgust. In chapter four, I argue that parents have a moral right to sometimes prioritize the interests of their children over the promotion of aggregate well-being, but I deny the popular claim that this parental prerogative is sufficient to establish a moral right to refuse all childhood vaccines. In chapter five, I argue that the state has the authority to coerce vaccination, though there are good reasons for it to use as little coercion as is necessary to achieve the goal of herd immunity. In chapter six, I argue that nonmedical vaccine exemptions are not required by liberal justice, concern for conscience, or pragmatic considerations. Finally, I conclude by identifying some ways in which this book's arguments might inform public policy debates about vaccine refusal.

Notes

1 Parents of children with compromised immune systems are often advised to refuse routine childhood vaccines (Centers for Disease Control and Prevention 1993; Centers for Disease Control and Prevention 2014b). Refusing vaccines for medical reasons does not raise the same questions about prudence, morality, and justice that nonmedical vaccine refusal raises.
2 The material in this paragraph draws upon *Vaccines*, the standard reference text for medical information about vaccines (Plotkin, Orenstein, and Offit 2012). I also draw upon material from the College of Physicians of Philadelphia (2014).
3 Yash Paul (2004) has argued that we should distinguish between 'herd immunity' and 'herd protection', and that we should use the term 'herd protection' to

denote what is usually meant by 'herd immunity'. On this view, 'herd protection' denotes the decreased chance of infection that nonimmune individuals within the group have because they are unlikely to be exposed to the disease. In contrast, 'herd immunity' refers to the decreased chance of infection that non-vaccinated persons within the group have because they have developed immunity through the "secondary spread of the agent used in the vaccination programme environment (by way of faecal matter from those who have been vaccinated)" (Dawson 2007, 162). I will follow conventional usage throughout this book and use 'herd immunity' to refer to what Paul calls 'herd protection'.

4 Of course, some cancers may be caused by communicable diseases, but the vaccines that prevent those diseases are *preventative* vaccines: they do not treat the cancer.

5 My discussion in the next two paragraphs benefits from American Academy of Pediatrics (2013); Centers for Disease Control and Prevention (2014b); and Centers for Disease Control and Prevention (2014d).

6 It is ironic that even if Wakefield's results were correct, he would have shown only that there is a very small risk of developing autism from vaccination. Parents would still have had overwhelming reason to vaccinate against measles, mumps, and rubella – which is what Wakefield said (John 2011, 499).

7 My discussion in the remainder of this section draws upon Durbach (2005); Poland and Jacobson (2011); Porter and Porter (1988); and Wolfe and Sharp (2002).

8 Freed et al. found that HPV was the most commonly refused vaccine, but this is not a routine early childhood vaccine, since ACIP recommends HPV for boys and girls who are 11 years old.

9 Dempsey et al. found that 13% of parents are using some kind of alternative vaccination schedule (Dempsey et al. 2011). Kempe et al. found that in a typical month over 90% of pediatricians meet with parents of young children who want to slow down the vaccine schedule (Kempe et al. 2015).

10 To be clear, I do not think Kahan would dispute any of these three points.

11 Mark Largent discusses the diverse political origins of vaccine denialism/refusal: "Left-leaning parents mingle concerns about vaccines with their environmental activism, health-conscious lifestyles, and anxieties about corporate power and profit motives. They are joined by rightwing libertarians who dislike governmental influence with what they consider personal decisions and by conspiracy theorists that see in vaccines a government plot to oppress or eliminate certain segments of the population" (Largent 2012, 16).

Bibliography

Abrams, Lindsay. 2014. "'The Daily Show': Anti-Vaxxers Are the Climate-Denying 'Nutjobs' of the Left." June 3. www.salon.com/2014/06/03/the_daily_show_anti_vaxxers_are_the_climate_denying_nutjobs_of_the_left/.

American Academy of Pediatrics. 2013. "Vaccine Safety: Examine the Evidence." Accessed June 11, 2015. www2.aap.org/immunization/families/faq/vaccinestudies.pdf.

Anderson, R. M., and R. M. May. 1985. "Vaccination and Herd Immunity to Infectious Diseases." *Nature* 318(6044): 323–329.

Australian Government – Department of Health. 2013. "Immunise – National Immunisation Program Schedule." July 1. www.immunise.health.gov.au/internet/immunise/publishing.nsf/Content/nips-ctn.

Baird, Gillian, Andrew Pickles, Emily Simonoff, Tony Charman, Peter Sullivan, Susie Chandler, Tom Loucas, et al. 2008. "Measles Vaccination and Antibody

Response in Autism Spectrum Disorders." *Archives of Disease in Childhood* 93(10): 832–837.

Behbehani, Abbas M. 1983. "The Smallpox Story: Life and Death of an Old Disease." *Microbiological Reviews* 47(4): 455.

Benin, A. L., D. J. Wisler-Scher, E. Colson, E. D. Shapiro, and E. S. Holmboe. 2006. "Qualitative Analysis of Mothers' Decision-Making about Vaccines for Infants: The Importance of Trust." *Pediatrics* 117(5): 1532–1541.

Berinksy, Adam. 2012. "Public Support for Vaccination Remains Strong." *YouGov: What the World Thinks.* December 5. http://today.yougov.com/news/2012/12/05/p ublic-support-vaccination-remains-strong/.

Bousquet, Jean, Richard Lockey, and Hans-Jorgen Malling. 1998. "Allergen Immunotherapy: Therapeutic Vaccines for Allergic Diseases. A WHO Position Paper." *Journal of Allergy and Clinical Immunology* 102(4): 558–562.

Brown, Katrina F., J. S. Kroll, M. J. Hudson, M. Ramsay, J. Green, S. J. Long, C. A. Vincent, G. Fraser, and N. Sevdalis. 2010. "Factors Underlying Parental Decisions about Combination Childhood Vaccinations Including MMR: A Systematic Review." *Vaccine* 28(26): 4235–4248.

Brown, Katrina F., Susannah J. Long, Mary Ramsay, Michael J. Hudson, John Green, Charles A. Vincent, J. Simon Kroll, Graham Fraser, and Nick Sevdalis. 2012. "UK Parents' Decision-Making about Measles–Mumps–Rubella (MMR) Vaccine 10 Years after the MMR-Autism Controversy: A Qualitative Analysis." *Vaccine* 30(10): 1855–1864.

Capeding, Maria Rosario, Josefina Cadorna-Carlos, May Book-Montellano, and Esteban Ortiz. 2008. "Immunogenicity and Safety of a DTaP-IPV//PRP≃T Combination Vaccine given with Hepatitis B Vaccine: A Randomized Open-Label Trial." *Bulletin of the World Health Organization* 86(6): 443–451.

Capozzola, Christopher. 2008. *Uncle Sam Wants You: World War I and the Making of the Modern American Citizen.* Oxford University Press.

Centers for Disease Control and Prevention. 1993. *Recommendations of the Advisory Committee on Immunization Practices (ACIP): Use of Vaccines and Immune Globulins in Persons with Altered Immunocompetence.* Accessed June 11, 2015. www.cdc. gov/mmwr/pdf/rr/rr4204.pdf.

Centers for Disease Control and Prevention. 2007. "Vaccine Information Statement: Diphtheria, Tetanus, and Pertussis – Vaccines – CDC." May 17. www.cdc.gov/ vaccines/hcp/vis/vis-statements/dtap.html.

Centers for Disease Control and Prevention. 2011. "CDC – Vaccine History – Vaccine Safety." February 8. www.cdc.gov/vaccinesafety/vaccine_monitoring/history.html.

Centers for Disease Control and Prevention. 2012a. "Vaccine Information Statement: MMR (Measles, Mumps, Rubella) – Vaccines – CDC." April 20. www. cdc.gov/vaccines/hcp/vis/vis-statements/mmr.html.

Centers for Disease Control and Prevention. 2012b. "CDC – Multiple Vaccines – Vaccine Safety." December 7. www.cdc.gov/vaccinesafety/vaccines/multipleva ccines.html.

Centers for Disease Control and Prevention. 2013a. "Vaccine Information Statement: Rotavirus – Vaccines – CDC." August 26. www.cdc.gov/vaccines/hcp/ vis/vis-statements/rotavirus.html.

Centers for Disease Control and Prevention. 2013b. *Morbidity and Mortality Weekly Report (MMWR)* 62. Accessed June 11, 2015. www.cdc.gov/mmwr/p review/mmwrhtml/mm6236a1.htm?s_cid=mm6236a1_w.

Centers for Disease Control and Prevention. 2014a. "CDC – Vaccines – Immunization Schedules Main Page." January 31. www.cdc.gov/vaccines/schedules/index.html.

Centers for Disease Control and Prevention. 2014b. "Possible Side-Effects from Vaccines." February 4. www.cdc.gov/vaccines/vac-gen/side-effects.htm.

Centers for Disease Control and Prevention. 2014c. "Notes from the Field: Measles – California, January 1–April 18, 2014." *Morbidity and Mortality Weekly Report (MMWR)*. April 25. www.cdc.gov/mmwr/preview/mmwrhtml/mm6316a 6.htm?s_cid=mm6316a6_w.

Centers for Disease Control and Prevention. 2014d. "Vaccine Information Statement: Home Page – Vaccines – CDC." June 11. www.cdc.gov/vaccines/hcp/vis/index.html.

Children's Hospital of Philadelphia. 2013. "History of Vaccine Schedule | The Children's Hospital of Philadelphia." *Vaccine Education Center*. Accessed July 31, 2015. www.chop.edu/service/vaccine-education-center/vaccine-schedule/history-of-vaccine-schedule.html.

College of Physicians of Philadelphia. 2014. "The History of Vaccines." Accessed July 13. www.historyofvaccines.org/.

Davis, Robert L., Piotr Kramarz, Kari Bohlke, Patti Benson, Robert S. Thompson, John Mullooly, Steve Black, et al. 2001. "Measles-Mumps-Rubella and Other Measles-Containing Vaccines Do Not Increase the Risk for Inflammatory Bowel Disease: A Case-Control Study from the Vaccine Safety Datalink Project." *Archives of Pediatrics & Adolescent Medicine* 155(3): 354–359.

Dawson, Angus. 2007. "Herd Protection as a Public Good: Vaccination and Our Obligations to Others." In *Ethics, Prevention, and Public Health*, edited by Angus Dawson and Marcel Verweij, 160–178. Clarendon Press.

Dempsey, Amanda F., L. M. Abraham, V. Dalton, and M. Ruffin. 2009. "Understanding the Reasons Why Mothers Do or Do Not Have Their Adolescent Daughters Vaccinated against Human Papillomavirus." *Annals of Epidemiology* 19(8): 531–538.

Dempsey, Amanda F., Sarah Schaffer, Dianne Singer, Amy Butchart, Matthew Davis, and Gary L. Freed. 2011. "Alternative Vaccination Schedule Preferences among Parents of Young Children." *Pediatrics* 128(5): 1–9.

DeStefano, Frank, Cristofer S. Price, and Eric S. Weintraub. 2013. "Increasing Exposure to Antibody-Stimulating Proteins and Polysaccharides in Vaccines Is Not Associated with Risk of Autism." *The Journal of Pediatrics* 163(2): 561–567.

Diekema, D. S. 2005. "Responding to Parental Refusals of Immunization of Children." *Pediatrics* 115(5): 1428–1431.

Downs, Julie S., Wändi Bruine de Bruin, and Baruch Fischhoff. 2008. "Parents' Vaccination Comprehension and Decisions." *Vaccine* 26(12): 1595–1607.

Dubé, Eve, Caroline Laberge, Maryse Guay, Paul Bramadat, Réal Roy, and Julie A. Bettinger. 2013. "Vaccine Hesitancy: An Overview." *Human Vaccines & Immunotherapeutics* 9(8): 1763–1773.

Durbach, Nadja. 2005. *Bodily Matters: The Anti-Vaccination Movement in England, 1853–1907*. Duke University Press.

Einsiedel, E. F. 2011. "Publics and Vaccinomics: Beyond Public Understanding of Science." *OMICS: A Journal of Integrative Biology* 15(9): 607–614.

Farrington, C., Elizabeth Miller, and Brent Taylor. 2001. "MMR and Autism: Further Evidence against a Causal Association." *Vaccine* 19(27): 3632–3635.

Fenner, Frank, Donald A. Henderson, Isao Arita, Zdenek Jezek, Ivan Danilovich Ladnyi. 1988. *Smallpox and Its Eradication.* World Health Organization.

Fine, Paul E. M. 1993. "Herd Immunity: History, Theory, Practice." *Epidemiologic Reviews* 15(2): 265–302.

Finn, Olivera J. 2008. "Cancer Immunology." *New England Journal of Medicine* 358(25): 2704–2715.

Fombonne, Eric, Rita Zakarian, Andrew Bennett, Linyan Meng, and Diane McLean-Heywood. 2006. "Pervasive Developmental Disorders in Montreal, Quebec, Canada: Prevalence and Links with Immunizations." *Pediatrics* 118(1): e139–150.

Freed, Gary L., Sarah J. Clark, Amy T. Butchart, Dianne C. Singer, and Matthew M. Davis. 2010. "Parental Vaccine Safety Concerns in 2009." *Pediatrics* 125(4): 654–659. doi:10.1542/peds.2009–1962.

Glanz, Jason M., D. L. McClure, D. J. Magid, M. F. Daley, E. K. France, D. A. Salmon, and S. J. Hambidge. 2009. "Parental Refusal of Pertussis Vaccination Is Associated with an Increased Risk of Pertussis Infection in Children." *Pediatrics* 123(6): 1446–1451.

Glanz, Jason M., Sophia R. Newcomer, Komal J. Narwaney, Simon J. Hambidge, Matthew F. Daley, Nicole M. Wagner, David L. McClure, et al. 2013. "A Population-Based Cohort Study of Undervaccination in 8 Managed Care Organizations across the United States." *JAMA Pediatrics* 167(3): 274–281.

Gust, D. A., N. Darling, A. Kennedy, and B. Schwartz. 2008. "Parents with Doubts about Vaccines: Which Vaccines and Reasons Why." *Pediatrics* 122(4): 718.

Healy, C. Mary, and Larry K. Pickering. 2011. "How to Communicate with Vaccine-Hesitant Parents." *Pediatrics* 127 (Supplement 1): S127–133.

Henderson, Donald. 2009. *Smallpox: The Death of a Disease: The Inside Story of Eradicating a Worldwide Killer.* Prometheus Books.

Heron, Jon, Jean Golding, and the ALSPAC Study Team. 2004. "Thimerosal Exposure in Infants and Developmental Disorders: A Prospective Cohort Study in the United Kingdom Does Not Support a Causal Association." *Pediatrics* 114(3): 577–583.

Hviid, Anders, Michael Stellfeld, Jan Wohlfahrt, and Mads Melbye. 2003. "Association between Thimerosal-Containing Vaccine and Autism." *JAMA: The Journal of the American Medical Association* 290(13): 1763–1766.

Jacobson, R. M., P. V. Targonski, and G. A. Poland. 2007. "A Taxonomy of Reasoning Flaws in the Anti-Vaccine Movement." *Vaccine* 25(16): 3146–3152.

Jenner, Edward. 1798. *An Inquiry into the Causes and Effects of the Variolæ Vaccinæ.* Sampson Low.

John, Stephen. 2011. "Expert Testimony and Epistemological Free-Riding: The MMR Controversy." *The Philosophical Quarterly* 61(244): 496–517.

Kahan, Dan M. 2013. "A Risky Science Communication Environment for Vaccines." *Science* 342(6154): 53–54.

Kahan, Dan M. 2014. *Vaccine Risk Perceptions and Ad Hoc Risk Communication: An Empirical Assessment.* SSRN Scholarly Paper ID 2386034. Social Science Research Network. Accessed June 17, 2015. http://papers.ssrn.com/abstract=2386034.

Kahan, Dan M., and D. Braman. 2006. "Cultural Cognition and Public Policy." *Yale Law & Policy Review* 24: 149.

Kaye, James A., Maria del Mar Melero-Montes, and Hershel Jick. 2001. "Mumps, Measles, and Rubella Vaccine and the Incidence of Autism Recorded by

General Practitioners: A Time Trend Analysis." *British Medical Journal* 322 (7284): 460–463.

Kempe, Allison, Sean T. O'Leary, Allison Kennedy, Lori A. Crane, Mandy A. Allison, Brenda L. Beaty, Laura P. Hurley, Michaela Brtnikova, Andrea Jimenez-Zambrano, and Shannon Stokley. 2015. "Physician Response to Parental Requests to Spread Out the Recommended Vaccine Schedule." *Pediatrics* 135(4): 666–677

Klein, Nicola P., Laurie Aukes, Janelle Lee, Bruce Fireman, Stuart K. Shapira, Barbara Slade, Roger Baxter, and Marshall Summar. 2011. "Evaluation of Immunization Rates and Safety among Children with Inborn Errors of Metabolism." *Pediatrics* 127(5): e1139–1146.

Klein, Nicola P., Edwin Lewis, Roger Baxter, Eric Weintraub, Jason Glanz, Allison Naleway, Lisa A. Jackson, et al. 2012. "Measles-Containing Vaccines and Febrile Seizures in Children Age 4 to 6 Years." *Pediatrics* 129(5): 809–814.

Konner, Melvin. 2011. "Epidemiology: Epidemic of Panic." *Nature* 469(7331): 468–469.

Largent, M. A. 2012. *Vaccine: The Debate in Modern America.* Johns Hopkins University Press.

Leask, Julie, Paul Kinnersley, Cath Jackson, Francine Cheater, Helen Bedford, and Greg Rowles. 2012. "Communicating with Parents about Vaccination: A Framework for Health Professionals." *BMC Pediatrics* 12(1): 154.

Leung, Angela Ki Che. 2011. "'Variolation' and Vaccination in Late Imperial China, Ca 1570–1911." In S. A. Plotkin ed. *History of Vaccine Development*, 5–12. Springer.

Luyten, Jeroen, Pieter Desmet, Veronica Dorgali, Niel Hens, and Philippe Beutels. 2013. "Kicking against the Pricks: Vaccine Sceptics Have a Different Social Orientation." *The European Journal of Public Health* 24(2): 310–314.

MacKenzie, Debora. 2010. "How to Be a Denialist." *New Scientist* 206(2760): 38–41.

Mäkelä, Annamari, J. Pekka Nuorti, and Heikki Peltola. 2002. "Neurologic Disorders after Measles-Mumps-Rubella Vaccination." *Pediatrics* 110(5): 957–963.

May, T., and R. D. Silverman. 2003. "'Clustering of Exemptions' as a Collective Action Threat to Herd Immunity." *Vaccine* 21(11–12): 1048–1051.

May, T., and R. D. Silverman. 2005. "Free-Riding, Fairness and the Rights of Minority Groups in Exemption from Mandatory Childhood Vaccination." *Human Vaccines* 1(1): 12–15.

Meissner, H. Cody, Peter M. Strebel, and Walter A. Orenstein. 2004. "Measles Vaccines and the Potential for Worldwide Eradication of Measles." *Pediatrics* 114(4): 1065–1069. doi:10.1542/peds.2004-0440.

Mnookin, Seth. 2011. *The Panic Virus: A True Story of Medicine, Science, and Fear.* Simon & Schuster.

National Health Service, N. H. S. 2014. "Vaccination Schedule – Vaccinations – NHS Choices." *NHS Choices.* April 4. www.nhs.uk/Conditions/vaccinations/Pages/vaccination-schedule-age-checklist.aspx.

National Vaccine Information Center. 2015. "About Us." Accessed February 23. http://www.nvic.org/about.aspx.

Nicholson, A. J., and J. Ramet. 2013. "Improving Immunisation Uptake across Europe." *Irish Medical Journal* 106(5): 280–282.

Ołpiński, Marian. 2012. "Anti-Vaccination Movement and Parental Refusals of Immunization of Children in USA." *Pediatria Polska* 87(4): 381–385. doi:10.1016/j.pepo.2012.05.003.

Omer, S. B., K. S. Enger, L. H. Moulton, N. A. Halsey, S. Stokley, and D. A. Salmon. 2008. "Geographic Clustering of Nonmedical Exemptions to School Immunization Requirements and Associations with Geographic Clustering of Pertussis." *American Journal of Epidemiology* 168(12): 1389–1396.

Omer, S. B., Jennifer Richards, Michelle Ward, and Robert Bednarczyk. 2012. "Vaccination Policies and Rates of Exemption from Immunization, 2005–2011." *New England Journal of Medicine* 367(12): 1170–1171.

Omer, S. B., D. A. Salmon, W. A. Orenstein, M. P. deHart, and N. Halsey. 2009. "Vaccine Refusal, Mandatory Immunization, and the Risks of Vaccine-Preventable Diseases." *New England Journal of Medicine* 360(19): 1981–1988.

Paul, Yash. 2004. "Herd Immunity and Herd Protection." *Vaccine* 22(3): 301–302.

Pebody, R. G., N. J. Gay, L. M. Hesketh, A. Vyse, P. Morgan-Capner, D. W. Brown, P. Litton, and E. Miller. 2002. "Immunogenicity of Second Dose Measles-Mumps-Rubella (MMR) Vaccine and Implications for Serosurveillance." *Vaccine* 20(7–8): 1134–1140.

Peltola, Heikki, Annamari Patja, Pauli Leinikki, Martti Valle, Irja Davidkin, and Mikko Paunio. 1998. "No Evidence for Measles, Mumps, and Rubella Vaccine-Associated Inflammatory Bowel Disease or Autism in a 14-Year Prospective Study." *The Lancet* 351(9112): 1327–1328.

Plotkin, Stanley A., Walter A. Orenstein, and Paul A. Offit. 2012. *Vaccines: Expert Consult.* 6th ed. Saunders.

Poland, G. A., and R. M. Jacobson. 2011. "The Age-Old Struggle against the Antivaccinationists." *New England Journal of Medicine* 364(2): 97–99.

Porter, D., and R. Porter. 1988. "The Politics of Prevention: Anti-Vaccinationism and Public Health in Nineteenth-Century England." *Medical History* 32(3): 231–252.

Price, Cristofer S., William W. Thompson, Barbara Goodson, Eric S. Weintraub, Lisa A. Croen, Virginia L. Hinrichsen, Michael Marcy, et al. 2010. "Prenatal and Infant Exposure to Thimerosal from Vaccines and Immunoglobulins and Risk of Autism." *Pediatrics* 126(4): 656–664.

Public Policy Polling. 2013. "Democrats and Republicans Differ on Conspiracy Theory Beliefs." Accessed June 11, 2015. www.publicpolicypolling.com/main/2013/04/democrats-and-republicans-differ-on-conspiracy-theory-beliefs.html.

Robison, Steve G., Holly Groom, and Collette Young. 2012. "Frequency of Alternative Immunization Schedule Use in a Metropolitan Area." *Pediatrics* 130(1): 32–38.

Sadaf, Alina, Jennifer L. Richards, Jason Glanz, Daniel A. Salmon, and Saad B. Omer. 2013. "A Systematic Review of Interventions for Reducing Parental Vaccine Refusal and Vaccine Hesitancy." *Vaccine* 31(40): 4293–4304.

Salathé, Marcel, and Sebastian Bonhoeffer. 2008. "The Effect of Opinion Clustering on Disease Outbreaks." *Journal of the Royal Society Interface* 5(29): 1505–1508.

Salmon, Daniel A., Lawrence H. Moulton, Saad B. Omer, M. Patricia deHart, Shannon Stokley, and Neal A. Halsey. 2005. "Factors Associated with Refusal of Childhood Vaccines among Parents of School-Aged Children: A Case-Control Study." *Archives of Pediatrics & Adolescent Medicine* 159(5): 470–476.

Schechter, R., and J. K. Grether. 2008. "Continuing Increases in Autism Reported to California's Developmental Services System: Mercury in Retrograde." *Archives of General Psychiatry* 65(1): 19–24.

Sears, R. 2007. *The Vaccine Book: Making the Right Decision for Your Child*. Little, Brown and Company.

Silverman, Kenneth. 2001. *The Life and Times of Cotton Mather*. Welcome Rain Publishers.

Sioud, Mouldy. 2007. "An Overview of the Immune System and Technical Advances in Tumor Antigen Discovery and Validation." In *Target Discovery and Validation Reviews and Protocols*, edited by Mouldy Sioud, 277–318. Springer.

Smeeth, Liam, Claire Cook, Eric Fombonne, Lisa Heavey, Laura C. Rodrigues, Peter G. Smith, and Andrew J. Hall. 2004. "MMR Vaccination and Pervasive Developmental Disorders: A Case-Control Study." *The Lancet* 364(9438): 963–969.

Smith, Michael J., and Gary S. Marshall. 2010. "Navigating Parental Vaccine Hesitancy." *Pediatric Annals* 39(8): 476.

Smith, Michael J., and Charles R. Woods. 2010. "On-Time Vaccine Receipt in the First Year Does Not Adversely Affect Neuropsychological Outcomes." *Pediatrics* 125(6): 1134–1141.

Smith, Philip J., Susan Y. Chu, and Lawrence E. Barker. 2004. "Children Who Have Received No Vaccines: Who Are They and Where Do They Live?" *Pediatrics* 114(1): 187–195.

Specter, Michael. 2009. *Denialism: How Irrational Thinking Hinders Scientific Progress, Harms the Planet, and Threatens Our Lives*. Penguin Press.

Spier, R. E. 1998. "Ethical Aspects of Vaccines and Vaccination." *Vaccine* 16(19): 1788–1794.

Tafuri, S., M. S. Gallone, M. G. Cappelli, D. Martinelli, R. Prato, and C. Germinario. 2014. "Addressing the Anti-Vaccination Movement and the Role of HCWs." *Vaccine* 32(38): 4860–4865.

Taylor, Brent, Elizabeth Miller, C. Paddy Farrington, Maria-Christina Petropoulos, Isabelle Favot-Mayaud, Jun Li, and Pauline A. Waight. 1999. "Autism and Measles, Mumps, and Rubella Vaccine: No Epidemiological Evidence for a Causal Association." *The Lancet* 353(9169): 2026–2029.

Thucydides. 1972. *History of the Peloponnesian War*. Translated by Rex Warner. Penguin Group.

Till, Stephen J., James N. Francis, Kayhan Nouri-Aria, and Stephen R. Durham. 2004. "Mechanisms of Immunotherapy." *Journal of Allergy and Clinical Immunology* 113(6): 1025–1034.

Van Panhuis, Willem G., John Grefenstette, Su Yon Jung, Nian Shong Chok, Anne Cross, Heather Eng, Bruce Y. Lee, Vladimir Zadorozhny, Shawn Brown, and Derek Cummings. 2013. "Contagious Diseases in the United States from 1888 to the Present." *New England Journal of Medicine* 369(22): 2152–2158.

Viens, A. M., C. M. Bensimon, and R. E. G. Upshur. 2009. "Your Liberty or Your Life: Reciprocity in the Use of Restrictive Measures in Contexts of Contagion." *Journal of Bioethical Inquiry* 6(2): 207–217.

Wagner, William. 2011. "God, Government, and Parental Rights." In *Vaccine Epidemic*, edited by Louise Kuo Habakus and Mary Holland, 45–48. Skyhorse Publishing.

Wakefield, Andrew J. 2011. *Callous Disregard: Autisms and Vaccines: The Truth Behind a Tragedy*. Skyhorse Publishing.

Wakefield, Andrew J., S. H. Murch, A. Anthony, J. Linnell, D. M. Casson, M. Malik, M. Berelowitz, et al. 1998. "RETRACTED: Ileal-Lymphoid-Nodular

Hyperplasia, Non-Specific Colitis, and Pervasive Developmental Disorder in Children." *The Lancet* 351(9103): 637–641.

Wei, F., J. Mullooly, M. Goodman, M. McCarty, A. Hanson, B. Crane, and J. Nordin. 2009. "Identification and Characteristics of Vaccine Refusers." *BMC Pediatrics* 9(1): 18.

Williams, S. Elizabeth, and Rebecca Swan. 2014. "Formal Training in Vaccine Safety to Address Parental Concerns Not Routinely Conducted in US Pediatric Residency Programs." *Vaccine* 32(26): 3175–3178.

Willrich, Michael. 2008. "'The Least Vaccinated of Any Civilized Country': Personal Liberty and Public Health in the Progressive Era." *Journal of Policy History* 20(1): 76–93.

Wolfe, R. M., and L. K. Sharp. 2002. "Anti-Vaccinationists Past and Present." *British Medical Journal* 325(7361): 430–432.

Wright, James A., and Clare Polack. 2006. "Understanding Variation in Measles–Mumps–Rubella Immunization Coverage – a Population-Based Study." *European Journal of Public Health* 16(2): 137–142.

Zhou, Fangjun, Abigail Shefer, Jay Wenger, Mark Messonnier, Li Yan Wang, Adriana Lopez, Matthew Moore, Trudy V. Murphy, Margaret Cortese, and Lance Rodewald. 2014. "Economic Evaluation of the Routine Childhood Immunization Program in the United States, 2009." *Pediatrics* 133(4): 577–585.

1 Gender, vaccine denialism, and resistant epistemic communities

"The physician-patient relationship, like so many other human relationships, requires an element of trust. I certainly neither want nor expect a return to the paternalistic 'doctor knows best' mindset of bygone years, but I do need to know that [a] patient's parents respect my training and expertise."

(Saunders 2014)

When parents trust pediatricians, they usually vaccinate their children (Benin et al. 2006; Larson et al. 2011). And when it comes to vaccine science, parents generally place more trust in pediatricians than they place anywhere else (Freed et al. 2011). So, we should pay attention when these trusting relationships break down, as they often do in the case of vaccine denialism.

Are vaccine denialists irrational, overly emotional, or insufficiently attentive to the evidence about vaccines their pediatricians offer? I don't think they are. But some advocates of routine childhood vaccination seem to embrace narratives that emphasize the supposed cognitive deficits of vaccine denialists. For example, Seth Mnookin writes for *The Atlantic* that vaccine denialism is characterized by "irrational rhetoric," and Michael Specter writes in *Denialism* that vaccine denialists are victims of "irrational thinking" (Mnookin 2011b; Specter 2009). An article in *Scrubs* (a magazine for nurses) provides advice for overcoming the "irrational fears" patients may have about vaccines, while a book reviewer for NewScientist.com frames the differences between advocates of mainstream medicine and vaccine denialists in terms of "vaccines vs. irrationality" (Mooney 2011; Pregerson 2011). Even some writers who have been more sympathetic with vaccine denialists claim vaccine denialists are unreasonable (Ropeik 2011). More troubling has been the occasional tendency of critics to ascribe a gendered idea of irrationality to vaccine denialists: hysteria. For example, both the *New York Post* and *National Public Radio* (NPR) have attributed decreased rates of childhood vaccination to 'vaccine hysteria' (Goldberg 2011; Moss-Coane 2011). One may invoke 'hysteria' without sexist intent, but that may not block worries about the gendered nature of that term's conception of irrationality, especially given the prominence of mothers among vaccine denialists.[1]

In this chapter, I argue that it may sometimes be reasonable for parents (especially mothers) to refuse to grant credibility to the testimony of pediatricians. This is for both general reasons and for reasons that are particular to parent-pediatrician interactions. Parents may be aware of physicians' historical and ongoing abuse of their (epistemic) power, and they may have been treated paternalistically by pediatricians. Furthermore, vaccine denialists sometimes participate in democratic communities of 'parent-researchers' that reject the authoritarianism of traditional medical practice. Accordingly, one reason vaccine denialists may disagree with vaccine proponents about the reasons to vaccinate is because they also disagree about the sorts of practices that are conducive to good reasoning about health care choices. In place of the priority mainstream medicine places on empirically grounded and peer-reviewed research, vaccine denialists often uncritically affirm their fellow parents' beliefs about their children's health, and they refuse to recognize differences in medical expertise and competence.[2]

My task in this chapter is both descriptive and evaluative. I describe the different epistemic practices and values that are present in communities of vaccine denialists. My work should also inform the judgments we make about vaccine denialists, by showing that some of the practices that lead to vaccine denialism are better than those which are prevalent in mainstream medicine, while some of them are much worse. The fact that vaccine denialists are motivated by a commitment to some good epistemic practices (such as non-authoritarian relationships between pediatricians and parents) is a reason for thinking that they are not as 'irrational' as many have claimed them to be. However, vaccine denialists are insufficiently committed to truth-oriented inquiry.[3] The poor epistemic practices prevalent in vaccine denialist communities prevent vaccine denialists from endorsing the well-established results of vaccine science.

Comments on method: epistemology, feminist philosophy, and testimony

It may help to make three preliminary points about this chapter's methodology. First, I assume an empirically grounded conception of medical knowledge, though I do not presuppose a particular epistemic theory.[4] Also, I take for granted that our dispositions and practices may do a better or worse job of orienting us towards medical knowledge. My use of terms such as 'epistemic virtue' and 'epistemic vice' should be understood in the context of these general presuppositions. Here, I draw on virtue epistemology, a tradition that goes back to Aristotle and which has recently received renewed interest. Virtue epistemologists are less interested in identifying 'necessary and sufficient' conditions for knowledge than in describing the dispositions that better orient knowers towards knowledge. These virtues include trustworthiness, credibility, and accuracy, among many others.[5] Accordingly, an 'epistemic virtue' relative to inquiry about medicine is a disposition which facilitates the acquisition of empirically grounded medical knowledge. In contrast, an 'epistemic vice' relative to inquiry about medicine is a disposition which inhibits the acquisition of empirically grounded medical knowledge. For example, I will argue that it is epistemically vicious for vaccine denialists to avoid interactions with mainstream pediatricians who may challenge their views. A disposition to avoid potentially productive epistemic 'friction' is not conducive to acquiring medical knowledge.

Second, I turn to feminist scholarship in this chapter (and elsewhere in the book) because the interactions that occur in mainstream pediatric practice and among vaccine denialists are often influenced by gender, and because they manifest the sorts of gender-related power inequalities that have often been the focus of feminist work.[6] For example, the work of caring for children is gendered feminine, as is parental care for children's health, e.g. 'doctor mom'. And mothers make most of the decisions about how children interact with medical professionals. A report from the Henry J. Kaiser Family Foundation found that, in around 80% of households with children, mothers take the children to the doctor and have primary responsibility for making decisions about medical interventions (Henry J. Kaiser Family Foundation 2013). The public faces of vaccine denialism and refusal are often the faces of mothers, such as Alicia Silverstone, Jenny McCarthy, and Barbara Loe Fisher (Silverstone 2014; Williams 2014). Their online communities often focus on mothers, such as the Thinking Moms' Revolution (2014) or Moms against Mercury (2014). And books and other media in the vaccine denialist/refuser world are often directed towards mothers, too, e.g. *Mother Warriors* (McCarthy 2008). In contrast, the epistemic practices of physicians are often gendered masculine (even though many physicians are women).[7] Therefore, interactions between parents and pediatricians surrounding vaccination decisions take place against the background of gender inequalities and gendered conceptions of the reasoning of physicians and parents.[8]

Third, this chapter's discussion of the epistemic virtues and vices of vaccine denialists draws on the autobiographical testimony of vaccine denialists. Vaccine denialists have firsthand knowledge of how they have been treated by physicians and how the internal practices of vaccine denialist communities differ from those that are prevalent in mainstream medical contexts. Furthermore, we sometimes have good reason to lend credibility to the reports of social subordinates about the conditions of their social subordination. Parents – and especially mothers – who believe that they have been treated disrespectfully by physicians are likely to know more about the conditions of their treatment than their pediatricians are likely to know.[9] Of course, parental testimony may be legitimately challenged by the testimony of others, including physicians. But, for my purposes, parental testimony is sufficient to illustrate both the virtuous and vicious epistemic dispositions to which vaccine denialists are prone.[10]

Reasonable skepticism

There are good reasons to question the consensus view that vaccine denialism results from parental (and especially maternal) irrationality.

First, the socially privileged have often attempted to quell dissent by impugning the rationality of those who have challenged distributions of power. Anti-labor employers such as Henry Ford famously thought unions were bad for workers and that workers were too blinded by their short-term interests to realize this putative fact (Ford 2013, chap. 18). Racists who defended Jim Crow frequently insulted the cognitive capacities of civil rights activists.[11] And advocates for patriarchy have long invoked the supposed irrationality of women as a justification for their cause. Today, some businesses make money by convincing the public that grassroots protestors are irrational. A company called Stratfor tells its clients that (for a fee) it can persuade (what it calls) the realists, idealists, and opportunists that radicals are unreasonable agitators, with the aim of delegitimizing otherwise popular resistance movements (Horn 2013).

Since I am especially interested in the relationship between mothers and pediatricians, it may be helpful to reflect on the history of the relationship between femininity and 'irrationality'. As early as Plato, ideals of reason were often tied to ideas of masculinity while conceptions of irrationality were tied to ideas of femininity. Philosophers including Susan Bordo, Virginia Held, and Genevieve Lloyd (among many others) have shown how the supposed dichotomy of the 'rational man' and the 'irrational woman' has often been constructed and invoked to deny women equal social and political status (Bordo 1987; Held 1990; Lloyd 1993). This history of 'irrationality' is a reason to resist the quick conclusion that mothers' vaccine denialism can be explained by scientific illiteracy or by their failure to exercise reasonable control over their emotions.

A second reason to resist the claim that mothers act irrationally when they refuse to defer to the (supposed) epistemic authority of medical experts is that medical authorities have often harmed women.[12] In particular, activists and scholars have revealed and criticized the tendency of physicians to treat women's bodies as mere objects on which to perform their craft (Sherwin 1992). Women have often been abused in medical contexts, including coercive (interventions in) pregnancy and childbirth, involuntary sterilization, and more general violations of women's autonomy and informed consent. Consider one regrettably contemporary example: non-consensual pelvic exams. In many countries, it has until recently been common, if unofficial, practice for rooms of medical students to perform non-consensual pelvic examinations on women who had been anesthetized for medical procedures. In many cases, pelvic exams were not indicated for the procedures women had consented to receive (Coldicott, Pope, and Roberts 2003; Dwyer and Rothstein 1993). In the context of these sorts of historical (and sometimes ongoing) abuses, it is not 'irrational' for mothers to refuse to blindly trust the testimony their children's pediatricians offer about vaccines.

We can find further support for the reasonableness of mothers' skepticism about the testimony of medical authorities by reflecting on the particular ways in which *mothers* have been subjected to medical abuses. It is common for mothers to report they were disrespected or coerced during their hospital birthing experiences. These violations range from the relatively mild – being tethered by fetal heart monitors or otherwise restricted in birthing positions – to the more severe, including unnecessary episiotomies and caesarean sections (Block 2007; Gaskin 2011; Wagner 2008). Maternal vigilance about childhood medical interventions is also reasonable given social tendencies to hold mothers (rather than fathers, public institutions, etc.) responsible for how children turn out (Alcorn 2013; Lerner 2010). Mothers are often the first people to be blamed for children's poor health. For a notable example, the history of autism began by pointing the finger at mothers (Mnookin 2011a, 76–77). Bruno Bettelheim famously wrote that (what would come to be called) autism resulted from dysfunctional early attachment between mother and child (Bettelheim 1959). In social contexts in which mothers are so often the object of abuse and blame, it makes sense for them to be hyper-vigilant about the safety of their children. Maternal caution about children's health care makes even more sense in societies that do not offer much assistance to mothers of children with serious health conditions. In the absence of state-financed health care, childcare, and intervention services for children with disabilities, mothers have good reason to be especially risk averse, and to refuse to quickly assent to a pediatrician's testimony about the safety of vaccines. In chapter four, I discuss whether this sort of maternal vigilance – what Stephen John calls "hyper-rational parenting" – involves parents in immoral forms of free-riding (John 2011, 507). For now, I want to emphasize that parental skepticism about the safety and efficacy of vaccines is more reasonable than it may initially appear to be.

Many historical and ongoing abuses of medical power may have little to do with gender, but they may nonetheless give mothers (and fathers) good reason to withhold quick assent to the testimony that pediatricians provide about vaccine safety. For example, consider the common practice of over-prescription, e.g. of stimulants and antipsychotics for children (Schiff et al. 2011); the troubling recalls of unsafe high-profile drugs, e.g. Vioxx (Epstein 2013; Intemann and de Melo-Martín 2014); and the (not unrelated) corporate cooptation of both pharmaceutical research and physician continuing education (Lexchin et al. 2003; Wazana 2000).

On a more general note, parents may be aware that 'medicine' has often been dangerous, even though medical professionals have consistently vouched for its safety. The practice of bloodletting continued through the 19th century (Kerridge and Lowe 1994); doctors prescribed mercury, arsenic, and silver well into the 20th century (Jolliffe 1993; Swiderski

2008). Women were told to douche with Lysol and were encouraged to give their infants morphine to help them sleep (Bause 2012; Ferranti 2010). And the history of vaccines has not been exempt from dangerous mistakes. Production errors at Cutter Laboratories in 1954–1955 led to the manufacture of Salk polio vaccine with non-attenuated live virus. (The virus was supposed to have been 'killed' during production.) This error caused 200 cases of paralytic polio and 10 deaths. In 1976 the federal government overreacted to initial reports about a potential swine flu epidemic by calling for a nationwide immunization effort. The swine flu killed just 1 person, but the vaccine caused 500 cases of Guillain–Barré syndrome and killed 25 (Neustadt, Califano, and Fineberg 1978; Offit 2007).[13] Parents who know this (sometimes recent) history may thereby have good reason to resist granting quick credibility to the testimony that their pediatricians offer about the safety and efficacy of vaccines. Their hesitancy to defer to the expertise of pediatricians is even more understandable if their pediatricians are unwilling to admit to this troubled history and to the reality of current risks.

Parents are right to resist a narrative that is popular among vaccine proponents, according to which errors in the production of vaccines (or in vaccine policy, more generally) are a thing of the past. On the contrary, basic inductive reasoning tells us to expect vaccines to have safety problems in the future and to believe that there are errors in today's vaccine policies. To paraphrase David Hume, we cannot help but believe that the future will resemble the past. Of course, this is not by itself a reason not to vaccinate, since we do not know when and where mistakes are being made. However, our knowledge of the history of medical abuses and mistakes gives us reason to be skeptical of the quick assurances about vaccine safety that pediatricians may offer.

Epistemic vice and testimonial injustice in mainstream medicine

So far, I have shown (at most) that vaccine hesitancy may be justified. Facts about gender oppression and medical abuses provide mothers with good reasons to be skeptical of physicians' assurances regarding the safety and efficacy of vaccines. But this is to say only that parents are right to demand that physicians provide accurate and adequate answers to their questions about vaccines, and that physicians should grant appropriate credibility to parental testimony about their children's health. What I have said does not justify vaccine denialism, though it does make it less unreasonable than it may first appear to be.[14]

Now, I want to introduce another reason to resist the conclusion that vaccine denialists are 'irrational': Vaccine denialists often report that their children's pediatricians failed to be respectful listeners or to offer adequate accounts of the usefulness or safety of vaccines. Consider the stories of two prominent vaccine denialists:

Barbara Loe Fisher "founded America's modern-day vaccine denialism movement" and created the National Vaccine Information Center (NVIC), "the most powerful anti-vaccine organization in America" (Specter 2009, 7, 60). Fisher became an activist after she concluded that physicians had lied to her about the possible side effects of the pertussis vaccine (Offit 2010, 81). Specifically, she claims that physicians were insufficiently attentive to her reports of her child's developmental regression in the aftermath of vaccination. It seemed to Fisher that her doctors were elitists and frauds and that their failure to be attentive to trustworthy parental testimony contributed to the harms some children experienced through vaccination. She has dedicated her life to building a social movement that can bring this 'truth' to light.

Jenny McCarthy, a model and actress, is a prominent advocate for 'vaccine safety'. She was a spokesperson and board member for Generation Rescue, an advocacy group that claimed vaccines contribute to autism. According to McCarthy, her child's pediatrician mocked her concerns about the existence of a link between the MMR vaccine and her child's behavioral regression (McCarthy 2008; McCarthy 2011; Mnookin 2011a, 250–260). As a result of these experiences, McCarthy committed herself to building and supporting a social movement that would empower parents to make informed choices about vaccines. In the words of Oprah Winfrey, Jenny McCarthy decided to become a leader of the vaccine denialism movement because she refused to "bow to authority" and insisted that her voice be heard (Mnookin 2011a, 253).

Other vaccine denialists tell stories similar to those of Fisher and McCarthy. Sherri Tenpenny has collected dozens of these stories on her webpage, entitled "Boycott Pediatrician Bullies" (Tenpenny 2014). The recurring theme is that pediatricians laugh and yell at parents, refuse to take their concerns seriously, and sometimes kick them out of the office when they do not agree to vaccinate. David Kirby, the author of *Evidence of Harm* (a book that reports favorably on vaccine denialism), says that many of the parents he interviewed became critical of vaccines after they had negative interactions with physicians (Kirby 2006). These parents report being talked down to, being "barked at," and feeling like they were "banished to a small corner of the room" when they raised critical questions about vaccines or when they shared their experiences of their children's developmental regression in the aftermath of vaccination (Kirby 2006, 13). According to Kirby, many vaccine denialists now think of pediatricians as sadists who "poked and prodded" children "like some pet science project" (Kirby 2006, 23). They believe physicians are so interested in preserving their power that they are unwilling to listen. More sympathetic portrayals of pediatricians also provide evidence of poor epistemic practices. For example, Andrea Kitta describes pediatricians who dread conversations with parents who want to talk about vaccine safety at office visits (Kitta 2012, 52–57). These physicians do not laugh or yell at parents, but they do wish parents would stop asking so many questions, and would just agree to let their kids get the shots.

It is a poor epistemic practice for pediatricians to be disrespectful and dismissive in response to parents' questions about vaccine safety, or to fail to grant appropriate credibility to parents' testimony about their children's responses to vaccinations. A disposition to engage in either of these behaviors is an epistemic vice since it makes pediatricians and parents less likely to arrive at true beliefs about both vaccination and children's health, more generally.[15] This is because parents and pediatricians are more likely to arrive at true beliefs about childhood vaccination when pediatricians treat parents as experts about their children's symptoms and medical histories, and when pediatricians treat parents' questions and concerns with respect.

A physician's epistemic viciousness may also be an instance of what Miranda Fricker has called *epistemic injustice* (Fricker 2007). A pediatrician's failure to grant credibility to parents becomes *unjust* when it results from group-based bias, e.g. about the epistemic credibility of non-professionals or women. In particular, this would be an example of *testimonial injustice*,[16] since prejudice can cause pediatricians "to give a deflated level of credibility to a speaker's word" (Fricker 2007, 1).[17] For example, pediatricians may discount or dismiss a mother's experiential or intuitive knowledge on the grounds that it lacks the rigor or objectivity of medical knowledge, or because it arises from the experiences of a non-professional (Fricker 2007, 90f). Hilde Lindemann writes that when a physician discounts a mother's "experiential testimony" because she is a woman (or a non-professional) the relationship between the two "stops being merely a hierarchy and becomes an oppressive hierarchy" (Lindemann 2007, 122–123).[18] It is oppressive because it "excludes the subject [the mother] from trustful conversation" on the basis of her membership in a disadvantaged social group (Fricker 2007, 53). An observation from Lorraine Code is apt in this context: Resistance to the epistemic authority of women often *increases* as women become more educated and more socially powerful (Code 1991). If Code is right, we would expect pediatricians to be even more dismissive when educated and assertive mothers consider vaccine denialism/refusal.

According to Miranda Fricker, being excluded from the respectful give-and-take of reasons is an especially grave offense. Participation in trustful conversation plays a central role in our lives. Being excluded from this activity causes moral harm to the victim of epistemic injustice and undermines the likelihood that inquiry will achieve its epistemic goals. Fricker stresses that testimonial injustice

> marginalizes the subject in her participation in the very activity [trustful conversation] that steadies the mind and forges an essential aspect of identity – two processes of fundamental psychological importance for the individual. Further, testimonial injustice is not

merely a moment of exclusion from this doubly psychologically valuable activity, it is a prejudicial exclusion.

(Fricker 2007, 53–54)

We all need to be able to participate in a respectful give-and-take of reasons with the people with whom we share our lives. Trustful conversation helps us to avoid mistaken ways of thinking, and it allows us to identify ourselves as valued participants in communities of knowing.

Pediatricians may commit acts of testimonial injustice because they are vulnerable to a set of epistemic vices to which privileged persons are often prone.[19] José Medina has identified three epistemic vices to which socially privileged persons (such as physicians) often succumb. First, pediatricians may be under the sway of *epistemic arrogance* if their power as physicians makes them so epistemically conceited that they "have a hard time learning from their mistakes, their biases, and the constraints and presuppositions of their position in the world" (Medina 2013, 30). Second, pediatricians may be subject to *laziness* if their social privilege causes a "habitual lack of curiosity [that] atrophies [their] cognitive attitudes and dispositions" (Medina 2013, 33). The repetitive and rushed nature of many pediatrician-parent interactions may encourage unconscious and mechanistic medical practice. Finally, pediatricians may have the vice of *closed-mindedness* if their failures to take maternal testimony seriously result from effortful attempts to ignore or hide information that might compromise their social position (or their self-image) (Medina 2013, 34). Getting clear about which of these epistemic vices contribute to particular instances of testimonial injustice depends on the details of each case. But these seem to be the sorts of epistemic vices that are operating in some of the cases vaccine denialists describe.

My focus on Fricker's work on epistemic injustice should not be taken to imply that she is the only (or the first) person to address this topic. Indeed, the exclusion of women from trusting conversation has long been a focus of feminist criticism. Consider Sandra Harding's observation of

the struggle we have had to get women's testimony about rape, wife battering, sexual harassment, and incest experiences accepted as reliable by police, the courts, employers, psychiatrists, other men and women, etc.

(Harding 1987, 77)

It is difficult to generate consensus in favor of widespread social and political changes if many members of one's society do not know what the problems are and if they cannot hear what the oppressed are saying. For these (and for other) reasons, feminist philosophers such as Lorraine Code and Helen Longino have often focused on the ways in which failures to properly respond to the testimony of the oppressed relate to the moral wrongs of gender oppression (Code 2004; Longino 2002). Philosophers who have written about race-based oppression, such as Charles Mills, José Medina, and Linda Martín Alcoff, have also often focused on the epistemological bases of racism and white supremacy. Accordingly, Fricker's work on epistemic injustice (and testimonial injustice) takes place against a background of widespread acceptance among philosophers of the significant role that epistemic deficits play in our evaluation of phenomena related to group-based oppression.

One reason to be disappointed about the breakdown in trusting relationships between vaccine denialist parents and pediatricians is that under optimal conditions, a pediatrician would be a parent's most-trusted authority on childhood vaccines. However, when a pediatrician refuses to respectfully respond to a mother's worries about the necessity or safety of vaccination, or when he refuses to take seriously her reports about her child's deteriorating health in the aftermath of vaccination, he may also undermine the trust *she* is willing to place in *his testimony* about vaccines.[20] His failure to treat her testimony appropriately shows that he does not make good judgments about the credibility of sources of (putative) knowledge. Therefore, a pediatrician's epistemic viciousness in his treatment of maternal testimony provides a mother with a reason to decrease the credibility she grants to the pediatrician's testimony, and this includes his testimony about the safety of vaccines. How much a mother is permitted to discount the credibility of her pediatrician's testimony depends on the severity of the epistemic vices the pediatrician displays. At the very least, the existence of an authoritarian pediatrician-parent relationship is a reason for a mother to be skeptical of her pediatrician's claims about vaccine science. Such a dysfunctional relationship also provides a reason for her to seek out communities of medical practice which better affirm her status as a knower.

Mothers who have been subjected to testimonial injustice by their children's pediatricians have good reason to find other health care providers for their children, specifically, pediatricians who will not subject them to testimonial injustice. (Victims of oppression have a right to escape oppressive conditions.) Even if they may be obligated to resist their oppression, the best way to resist one's oppression may sometimes be to abandon oppressive relationships and to create new forms of social life. It would be best for a mother who has faced epistemic injustice at the hands of a mainstream pediatrician to seek out another mainstream pediatrician, and to insist that the new pediatrician include her in trustful conversation. However, a mother who believes that testimonial injustices are prevalent among mainstream pediatricians may have a good reason (about *reasoning*) for abandoning mainstream pediatric practices in favor of communities of medical inquiry in which testimonial injustices are less common.

To be clear: The epistemic vices I have described in this section may not be prevalent among pediatricians. But stories about these vices are pervasive in the narratives that vaccine denialists provide. Furthermore, the blame for these poor practices surely does not rest entirely with individual pediatricians. Instead, the fact that pediatricians often have little time to meet with parents likely contributes to breakdowns in trustworthy communication (see e.g. Dugdale, Epstein, and Pantilat 1999; Halfon et al. 2011). The fact that pediatricians are often underprepared to deal with patients (and parents) who expect to be informed and active participants in their medical care does not help either.[21] We also should not be too quick to conclude that pediatricians who are paternalistic (and otherwise disrespectful) are consciously biased against mothers, i.e. as women or non-professionals. I assume that few pediatricians think of themselves as sexists or classists. Instead, many of the pediatricians who vaccine denialists describe could be responding to their *implicit biases*, that is, biases of which they are not aware.[22] Finally, I have so far uncritically accepted parents' testimony that their children's pediatricians have subjected them to experiences that can be accurately characterized as epistemic injustices. This testimony may turn out to be unreliable. However, even if the testimony of vaccine denialists is inaccurate, and even if their pediatricians have done them no (epistemic) harm, the fact that parents believe that they have been subjected to testimonial injustice is a reason to be concerned about the breakdown of trusting relationships between parents and pediatricians.

Resistant communities of medical inquiry

Parents who believe they have been subjected to testimonial injustice by their pediatricians may have good reason to join (or form) resistant epistemic communities since these communities may be relatively free of the paternalistic and authoritarian dynamics that are more common in mainstream medical contexts. However, these alternative epistemic spaces may cultivate their own epistemic vices, which may prevent the members of these communities from acquiring accurate information about vaccines. In order to make informed judgments about the epistemic virtues and vices of vaccine denialists, I want to say more about how these communities function. First, I want to place vaccine denialist communities in a broader historical and social context.

There have been resistant communities of medical inquiry for as long as medicine has been a profession. Women have often been at the forefront of these communities. In fact, we may view the history of alternative medical communities (including the history of vaccine denialist communities) as part of a continuous tradition of resistance against the ways in which post-19th-century medicine pushed women healers to the sidelines. In the pre-modern (and pre-scientific) period, much of the practice of healing was carried out by women, both through informal care for family and community members, and through more formal social roles, such as that of midwives (Achterberg 1991; Ehrenreich and English 2010; Green 1989). This is not to suggest that medical practice was egalitarian, but that it was pluralistic, and that there were important roles for women healers to play in various communities of medical practice, even in the face of institutionalized gender oppression. However, the professionalization of medicine, with its emphasis on uniform technique and medical technology, admitted of much less pluralism in medical practice. To be clear, professionalized science-based medicine was able to solve problems that vexed healers for millennia. The end of the 19th century and the beginning of the 20th century witnessed the introduction of antiseptic and aseptic techniques, safe blood transfusion, diagnostic X-ray technology, and sulfa antibiotics, in addition to vaccines against rabies, cholera, and diphtheria. It is surely a good thing that these science-based medical successes occurred and that they went quickly into widespread use. However, it is understandable that 'alternative healers' formed resistant communities, and we may reasonably regret that the professionalization of medicine conspired with patriarchy to drive women from the center of mainstream medical research and practice (with the exception of nursing) until the women's rights movements of the mid-20th century began to offer effective resistance. Given this historical context, we may come to believe that it was reasonable for women (and for other non-mainstream healers) to form resistant communities of medical inquiry and practice.

Consider some examples of women's leadership in alternative communities of medical inquiry: Mary Baker Eddy founded Christian Science and published *Science and Health with Key to the Scriptures* in 1875 (Eddy 2009). In the years since that time, millions of people have practiced her religion. They have adopted her belief that illness is an illusion of the material world and that prayer can help us to correct the false beliefs that give rise to illness. For another example, consider the story that Arthur Allen tells about Lora Little, one of the leaders of the early 20th century natural health movement. Little was

> [t]he most charismatic spokesperson for the new movement ... [She was a] feisty opponent of the medical establishment, ... a sort of granola-belt Mother Jones who promoted whole foods and naturopathy and denounced white sugar and white male medical practitioners before it was fashionable to do so.
>
> (Allen 2007, 104)

Another woman who preached the importance of diet and lifestyle for health was Sister Elizabeth Kenny. Kenny and her followers pioneered what would come to be called 'physical therapy' when they showed that some patients suffering from polio could avoid permanent paralysis if their limbs were kept in motion, rather than placed in braces or casts (Oshinsky 2006, 73f). She was such a prominent personality that for almost a decade she placed second (behind only Eleanor Roosevelt) in Gallup's poll of the "Most Admired Woman in America."

Finally, the Women's Health Movement gave voice to many of the values of the women's rights movements of the mid- to late 20th century. Participants in this movement attended 'self-help' seminars to learn about their bodies and their health. These seminars sometimes featured guided self-investigations of the vulva, vagina, and cervix (Murphy 2004). Nancy Tuana writes that the Women's Health Movement "aimed to take our bodies back from the institutions of medicine and reframe our knowledge and experiences of our bodies in ways not configured by sexism and andro-centrism" (Tuana 2006, 2). In 1973, The Boston Women's Health Book Collective published *Our Bodies, Ourselves* (Boston Women's Health Book Collective and Norsigian 2011). This book featured the testimony of a collection of women about their health experiences, and it focused on topics that were often ignored or shortchanged in mainstream medical contexts, including abortion and sexual pleasure.

La Leche League as a resistant epistemic community

La Leche League (LLL) is a breastfeeding support group. It manifests the same epistemic virtues as other resistant epistemic communities (including those formed by vaccine denialists). I discuss LLL to draw attention to the epistemic virtues I will discuss in greater detail in the next section.

At the turn of the 20th century, most young infants in the United States were exclusively breastfed (Fomon 2001). By the 1960s this would be true of fewer than one in three (Riordan and Countryman 1980). But in the early 1900s, mothers of infants turned to their mothers, sisters, cousins, and community members when they had trouble breastfeeding. These networks offered expert knowledge about how to maintain suc-cessful breastfeeding, and they provided support for solving common problems, such as tongue-ties. However, as individuals and nuclear families moved to urban centers for work and other opportunities, these familial knowledge communities became less accessible, if they continued to exist at all (Wolf 2003). Isolated mothers often struggled with breast-feeding and sometimes came to rely on (easily available) cow's milk to feed their babies. However, poor or nonexistent refrigeration meant that cow's milk occasionally went bad, and the infants who consumed it sometimes became sick or died. Industry and professional medicine were, therefore, responding to a real problem when they developed and pro-moted artificial infant formula. (Industry was also, of course, acting on the basis of its profit motive.) Physicians and industry, including large corporations such as Nestlé, promoted evaporated milk-based formulas as a healthy alternative to breast milk, and they played on mothers' fears and insecurities surrounding breastfeeding to promote the use of these products (Greer and Apple 1991). Soon, large majorities of mothers were feeding their babies with formula.

In 1956 a group of seven women formed LLL to offer support for breastfeeding mothers. They published *The Womanly Art of Breastfeeding* in 1958, and went on to lead a social movement that contributed to the re-normalization of breastfeeding by the turn of the 21st century (Hausman 2003; Weiner 1994; Wiessinger, West, and Pitman 2010). LLL (later to become La Leche League International, LLLI) was a resistant epistemic community. Its efforts have been so successful that it may not be so 'resistant' any longer. It promoted breastfeeding by forming and supporting groups of mothers, where each participant could offer guidance to the others based on her knowledge and experiences. As LLL grew, it sponsored and distributed original scientific research on the benefits of breastfeeding. LLL contributed to a shift in mainstream medical thinking about breast-feeding. Many hospitals have now refused to distribute the formula samples industry provides to them. Hospitals have also hired breastfeeding con-sultants to visit and work with new mothers, and they offer institutional support to LLL groups (Hannula, Kaunonen, and Tarkka 2008).

LLL is not a perfect organization and it has been criticized (justly, I think) for promoting an excessively child-focused approach to mothering (Kukla 2006). I acknowledge this criticism, but I focus on some positive features of LLL by way of segueing to my discussion of the epistemic virtues of vaccine denialist communities in the next section of this chapter. First, LLL groups are resistant epistemic communities. They collect and distribute knowledge to help mothers resist (once) dominant mothering practices, e.g. using infant formula and practicing early weaning. Second, LLL groups are democratic communities. LLL leaders undergo some training and they help run meetings, but their primary role is to encourage open conversa-tion among mothers, conversations which welcome everyone's views and experiences. The Mission Statement of LLLI illustrates the group's commitment to these epistemic virtues:

> Our Mission: To help mothers worldwide to breastfeed through mother-to-mother support, encouragement, information, and education, and to promote a better understanding of breastfeeding as an important element in the healthy development of the baby and mother.
>
> (Wiessinger, West, and Pitman 2010, 440)

In the next section, I argue that vaccine denialist communities often manifest the same epistemic virtues as does LLL.

Epistemic virtues of vaccine denialist communities

Vaccine denialists often do much more than reject vaccine science. They frequently participate in alternative communities of knowers. Indeed, parental social networks – both online and in-person – play a much larger role in the decision making of parents who refuse vaccines than they do for parents who vaccinate (Brunson 2013). But the social networks in which vaccine refusers participate often treat inquiry about medical science very differently than mainstream medical institutions do. Some of these differences may foster truth-oriented inquiry. One epistemic virtue of vaccine denialist communities is that they are spaces in which otherwise silent or sidelined voices can be heard. These communities allow people to engage in inquiry about childhood vaccines, regardless of their profession or education. This is a good thing. Consider what José Medina says about the importance of hearing what he calls "alien experiences" (Medina 2013, 46). In Medina's view there is a "critical and subversive potential" to the insights of members of relatively disadvantaged groups (Medina 2013, 47). Medina says that when we cultivate "consciousness from elsewhere," this can provide "insight into the cognitive limitations and obstacles of our perspectives" (Medina 2013, 200). The experiences and concerns of non-physician parents have epistemic value. Advocates of truth-oriented inquiry should be glad that there are spaces where their voices can be heard.

Another epistemic virtue of vaccine denialist communities is that they often practice democratic norms for allocating epistemic authority.[23] Vaccine denialist communities manifest this epistemic virtue in three ways. First, these are online and in-person communities in which anyone may access and contribute information about vaccination. An article from *The Lancet* observes that vaccine denialists

> have changed the environment around vaccines from top-down, expert-to-consumer (vertical) communication towards non-hierarchical, dialogue-based (horizontal) communication, through which the public increasingly questions recommendations of experts and public institutions on the basis of their own, often web-based, research.
>
> (Larson et al. 2011, 528)

One need not have a medical degree to enter into inquiry among vaccine denialists. For example, Jenny McCarthy reports that "[t]he University of Google is where I got my degree from" (Mnookin 2011a, 253). Like many vaccine denialists, McCarthy used the Internet to seek out information about vaccines. She developed online relationships with other parents who had similar experiences and worries surrounding childhood vaccination. One place that fosters these sorts of relationships is the online message board sponsored by *Mothering* magazine, which now contains over 30,000 conversations (and almost 350,000 posts) on the topic of childhood vaccination (Mothering 2015).[24] Many other communities – both online and in-person – support parents in resisting routine childhood vaccination. Like the *Mothering* magazine forums, these communities do not usually focus exclusively on vaccination. They also offer support to mothers who are committed to some combination of other parenting practices, including home-birthing, breastfeeding, cloth-diapering, co-sleeping, baby-wearing, and other aspects of 'natural' or 'attachment' parenting.[25] (In chapter three I will say more about the role that the idea of 'the natural' plays in vaccine denialism/refusal.)

On a personal note, my partner is a member of a local organization that is organized around the idea of attachment parenting. Many members of her group do not vaccinate or they selectively vaccinate, and they support each other in this decision through online and in-person discussions, even though the group's focus extends far beyond vaccination-related practices, and even though many members of the group vaccinate. (Our children are fully vaccinated.) For some indication of how significant these online communities have become for vaccine denialism, consider that the pharmaceutical giant GlaxoSmithKline has been monitoring online discussion forums to learn why so many parents have false beliefs about the safety and efficacy of its vaccines (Schectman 2013).

Some parents become so involved in vaccine-related inquiry that they call themselves "parent-researchers" (Mnookin 2011a, 135). In *The Panic Virus*, Seth Mnookin tells how the most active vaccine denialists have developed an alternative industry of labs and journals, where the relevant evidence consists of compilations of the "parental reports of autistic children" (Mnookin 2011a, 143–144).[26] These parent-researchers have sometimes attempted to engage with mainstream medical authorities. For example, David Kirby describes what happened when a group of parents attended a presentation about vaccine safety put on by the National Institutes of Health. At one point in the presentation, a parent interrupted the lecture:

> "Many of us here are not just parents, but researchers as well," she said. "We have come up with great ideas for controlled studies to look at immune panels, food allergies, nutritional deficiencies, gastrointestinal problems, and so on … How *dare* you patronize us with this kind of information … We are not stupid! We are educated, informed parents who have done thousands of hours of research in autism. We did not come here to be lectured to. We came to be listened to."
>
> (Kirby 2006, 104, emphasis in original)

Parents who participate in vaccine denialist communities are not just receiving information. They have become sources of information about vaccines, and they believe that they have something to offer to mainstream medical researchers.

Another way in which vaccine denialists promote the democratic allocation of epistemic authority is through collaborative relationships between pediatricians and parents. Physicians who are vaccine denialists, or who are willing to treat the children of vaccine denialists, often present themselves as co-equal participants with parents.[27] They may view themselves as correctives against (what they perceive to be) other physicians' paternalistic abuses of medical authority. For example, Andrew Wakefield explains that his involvement in vaccine denialism was a response to

[attempts to] dismiss parents' claims of a link between their child's disorder and MMR without due investigation, in breach of the most fundamental rules of clinical medicine ... When parents have their claims dismissed, out of hand ... they create frustration, resentment, and distrust; similarly disaffected parents form into self help groups.

(Wakefield 2011, 85)

Wakefield presents himself, and his work, as an antidote to the disrespectful and dismissive treatment many vaccine denialist parents claim to have received from their children's pediatricians. Jenny McCarthy writes that Andrew Wakefield "did the sort of thing most of us expect out of our doctors ... he listened closely to the stories of parents and he told the truth" (Wakefield 2011, iii). Wakefield's work on vaccine safety has more recently been exposed as unethical and fraudulent (there's more about this in the next section) (Deer 2011; General Medical Council 2010; Godlee, Smith, and Marcovitch 2011). However, there is no essential connection between the moral and academic lapses that led to the retraction of Wakefield's research (and to his disbarment from the medical profession), and the patient and respectful interactions Wakefield has had with parents. One can applaud Wakefield's epistemic and moral virtues without embracing his epistemic and moral vices.[28]

A final way in which vaccine denialist communities practice a democratic allocation of epistemic authority is that they place members of otherwise subordinate groups in leadership. Non-physician mothers have consistently been at the forefront of contemporary vaccine denialism's leadership. Lea Thompson helped spark the contemporary vaccine denialism movement with her 1982 NBC broadcast, *DPT: Vaccine Roulette* (Thompson and Nuell 1982). Along with Barbara Loe Fisher, Thompson helped promote the National Childhood Vaccine Injury Act of 1986 (Offit 2010, 60). Senator Paula Hawkins, who was the first (and still the only) woman senator from Florida, chaired the first congressional hearings on whether vaccines cause brain damage. The current executive director of NVIC, the largest advocacy group for vaccine safety, is a woman (as is a super-majority of its board and staff) (National Vaccine Information Center 2015). Jenny McCarthy has been called "America's most recognized anti-vaccine activist," with books, a television show, and numerous television and print interviews (Offit 2010, 151). McCarthy's work has been promoted by Oprah Winfrey, who is one of the most powerful media personalities of our day. The prominence of these women signals to other non-physician mothers that their experiences, questions, and advice will be welcome in vaccine denialist communities.

We have good reason to seek out communities that engage in good epistemic practices. Therefore, parents who have been attracted to vaccine denialism by its epistemic virtues may have good reasons (about reasoning) for participating in vaccine denialism.

Epistemic vices of vaccine denialists

Vaccine denialist communities are committed to some good epistemic practices, but they are disposed to poor epistemic practices, too. These include the pursuit of an uncritical affirmation of their existing beliefs and a failure to show appropriate regard for differences in expertise or competence. Parents who have been attracted to vaccine denialism by these (or other) epistemic vices are responding to bad reasons (about reasoning).

Uncritical affirmation

It is epistemically vicious to pursue uncritical affirmation of your current beliefs. Vaccine denialists manifest this epistemic vice when they try to avoid engaging in the giving and taking of reasons with their pediatricians. Some vaccine denialists go to great lengths to prevent themselves from being challenged. They may replace their children's pediatricians with naturopaths, homeopaths, and chiropractors, i.e. medical professionals whose training in alternative therapies often leaves them un(der)prepared to understand research science, and who are predisposed to reject evidence-based forms of medicine (Ernst 2001). The fact that alternative medical practices are not usually covered by public and private health insurance programs means that alternative practitioners have strong incentives to develop and maintain their 'customer base', where this can include telling their 'customers' what they want to hear. But alternative practitioners need not have mercenary motives to reject vaccine science. At the core of many alternative forms of medical practice is the idea that patients are experts about their own health and health care, and the idea that medical professionals are partners whose job is to work alongside their patients. I just argued, in the previous section, that all pediatricians ought to treat parents as partners. But they ought not to treat parents' prejudices about vaccine science as authoritative. Instead, they ought to embrace (roughly) the same scientifically established set of beliefs about diseases and treatments as do other mainstream medical professionals. This is the promise of evidence-based medicine (Sackett et al. 1996). In contrast, alternative medical practitioners seem more likely to tailor diagnoses and treatments to suit the pre-existing beliefs of their patients. Parents who seek out alternative practitioners for this reason manifest epistemic vice.

Even when vaccine denialists engage with mainstream pediatricians, they often seek out practitioners who will not challenge them. And vaccine denialist communities frequently offer support to mothers who are 'shopping' for compliant physicians, or who are looking for strategies to shut down pro-vaccination narratives their pediatricians might provide. Consider the following advice that a user of the *Mothering* magazine online discussion forums provides to mothers who are looking for health care professionals:

> [A]s their mother ... you are there [sic] doctor! No one knows your kids better than you. Doctors are just human being [sic] who make a lot [sic] money. Find a doctor who won't give you hell about not vaxing ... do all your own research ... and find a naturopath there for assistance when necessary.
>
> (Mothering 2009)

This passage packs a lot of epistemic vice into a short space. We learn that parents are medical experts when it comes to their own children, doctors are businesspeople rather than medical experts, parents should find doctors who will not challenge them, and parents who are unable to find compliant physicians should turn to alternative practitioners – such as naturopaths, homeopaths or chiropractors – since these people will tell vaccine denialist parents what they want to hear.

A patient should not treat her physician like a kind of medical vending machine that she can use to get whatever treatment she has antecedently decided upon. Instead, patients should generally defer to physicians' expert judgments about the likely outcomes of various options. But, at least in the case of pediatric care, the scope of deference should be even larger: Parents should generally defer to physicians' value judgments about which medical interventions would be best for children. Of course, patients (and parents) should have some autonomy surrounding health care choices (though I will argue in chapters four and five that this value is not as relevant to vaccination choices as many people believe). But autonomous action should be *informed* action, and pediatricians are generally experts about both biomedical science and various values surrounding childhood health and well-being. Accordingly, I think pediatricians ought to be allowed to lead parents through deliberations about the medical choices for their child. And a person who is so resistant to adversarial deliberation about vaccines that she seeks out only practitioners who will accede to her existing beliefs and preferences, has taken one of the virtues of vaccine denialist communities and transformed it into a vice.

It is a sign of epistemic virtue that vaccine denialists refuse to have their views silenced. It is also a sign of epistemic virtue that vaccine denialists join with others to form resistant epistemic communities. But the drive to protect spaces in which mothers' voices can be heard stops being virtuous (and starts being vicious) when it manifests a resistance to the voices of mainstream medicine. Physicians are experts and experts ought to be heard, and resistant medical communities that avoid bringing parents into conversations with physicians are not preparing parents to reason well. Furthermore, a disposition towards unjustified self-confidence is an epistemic vice, perhaps the central epistemic vice. (In the next chapter, I discuss some causes and consequences of excessive epistemic self-reliance among vaccine denialists.) The reason to make space for mothers' concerns, questions, and experiences is so that these concerns, questions, and experiences can be brought into creative tension with the views of experts about vaccine science and pediatric medicine. Resistant epistemic communities should not promote epistemic closure, but should stimulate productive engagement across boundaries that might otherwise be difficult to cross.

There are a number of reasons to temper the blame we assign to parents who refuse to meet with mainstream pediatricians. The fact that pediatricians have subjected some parents (and especially mothers) to disrespectful (even abusive) treatment may make parental resistance to reasoning with pediatricians less blameworthy. Also, many of the parents who do not want to reason with physicians may have developed con-fidence about their views after online investigations and in-person dis-cussions. They may believe they have already given sufficient consideration to the reasons in favor of vaccination. Finally, parents whose children have serious disorders, such as autism, are likely to be exhausted by caring for their children. They are also more likely to have had a long series of hostile interactions with physicians and other public (health) officials. Accordingly, it may be less blameworthy for the parents of such children to avoid epistemic 'friction' with mainstream health care providers.

Another reason to mitigate the blame we assign to vaccine denialists is that testimonial injustice can be self-fulfilling.[29] When a pediatrician treats a mother as if she were incapable of understanding vaccine science, or as if she were unable to provide reliable testimony regarding her child's health, these interactions may make it more difficult for a mother to under-stand vaccine science or to provide reliable testimony. This is because testimonial injustice may occasion *stereotype threat*, i.e. when a member of a disadvantaged group instantiates a negative stereotype of her group after she has been made anxious or frustrated under conditions when she has the potential to confirm that negative stereotype (C. M. Steele 2010). When a mother is confronted by a pediatrician who assumes that she does not or cannot understand the science of vaccines, the anxiety or anger that this confrontation generates may, in turn, undermine the mother's ability to understand the relevant science. Women in sexist societies are frequently subjected to this kind of stereotype threat, and long-term exposure to stereotype threat in a particular domain can encourage people to avoid the domains in which they experience that stereotype threat.[30] For example, women who have frequently been subjected to stereotype threat under conditions which require them to demonstrate scientific knowledge may attempt to avoid conditions which require the demonstration of scientific knowledge. Instead, they may seek out supportive online communities (which often promote vaccine denialism) to avoid confrontations with pediatricians about the science of vaccines. And when these mothers find a medical professional who fosters a comfortable clinical space, as Andrew Wakefield supposedly did, they may be especially reluctant to recognize this person's epistemic and moral failures.

Disregarding differences in expertise and competence

Some vaccine denialists seem unwilling to recognize that physicians and medical researchers are more likely than non-physician parents to (be able to) well understand immunology, epidemiology, and other topics related to vaccination. This vicious tendency is distinct from a vicious tendency to avoid interactions with pediatricians, since parents can try to avoid confrontations with people who they nonetheless recognize as experts, and because parents may be willing to be challenged by physicians who they fail to recognize as experts about children's health care.

I argued earlier that mothers have some expert knowledge about their children, including knowledge about their medical histories and their current symptoms. Also, mothers' questions ought to be heard and responded to, and mothers ought to be recognized as persons who are capable of understanding and reasoning about vaccines. However, we should not overstate parental epistemic authority: Physicians, scientific researchers, and public health authorities possess forms of competence and expertise that most parents do not. A failure to recognize real differences in epistemic authority is a vicious overdevelopment of an otherwise virtuous tendency to allocate epistemic authority more democratically.

The case of Andrew Wakefield is an evocative example of vaccine denialists' failure to recognize differences in expertise or competence. Recall that Wakefield was the lead author of a paper that claimed to find a link between MMR vaccine, bowel disorders, and forms of behavioral regression that are common in autistic children (Wakefield et al. 1998). The publication of this paper contributed to public sentiment that vaccines were not as safe as mainstream medical authorities had promised. In the United Kingdom, the conservative media politicized this issue: It used the Wakefield study to raise questions about the ways in which the Labour government was running the National Health Service (Fitzpatrick 2012). As a result of the prominence that the *Lancet* paper (and its publicity) afforded him, Wakefield became a celebrated leader of the vaccine denialism movement, headlining conferences and serving as a model for vaccine denialists of 'a physician who listens to parents'.[31] However, the *British Medical Journal* later confirmed that the 1998 study was fraudulent, and that Wakefield had various conflicts of interest (Deer 2011; Godlee, Smith, and Marcovitch 2011). For example, Wakefield had applied for patents for alternative methods of delivering the vaccines that were contained in the MMR vaccine that he criticized in the *Lancet* paper. Also, Wakefield did not disclose that he was paid by attorneys whose clients were seeking compensation for supposed vaccine complications. Furthermore, the General Medical Council found Wakefield guilty of many serious ethical lapses, including ordering medically unnecessary and dangerous procedures for his research purposes. For that reason it barred him from practicing medicine in Great Britain (General Medical Council 2010).

Many vaccine denialists have rallied around Wakefield. Major autism activist groups continue to support him, and have denounced those who have criticized him (Age of Autism et al. 2011; Stone 2015). Wakefield's 2011 book, *Callous Disregard*, was well-reviewed by high-profile members of the vaccine denialism movement. Consider the following selection from a review of the book by Mary Holland, a co-founder of the Elizabeth Birt Center for Autism Law and Advocacy:

> Dr. Wakefield sets the record straight. It was not he who showed callous disregard towards vulnerable, sick children with autism. It was the British medical establishment, the General Medical Council, the media and the pharmaceutical industry that threw the children under the bus to protect the vaccine program.
>
> (Holland 2011, iii)

Parents who continue to put their trust in the views of Andrew Wakefield do not grant sufficient credibility to the processes by which academic journal articles are retracted or by which physicians are stripped of their licenses to practice. These vaccine denialists have granted insufficient epistemic weight to medical and academic experts.

Vaccine denialists also fail to acknowledge differences in competence and expertise when they rely on alternative medical practitioners to treat and prevent childhood diseases. While some alternative medical practices may be effective, many are not. Homeopathic 'vaccines' contain nothing but water, chiropractic spinal manipulation neither prevents nor cures measles, and a naturopath's prescription of a healthy diet and exercise will not prevent a child from getting polio. Also, vaccine denialists often see *themselves* as experts about the prevention and treatment of routine childhood diseases. It's true that vaccine denialists are, on average, better educated than parents who vaccinate their children (as I mentioned in the Introduction). However, vaccine denialists are not usually able to understand, diagnose, treat, or prevent childhood diseases as well as mainstream medical professionals can.

My objection may seem unwarranted since vaccine denialists and refusers often defer to alternative medical practitioners. But here, vaccine refusers and denialists unjustifiably claim a different form of expertise: They claim to be able to identify who the medical experts are, without deferring to the consensus views of science-backed mainstream medical institutions and authorities. One reason why vaccine denialists fail to defer to the medical expertise of mainstream pediatricians is because they do not defer to what the *meta-experts* (experts about who is an expert) say through peer-reviewed journal articles, degree-granting institutions, licensing organizations, and regulatory agencies. I acknowledge that it can sometimes be difficult for epistemic novices to decide who the experts are, especially when the putative experts disagree. But Alvin Goldman is right that novices can (and should) benefit from the appraisals of meta-experts, such as the ones I list above (Goldman 2001).[32] When they disregard this information, they have not reasoned well.[33]

One reason vaccine denialists fail to recognize differences in competence or expertise is because they sometimes endorse beliefs about vaccines for (the wrong) non-epistemic reasons.[34] For example, consider the belief that *toxins* in vaccines cause diseases and disorders, including autism. At one point vaccine denialists claimed that autism was caused by the mercury (thimerosal/thiomersal) in some vaccines (Kennedy 2005; Kirby 2006). Later, in the face of scientific studies which showed no evidence of a link between thimerosal/thiomersal and autism, vaccine denialists largely abandoned this claim. However, they went on to claim that other ingredients in vaccines (e.g. formaldehyde, aluminum) cause autism (Fombonne 2008; Gerber and Offit 2009).

It is commendable that vaccine denialists have been willing to abandon their confident beliefs about the etiology of autism in the face of overwhelming contradictory evidence. The problem is that vaccine denialists have a history of moving from unjustified confidence in one supposed vaccine-related cause of autism to unjustified confidence in another supposed vaccine-related cause of that disorder. This is not a practice of truth-oriented inquiry. Instead, it seems driven by a deep desire on the part of some parents of autistic children to identify a cause of their children's disorder and to believe there is something they can do to prevent other children from developing autism.[35] These motivations are understandable and praiseworthy. But the desire to make some sense out of a difficult situation, and the related desire to believe that there is something one can do to prevent similar difficulties for others, is not a reason to believe particular claims about what has caused one's difficulties. Inasmuch as such desires are among the reasons why vaccine denialists have decided that vaccines are unsafe, we have evidence that vaccine denialists sometimes assent to claims about vaccine safety for (irrelevant) non-epistemic reasons.

There may seem to be a tension in my view. On one hand, I criticize vaccine denialists for their failure to recognize the authority of medical experts. On the other hand, I advocate more democratic allocations of epistemic authority in pediatric practice. How could democratic allocations of epistemic authority be consistent with the recognition of differences of expertise or competence? According to some critics, advocating for inclusive and egalitarian communities of knowers (as feminist epistemologists often do) is inconsistent with recognizing hierarchies of expertise and competence. Therefore (this objection proceeds), feminist epistemology (and, by extension, my work) must fail to distinguish epistemic reasons from irrelevant considerations, which is to say that this is not a kind of epistemology worth taking seriously (see e.g. Pinnick, Koertge, and Almeder 2003).[36] Maybe hierarchical forms of medical practice are required if we are to ground medical beliefs in truth-responsive reasons. Perhaps we must reconcile ourselves to authoritarian pediatrician-parent relationships.

I have two replies to this worry. First, we can acknowledge that parents are generally experts on many topics, without denying that pediatricians are experts about vaccine science. For example, parents are experts about their children's symptoms, general dispositions, and medical histories. Of course, parental reports on these topics are fallible, but the fact that parents spend so much time with their children (and are generally attentive to them) means that parents should be granted at least as much epistemic authority on these topics as is granted to pediatricians, who usually see their patients only infrequently. This sort of *substantive epistemic egalitarianism* is consistent with the recognition that pediatricians are experts in most other domains of childhood health. Second, pediatricians should treat parents as partners in deliberations about health care choices for their children. This is not only because parents possess expert knowledge on some topics. It is also because of the epistemic harms pediatricians may cause to parents when they refuse to listen to parental reports or when they fail to respond respectfully to parents' questions and concerns. When pediatricians act from paternalistic motives or with a tone of condescension, they may thereby prevent parents from acquiring the epistemic benefits that might be generated by more respectful exchanges. This sort of *procedural epistemic egalitarianism* is also consistent with the recognition that pediatricians possess expert knowledge about children's health care.

Looking forward: gender justice and public health

I have argued that vaccine denialists sometimes reject the practices of reasoning that are prevalent in mainstream medical contexts. Furthermore, vaccine denialist communities have, in some ways, improved on mainstream medicine's status quo. Therefore, it is overly simplistic to claim that vaccine denialists are 'irrational'. However, vaccine denialists are also sometimes disposed to epistemic vices. These include a disposition to pursue uncritical affirmation of their existing beliefs and a tendency to fail to recognize differences in expertise or competence. Even if vaccine denialists are not 'irrational', they are not committed to the best practices for inquiry. Furthermore, individual pediatricians and parents are not entirely to blame for their poor epistemic practices. They bear some responsibility for their shortcomings, but the institutional practices of mainstream medicine, along with social and political forms of gender inequality, may also contribute to the formation and resilience of these epistemic vices. For these reasons, it is unlikely to be productive to focus on the epistemic failures of individual parents and pediatricians.

In my view, public health efforts to increase rates of routine childhood vaccination would do well to not focus exclusively on efforts to educate parents about the safety and efficacy of vaccines. Such efforts also ought to aim to undermine the epistemic vices that exist in mainstream medical communities, with any eye towards replicating the epistemic virtues present in vaccine denialist communities. In particular, advocates of routine childhood vaccination programs should work to root out practices of testimonial injustice (and epistemic injustice, more generally) in mainstream medical contexts, and to replace them with more democratic practices for allocating epistemic authority among parents and pediatricians. This would require major changes to the ways in which medicine is often practiced, and in which medical professionals are trained. For example, parents and pediatricians would need time to develop the trusting relationships which make the informed and respectful giving and taking of reasons possible. Robert Chen, the former head of Centers for Disease Control and Prevention's (CDC) Immunization Safety Branch, suggests that we might "prevent creating anti-vaccine activists" by promoting a "shift from traditional paternalistic to a shared decision making model" (R. Chen 1999, S44).[37] But it has been well-documented that current models of managed medical care can make it difficult to achieve this goal (Dugdale, Epstein, and Pantilat 1999; Largent 2012, 169–171). The fact that medical students lose their empathy for patients as their education progresses (D. Chen et al. 2007), and the fact that a capacity for empathy is central to effective recognition of the epistemic authority of persons who are different from oneself (Stueber 2006), means that significant reforms to medical education may be necessary.

One of this chapter's most surprising conclusions is that achieving greater social and political equality for women may help to rid mainstream medicine of some of the epistemic vices which vaccine denialists report. Recall that epistemic injustices, including testimonial injustice, are parasitic on broader forms of social and political inequality. Inasmuch as prejudices rooted in gender inequalities contribute to the epistemic injustices to which vaccine denialists claim to have been subjected, increased gender equality is likely to contribute to informed and respectful communication between mothers and pediatricians. Of course, public health advocates cannot hope to defeat sexism by themselves. However, the fact that sexism may contribute to vaccine denialism, even indirectly, should motivate those who care about public health to commit themselves to broader struggles for gender justice.

Finally, public health authorities and medical researchers should work to find ways to bring parent groups into mainstream conversations about vaccine risks. The most radical vaccine denialists may be unwilling to engage in an honest give-and-take of reasons. Their epistemic vices may go too deep. But some vaccine denialists may welcome the opportunity to engage in discussion with medical experts. The mainstream medical community owes it to these parents – and to everyone else – to make space for them in discussions about the safety and efficacy of vaccines.

Notes

1 On the history of 'hysteria', see Micale (1995).
2 This is evidence that Tim Dare is right to think disagreements between vaccine advocates and vaccine denialists are 'deep', rather than merely 'complex', since parties to these disagreements lack shared background standards and beliefs, and therefore cannot proceed to argue rationally about vaccines (Dare 2014).
3 For an account of the reasoning flaws of vaccine denialists that is broader than the one I discuss here, see Jacobson, Targonski, and Poland (2007).
4 This presupposition about medical knowledge is consistent with the possibility that non-empiricist methods of inquiry are appropriate in other contexts. It entails only the falsity of conceptions of *medical* knowledge that do not prioritize the results of empirical research, e.g. 'metaphysical' forms of medicine, such as traditional naturopathy or homeopathy.
5 For a longer list of epistemic virtues, and a broader account of virtue epistemology, see Zagzebski (1996).
6 This includes the impact of gendered power differences on inquiry, which has been a major focus of feminist work in epistemology (Alcoff and Potter 1993).
7 On the ways in which the language and practice of scientific enterprises (such as medicine) are gender symbolized as masculine, see Rooney (1991). We may hope that the increasing number of women in pediatric practice (e.g. 70% of medical residents in pediatrics are women) will mitigate the gendered dynamics of pediatric medicine (Women Chairs of the Association of Medical School Pediatric Department Chairs 2007).
8 It is notable that many of the social scientific studies of vaccine refusal/denialism have focused exclusively on mothers (Benin et al. 2006; Brown et al. 2012; Dempsey et al. 2009).
9 On standpoint epistemology, see Hartsock (2003).
10 For feminist defenses of reliance on testimony, see Campbell (2003).
11 On the trope of 'irrationality' in race-based oppression, see Blum (2002) and Haslanger (2000).
12 Hilde Lindemann writes that "[t]he primary contribution of feminism to bioethics is to note how imbalances of power in the sex-gender system play themselves out in medical practice and in the theory surrounding the practice" (Lindemann 2007).
13 The 1976 mass immunization program had some benefits. Those who were vaccinated maintained resistance against swine flu decades later, and have been much less likely to become infected in subsequent swine flu outbreaks (McCullers et al. 2010).

14 The fact that a physician believes he is giving accurate and adequate answers to patients is not sufficient reason for concluding that he is doing so. Physicians can be mistaken. But the occasional failures of individual physicians and medical institutions do not justify vaccine denialism.

15 When pediatricians act in ways that manifest this epistemic vice, they may commit moral wrongs, too, e.g. by violating patient autonomy. I say more about these moral ideals and their relevance for vaccine refusal in chapters four and five.

16 I have focused on instances of testimonial injustice, but the fact that pediatricians have also been unwilling to answer questions or to seriously consider objections is a reason for thinking that they may have subjected parents to other forms of epistemic injustice, too. For discussion of forms of epistemic injustice that extend beyond testimonial injustice, see Hookway (2010).

17 The term 'epistemic injustice' has been popularized by Miranda Fricker (2003, 2007). However, the idea it denotes has been explored in earlier work in feminist social epistemology (e.g. Addelson 1983).

18 For discussion of the way in which the professional/non-professional hierarchy can become oppressive, see Young (1990, 56–58).

19 For further discussion of epistemic injustice in health care contexts, see Carel and Kidd (2014).

20 On the vulnerability of the oppressed to the power of experts, see Code (1991) and Sherwin (1992).

21 These norms are not novel, but patients' invocation of these norms in medical practice is becoming increasingly widespread. See Faden, Beauchamp, and King (1986) on the historical development of these ideas. On the specific intersection of issues of patient autonomy, informed consent, and childhood vaccination, the following passage from Dr. Robert Sears is instructive: "In the old days, most parents simply followed their doctor's advice and automatically got their children vaccinated. But now virtually every parent has heard that there may be some side effects and other problems with vaccines, and they are confused" (R. Sears 2007, xi).

22 The contemporary idea of implicit bias results from work in social psychology on 'implicit cognition' and from the results of the Implicit Association Test (IAT) (Greenwald, McGhee, and Schwartz 1998). One famous experiment on implicit bias (that did not rely upon the IAT) showed that when identical fictitious resumes were sent in response to job ads, those resumes to which 'white' names were attached were 50% more likely to generate interviews than the resumes to which 'black' names were attached (Bertrand and Mullainathan 2004).

23 On the importance of egalitarian norms for allocating epistemic authority, see Anderson (1995) and Longino (2002).

24 *Mothering* magazine (both print and online) has been identified as a significant contributor to vaccine denialism/refusal. See e.g. Benin et al. (2006) and Kata (2012).

25 On 'attachment parenting', see William Sears et al. (2013).

26 For one example of 'research' into vaccine safety based on the reports of parents, see Bernard et al. (2001). The following comment from the editors of the journal in which this 'research' appears is instructive: "The purpose of *Medical Hypotheses* is to publish interesting theoretical papers. The journal will consider radical, speculative and non-mainstream scientific ideas provided they are coherently expressed" (Medical Hypotheses 2012). It seems likely that some of these 'alternative' forms of research are not so much manifestations of (the epistemic virtue of) egalitarian practices of inquiry, as they are the result of (the epistemic vice of) a failure to recognize differences in medical

expertise. I discuss this vice, and the tension between the epistemic virtues and vices present in vaccine denialist communities, in the following sections of the chapter.

27 The medical professionals who agree to treat vaccine denialists are not always vaccine denialists themselves. Instead, many of the physicians who treat non-vaccinated children have a high opinion of vaccines, though they also tend to believe that CDC understates the side effects of vaccination (Glanz et al. 2009; Salmon et al. 2008).

28 Another reason parents may love Wakefield (and doctors like him) is that Wakefield tells them what they want to hear, and because both our affect and our assessment of expertise are influenced by our pre-existing factual and cultural commitments. (I take up these common features of our cognition, and their role in vaccine denialism, in chapter two.)

29 Miranda Fricker describes this phenomenon: "[T]he prejudice operating against the speaker may have a self-fulfilling power, so that the subject of the injustice is socially *constituted* just as the stereotype depicts her (that's what she counts as socially), and/or she may be actually *caused* to resemble the prejudicial stereotype working against her (that's what she comes in some measure to be)" (Fricker 2007, 55, emphasis in original).

30 A common example is of girls and women who, after facing chronic stereotype threat in contexts that require the demonstration of mathematical knowledge, decide to avoid contexts that require the demonstration of mathematical knowledge (J. Steele, James, and Barnett 2002).

31 For example, Wakefield was the headline speaker at both the NVIC's 2009 annual conference and the International Chiropractors Association's 2008 annual conference.

32 See also Anderson (2011).

33 However, Kahan, Jenkins-Smith and Braman argue that people are likely to identify people as experts who they believe share their values (Kahan, Jenkins-Smith, and Braman 2011). So, even people who are willing to defer to experts may fail to defer to people who are actually experts, if they perceive that the real experts do not share their values. I discuss the role of groupishness – and 'cultural cognition' in particular – in the next chapter.

34 As I discuss in chapters two and three, non-epistemic values may sometimes play a legitimate role in shaping our views about science-informed policy. Indeed, as Heather Douglas has convincingly argued, it would be impossible for scientific judgments about subjects we care about *not* to be informed by non-epistemic values (Douglas 2009). (Here, I acknowledge Phyllis Rooney's argument that the divide between epistemic and non-epistemic values is not always clear, but I take for granted that we can sometimes meaningfully use this distinction.) (Rooney 1992). So, the problem is not that vaccine denialists allow value judgments to influence their response to the scientific consensus, but that they may be motivated by the *wrong* values. In particular, a desire to explain the origins of one's suffering is not a good reason to reject consensus views about the safety of vaccines.

35 For an illustration of the comfort and hope parents may experience as a result of 'learning' that their children's autism was caused by vaccines, see McCarthy (2008).

36 For a critical response to this book's dismissal of feminist epistemology, see Anderson (2012).

37 A study by Opel et al. might seem to give us reason to worry about the effectiveness of a 'shared decision making model' for lowering rates of vaccine refusal/denialism (Opel et al. 2013). Opel et al. found that parents are more likely to agree to vaccinate their children when pediatricians initiate interactions with

the presumption that children will be vaccinated. And they found that fewer parents agree to vaccinate their children when pediatricians begin with open-ended questions about whether parents would like to vaccinate. I am not worried about this result, since a presumption in favor of vaccination is consistent with pediatricians treating parents with appropriate epistemic respect. Pediatricians may respond respectfully to parental questions and concerns even when they begin their interactions by presuming to follow a typical standard of care.

Bibliography

Achterberg, Jeanne. 1991. *Woman as Healer*. Reprint. Shambhala.

Addelson, Kathryn. 1983. "The Man of Professional Wisdom." In *Discovering Reality*, edited by Sandra Harding and Merrill Hintikka, 165–186. Kluwer.

Age of Autism, Autism Action Network, Autism Media Channel, Autism One, Autism File Global, Autism Research Institute, Elizabeth Birt Center for Autism Law and Advocacy, et al. 2011. "Autism Advocacy Organizations and Parent Groups Support Dr. Andrew Wakefield." January 12. www.prnews wire.com/news-releases/autism-advocacy-organizations-and-parent-groups-supp ort-dr-andrew-wakefield-113355509.html.

Alcoff, Linda Martín, and Elizabeth Potter, eds. 1993. *Feminist Epistemologies*. Routledge.

Alcorn, Katrina. 2013. *Maxed Out: American Moms on the Brink*. Seal Press.

Allen, Arthur. 2007. *Vaccine: The Controversial Story of Medicine's Greatest Lifesaver*. W. W. Norton & Company.

Anderson, Elizabeth. 1995. "The Democratic University: The Role of Justice in the Production of Knowledge." *Social Philosophy and Policy* 12(2): 186–219.

Anderson, Elizabeth. 2011. "Democracy, Public Policy, and Lay Assessments of Scientific Testimony." *Episteme* 8(2): 144–164.

Anderson, Elizabeth. 2012. "How Not to Criticize Feminist Epistemology: Review of Pinnick, Koertge, and Almeder." Accessed June 14. www-personal.umich. edu/%7Eeandersn/hownotreview.html.

Bause, George S. 2012. "Mrs. Winslow's Soothing Syrup:" *Anesthesiology* 116(1): 8. doi:10.1097/ALN.0b013e318244c10a.

Benin, A. L., D. J. Wisler-Scher, E. Colson, E. D. Shapiro, and E. S. Holmboe. 2006. "Qualitative Analysis of Mothers' Decision-Making about Vaccines for Infants: The Importance of Trust." *Pediatrics* 117(5): 1532–1541.

Bernard, S., A. Enayati, L. Redwood, H. Roger, and T. Binstock. 2001. "Autism: A Novel Form of Mercury Poisoning." *Medical Hypotheses* 56(4): 462–471.

Bertrand, M., and S. Mullainathan. 2004. "Are Emily and Greg More Employable than Lakisha and Jamal? A Field Experiment on Labor Market Discrimination." *American Economic Review* 94(4): 991–1013.

Bettelheim, Bruno. 1959. "Joey: A Mechanical Boy." *Scientific American* 200(3): 117–126.

Block, Jennifer. 2007. *Pushed: The Painful Truth about Childbirth and Modern Maternity Care*. Da Capo Lifelong.

Blum, L. A. 2002. *"I'm Not a Racist, But...": The Moral Quandary of Race*. Cornell University Press.

Bordo, Susan R. 1987. *The Flight to Objectivity: Essays on Cartesianism and Culture*. SUNY Press.

Boston Women's Health Book Collective and Judy Norsigian. 2011. *Our Bodies, Ourselves*. Touchstone.

Brown, Katrina F., Susannah J. Long, Mary Ramsay, Michael J. Hudson, John Green, Charles A. Vincent, J. Simon Kroll, Graham Fraser, and Nick Sevdalis. 2012. "UK Parents' Decision-Making about Measles–Mumps–Rubella (MMR) Vaccine 10 Years after the MMR-Autism Controversy: A Qualitative Analysis." *Vaccine* 30(10): 1855–1864.

Brunson, Emily K. 2013. "The Impact of Social Networks on Parents' Vaccination Decisions." *Pediatrics* 131(5): e1397–1404. doi:10.1542/peds.2012–2452.

Campbell, Sue. 2003. *Relational Remembering: Rethinking the Memory Wars*. Rowman & Littlefield Publishers.

Carel, Havi, and Ian James Kidd. 2014. "Epistemic Injustice in Healthcare: A Philosophical Analysis." *Medicine, Health Care and Philosophy*, April, 1–12.

Chen, Daniel, Robert Lew, Warren Hershman, and Jay Orlander. 2007. "A Cross-Sectional Measurement of Medical Student Empathy." *Journal of General Internal Medicine* 22(10): 1434–1438.

Chen, R. T. 1999. "Vaccine Risks: Real, Perceived and Unknown." *Vaccine* 17: S41–46.

Code, Lorraine. 1991. *What Can She Know? Feminist Theory and the Construction of Knowledge*. Cornell University Press.

Code, Lorraine. 2004. "The Power of Ignorance." *Philosophical Papers* 33(3): 291–308.

Coldicott, Y., C. Pope, and C. Roberts. 2003. "The Ethics of Intimate Examinations – Teaching Tomorrow's Doctors." *British Medical Journal* 326: 97–101.

Dare, Tim. 2014. "Disagreement Over Vaccination Programmes: Deep or Merely Complex and Why Does It Matter?" *HEC Forum* 26(1): 43–57.

Deer, B. 2011. "How the Vaccine Crisis Was Meant to Make Money." *British Medical Journal* 342: c5258. www.bmj.com/content/342/bmj.c5258.

Dempsey, A. F., L. M. Abraham, V. Dalton, and M. Ruffin. 2009. "Understanding the Reasons Why Mothers Do or Do Not Have Their Adolescent Daughters Vaccinated against Human Papillomavirus." *Annals of Epidemiology* 19(8): 531–538.

Douglas, Heather E. 2009. *Science, Policy, and the Value-Free Ideal*. University of Pittsburgh Press.

Dugdale, David C., Ronald Epstein, and Steven Z. Pantilat. 1999. "Time and the Patient–Physician Relationship." *Journal of General Internal Medicine* 14(S1): 34–40. doi:10.1046/j.1525–1497.1999.00263.x.

Dwyer, J., and J. Rothstein. 1993. "Case Study: One More Pelvic Exam." *The Hastings Center Report* 23(6): 27–29.

Eddy, Mary. 2009. *Science and Health*. Reprint. Applewood Books.

Ehrenreich, Barbara, and Deirdre English. 2010. *Witches, Midwives, & Nurses: A History of Women Healers*. Feminist Press at the City University of New York.

Epstein, Richard A. 2013. "Regulatory Paternalism in the Market for Drugs: Lessons from Vioxx and Celebrex." *Yale Journal of Health Policy, Law, and Ethics* 5(2): 6.

Ernst, E. 2001. "Rise in Popularity of Complementary and Alternative Medicine: Reasons and Consequences for Vaccination." *Vaccine* 20: S90–93.

Faden, R. R., T. L. Beauchamp, and N. M. P. King. 1986. *A History and Theory of Informed Consent*. Oxford University Press.

Ferranti, Michelle. 2010. "From Birth Control to That 'Fresh Feeling': A Historical Perspective on Feminine Hygiene in Medicine and Media." *Women & Health* 49(8): 592–607.

Fitzpatrick, Michael. 2012. *MMR and Autism: What Parents Need to Know.* Routledge.

Fombonne, E. 2008. "Thimerosal Disappears but Autism Remains." *Archives of General Psychiatry* 65(1): 15–16.

Fomon, Samuel J. 2001. "Infant Feeding in the 20th Century: Formula and Beikost." *The Journal of Nutrition* 131(2): 409–420S.

Ford, Henry. 2013. *My Life and Work.* Create Space Independent Publishing Platform.

Freed, G. L., S. J. Clark, A. T. Butchart, D. C. Singer, and M. M. Davis. 2011. "Sources and Perceived Credibility of Vaccine-Safety Information for Parents." *Pediatrics* 127 (Supplement): S107–112.

Fricker, Miranda. 2003. "Epistemic Justice and a Role for Virtue in the Politics of Knowing." *Metaphilosophy* 34(1–2): 154–173.

Fricker, Miranda. 2007. *Epistemic Injustice: Power and the Ethics of Knowing.* Oxford University Press.

Gaskin, Ina May. 2011. *Birth Matters: A Midwife's Manifesta.* Seven Stories Press.

General Medical Council. 2010. *Fitness to Practice Panel Hearing, Andrew Wakefield, Determination of Serious Professional Misconduct.* Accessed June 11, 2015. www.nhs.uk/news/2010/01january/documents/facts%20wwsm%20280110%20final%20complete%20corrected.pdf.

Gerber, Jeffrey S., and Paul A. Offit. 2009. "Vaccines and Autism: A Tale of Shifting Hypotheses." *Clinical Infectious Diseases: An Official Publication of the Infectious Diseases Society of America* 48(4): 456–461.

Glanz, J. M., D. L. McClure, D. J. Magid, M. F. Daley, E. K. France, D. A. Salmon, and S. J. Hambidge. 2009. "Parental Refusal of Pertussis Vaccination Is Associated with an Increased Risk of Pertussis Infection in Children." *Pediatrics* 123(6): 1446–1451.

Godlee, F., J. Smith, and H. Marcovitch. 2011. "Wakefield's Article Linking MMR Vaccine and Autism Was Fraudulent." *British Medical Journal* 342: c7452. www.bmj.com/content/342/bmj.c7452.

Goldberg, Robert. 2011. "A Deadly Hysteria." *New York Post*, September 13, sec. Columnists. www.nypost.com/p/news/opinion/opedcolumnists/deadly_hysteria_cQ6rr4Fm6nmNL20tPqnVxO.

Goldman, A. I. 2001. "Experts: Which Ones Should You Trust?" *Philosophy and Phenomenological Research* 63(1): 85–110.

Green, Monica. 1989. "Women's Medical Practice and Health Care in Medieval Europe." *Signs* 14(2): 434–473.

Greenwald, A. G., D. E. McGhee, and J. L. K. Schwartz. 1998. "Measuring Individual Differences in Implicit Cognition: The Implicit Association Test." *Journal of Personality and Social Psychology* 74(6): 1464–1480.

Greer, Frank R., and Rima D. Apple. 1991. "Physicians, Formula Companies, and Advertising: A Historical Perspective." *American Journal of Diseases of Children* 145(3): 282–286.

Halfon, Neal, Gregory D. Stevens, Kandyce Larson, and Lynn M. Olson. 2011. "Duration of a Well-Child Visit: Association with Content, Family-Centeredness, and Satisfaction." *Pediatrics* 128(4): 657–664. doi:10.1542/peds.2011-0586.

Hannula, Leena, Marja Kaunonen, and Marja-Terttu Tarkka. 2008. "A Systematic Review of Professional Support Interventions for Breastfeeding." *Journal of Clinical Nursing* 17(9): 1132–1143.

Harding, Sandra. 1987. "Ascetic Intellectual Opportunities: Reply to Alison Wylie." In *Science, Morality and Feminist Theory*, edited by M. Hanen and K. Nielson, 75–85. University of Calgary Press.

Hartsock, Nancy. 2003. "The Feminist Standpoint: Developing the Ground for a Specifically Feminist Historical Materialism." In *Feminist Perspectives on Epistemology, Metaphysics, Methodology, and the Philosophy of Science*, edited by Sandra Harding and Merrill Hintikka, 2nd ed., 283–310. Springer.

Haslanger, Sally. 2000. "Gender and Race: (What) Are They? (What) Do We Want Them to Be?" *Nous* 34(1): 31–55.

Hausman, Bernice L. 2003. *Mother's Milk: Breastfeeding Controversies in American Culture*. Routledge.

Held, V. 1990. "Feminist Transformations of Moral Theory." *Philosophy and Phenomenological Research* 50: 321–344.

Henry J. Kaiser Family Foundation. 2013. *Kaiser Women's Health Survey*. Henry J. Kaiser Family Foundation. Accessed June 11, 2015. http://files.kff.org/attachm ent/balancing-on-shaky-ground-women-work-and-family-health-data-note.

Holland, Mary. 2011. "Callous Disregard." Accessed June 11, 2015. www.ca llous-disregard.com/reviews.htm.

Hookway, C. 2010. "Some Varieties of Epistemic Injustice: Reflections on Fricker." *Episteme* 7(2): 151–163.

Horn, Steve. 2013. "How to Win the Media War against Grassroots Activists: Stratfor's Strategies." July 29. www.mintpressnews.com/stratfor-strategies-how-to-win-the-media-war-against-grassroots-activists/166078/.

Intemann, Kristen, and Inmaculada de Melo-Martín. 2014. "Addressing Problems in Profit-Driven Research: How Can Feminist Conceptions of Objectivity Help?" *European Journal for Philosophy of Science* 4(2): 135–51.

Jacobson, R. M., P. V. Targonski, and G. A. Poland. 2007. "A Taxonomy of Reasoning Flaws in the Anti-Vaccine Movement." *Vaccine* 25(16): 3146–3152.

John, Stephen. 2011. "Expert Testimony and Epistemological Free-Riding: The MMR Controversy." *The Philosophical Quarterly* 61(244): 496–517.

Jolliffe, D. M. 1993. "A History of the Use of Arsenicals in Man." *Journal of the Royal Society of Medicine* 86(5): 287.

Kahan, Dan M., H. Jenkins-Smith, and D. Braman. 2011. "Cultural Cognition of Scientific Consensus." *Journal of Risk Research* 14(2): 147–174.

Kata, Anna. 2012. "Anti-Vaccine Activists, Web 2.0, and the Postmodern Paradigm – An Overview of Tactics and Tropes Used Online by the Anti-Vaccination Movement." *Vaccine* 30(25): 3778–3789.

Kennedy, Robert F. 2005. "Deadly Immunity." *Rolling Stone*, July 14.

Kerridge, I. H., and M. Lowe. 1994. "Bloodletting: The Story of a Therapeutic Technique." *The Medical Journal of Australia* 163(11–12): 631–633.

Kirby, David. 2006. *Evidence of Harm: Mercury in Vaccines and the Autism Epidemic: A Medical Controversy*. St. Martin's Griffin.

Kitta, Andrea. 2012. *Vaccinations and Public Concern in History*. Routledge.

Kukla, Rebecca. 2006. "Ethics and Ideology in Breastfeeding Advocacy Campaigns." *Hypatia* 21(1): 157–180.

Largent, M. A. 2012. *Vaccine: The Debate in Modern America*. Johns Hopkins University Press.

Larson, H. J., L. Z. Cooper, J. Eskola, S. L. Katz, and S. Ratzan. 2011. "Addressing the Vaccine Confidence Gap." *The Lancet* 378(9790): 526–535.

Lerner, Sharon. 2010. *The War on Moms: On Life in a Family-Unfriendly Nation.* John Wiley & Sons.

Lexchin, Joel, Lisa A. Bero, Benjamin Djulbegovic, and Otavio Clark. 2003. "Pharmaceutical Industry Sponsorship and Research Outcome and Quality: Systematic Review." *British Medical Journal* 326(7400): 1167–1170.

Lindemann, Hilde. 2007. "Feminist Bioethics: Where We've Been, Where We're Going." In *Feminist Philosophy*, edited by Linda Alcoff and Eva Kittay, 116–130. Blackwell Publishing.

Lloyd, Genevieve. 1993. *Man of Reason: "Male" and "Female" in Western Philosophy.* 2nd ed. University of Minnesota Press.

Longino, Helen E. 2002. *The Fate of Knowledge.* Princeton University Press.

McCarthy, Jenny. 2008. *Mother Warriors: A Nation of Parents Healing Autism Against All Odds.* Dutton Adult.

McCarthy, Jenny. 2011. "Foreword." In *Callous Disregard*, by Andrew J. Wakefield, iii. Skyhorse Publishing.

McCullers, Jonathan A., Lee-Ann Van De Velde, Kim J. Allison, Kristen C. Branum, Richard J. Webby, and Patricia M. Flynn. 2010. "Recipients of Vaccine Against the 1976 'Swine Flu' Have Enhanced Neutralization Responses to the 2009 Novel H1N1 Influenza Virus." *Clinical Infectious Diseases* 50(11): 1487–1492.

Medical Hypotheses. 2012. "Medical Hypotheses – Guide for Authors." Accessed June 8. www.elsevier.com/wps/find/journaldescription.cws_home/623059/autho rinstructions.

Medina, José. 2013. *The Epistemology of Resistance: Gender and Racial Oppression, Epistemic Injustice, and Resistant Imaginations.* Oxford University Press.

Micale, Mark S. 1995. *Approaching Hysteria: Disease and Its Interpretations.* Princeton University Press.

Mnookin, Seth. 2011a. *The Panic Virus: A True Story of Medicine, Science, and Fear.* Simon & Schuster.

Mnookin, Seth. 2011b. "What Drives Irrational Rhetoric? The Case of Childhood Vaccinations." *The Atlantic.* January 11. www.theatlantic.com/national/archive/ 2011/01/what-drives-irrational-rhetoric-the-case-of-childhood-vaccinations/69291/.

Moms against Mercury. 2014. Accessed June 11, 2015. www.momsagainstm ercury.org/.

Mooney, Chris. 2011. "Irrationality vs Vaccines: Fighting for Reality." *New Scientist: CultureLab.* January 13. www.newscientist.com/blogs/culturelab/2011/01/irra tionality-vs-vaccines-fighting-for-reality.html.

Moss-Coane, Marty. 2011. "The History and Hysteria around Vaccines." *Radio Times.* WHYY. Accessed June 11, 2015. http://whyy.org/cms/radiotimes/2011/ 03/01/the-history-of-and-hysteria-around-vaccines/.

Mothering. 2009. "Mothering Forums > Baby > Baby Health >Vaccinations > I'm Not Vaccinating > Give Me Strength." *Mothering.* September 22. www.mother ing.com/forum/443-i-m-not-vaccinating/1135869-give-me-strength.html.

Mothering. 2015. "Forums." *Mothering.* Accessed February 17. www.mothering. com/forum/index.php.

Murphy, Michelle. 2004. "Immodest Witnessing: The Epistemology of Vaginal Self-Examination in the US Feminist Self-Help Movement." *Feminist Studies* 30(1): 115–147.

National Vaccine Information Center. 2015. "About Us." Accessed February 23. www.nvic.org/about.aspx.

Neustadt, Richard Elliott, Joseph Anthony Califano, and Harvey V. Fineberg. 1978. *The Swine Flu Affair*. US Government Printing Office.

Offit, Paul A. 2007. *The Cutter Incident: How America's First Polio Vaccine Led to the Growing Vaccine Crisis*. Yale University Press.

Offit, Paul A. 2010. *Deadly Choices: How the Anti-Vaccine Movement Threatens Us All*. Basic Books.

Opel, Douglas J., John Heritage, James A. Taylor, Rita Mangione-Smith, Halle Showalter Salas, Victoria DeVere, Chuan Zhou, and Jeffrey D. Robinson. 2013. "The Architecture of Provider-Parent Vaccine Discussions at Health Supervision Visits." *Pediatrics* 132(6): 1–10. doi:10.1542/peds.2013–2037.

Oshinsky, David M. 2006. *Polio: An American Story*. Oxford University Press.

Pinnick, C. L., N. Koertge, and R. F. Almeder, eds. 2003. *Scrutinizing Feminist Epistemology: An Examination of Gender in Science*. Rutgers University Press.

Pregerson, Brady. 2011. "Patients with an Irrational Fear of Vaccinations." *Scrubs*. September 2. http://scrubsmag.com/patients-with-an-irrational-fear-of-vaccinations/.

Riordan, Jan, and Betty Ann Countryman. 1980. "Infant Feeding Patterns Past and Present." *Journal of Obstetric, Gynecologic, & Neonatal Nursing* 9(4): 207–210.

Rooney, Phyllis. 1991. "Gendered Reason: Sex Metaphor and Conceptions of Reason." *Hypatia* 6(2): 77–103.

Rooney, Phyllis. 1992. "On Values in Science: Is the Epistemic/Non-Epistemic Distinction Useful?" In *PSA: Proceedings of the Biennial Meeting of the Philosophy of Science Association*, edited by D. Hull, M. Forbes, and K. Okruhlik,1: 13–22. Philosophy of Science Association.

Ropeik, David. 2011. "The Perception Gap: An Explanation for Why People Maintain Irrational Fears." *Scientific American*. February 3. http://blogs.scientificamerican.com/guest-blog/2011/02/03/the-perception-gap-an-explanation-for-why-people-maintain-irrational-fears/.

Sackett, David L., William M. Rosenberg, J. A. Gray, R. Brian Haynes, and W. Scott Richardson. 1996. "Evidence Based Medicine: What It Is and What It Isn't." *British Medical Journal* 312(7023): 71.

Salmon, D. A., W. K. Y. Pan, S. B. Omer, A. M. Navar, W. Orenstein, E. K. Marcuse, J. Taylor, et al. 2008. "Vaccine Knowledge and Practices of Primary Care Providers of Exempt vs. Vaccinated Children." *Human Vaccines* 4(4): 286–291.

Saunders, Russell. 2014. "Pediatrician: Vaccinate Your Kids – Or Get Out of My Office." *The Daily Beast*. January 30. www.thedailybeast.com/articles/2014/01/30/the-real-reason-pediatricians-want-you-to-vaccinate-your-kids.html.

Schectman, Joel. 2013. "Glaxo Mined Online Parent Discussion Boards for Vaccine Worries." May 1. http://blogs.wsj.com/cio/2013/05/01/glaxo-mined-online-parent-discussion-boards-for-vaccine-worries/?mod=WSJ_hpp_sections_cio.

Schiff, Gordon D., William L. Galanter, Jay Duhig, Amy E. Lodolce, Michael J. Koronkowski, and Bruce L. Lambert. 2011. "Principles of Conservative Prescribing." *Archives of Internal Medicine* 171(16): 1433–1440.

Sears, R. 2007. *The Vaccine Book: Making the Right Decision for Your Child*. Little, Brown and Company.

Sears, William, Martha Sears, Robert Sears, and James Sears. 2013. *The Baby Book, Revised Edition: Everything You Need to Know About Your Baby from Birth to Age Two*. Hachette Digital.

Sherwin, S. 1992. *No Longer Patient: Feminist Ethics and Health Care*. Temple University Press.

Silverstone, Alicia. 2014. *The Kind Mama: A Simple Guide to Supercharged Fertility, a Radiant Pregnancy, a Sweeter Birth, and a Healthier, More Beautiful Beginning.* Rodale Books.

Specter, Michael. 2009. *Denialism: How Irrational Thinking Hinders Scientific Progress, Harms the Planet, and Threatens Our Lives.* Penguin Press.

Steele, Claude M. 2010. *Whistling Vivaldi: And Other Clues to How Stereotypes Affect Us.* W. W. Norton & Company.

Steele, J., J. B. James, and R. C. Barnett. 2002. "Learning in a Man's World: Examining the Perceptions of Undergraduate Women in Male-Dominated Academic Areas." *Psychology of Women Quarterly* 26(1): 46–50.

Stone, John. 2015. "The Washington Post Whips Up Fear and Blames Andrew Wakefield – Age of Autism." January 25. www.ageofautism.com/2015/01/the-washington-post-whips-up-fear-and-blames-andrew-wakefield.html.

Stueber, Karsten R. 2006. *Rediscovering Empathy: Agency, Folk Psychology, and the Human Sciences.* Cambridge University Press.

Swiderski, Richard M. 2008. *Quicksilver: A History of the Use, Lore and Effects of Mercury.* McFarland.

Tenpenny, Sherri J. 2014. "Boycott Pediatrician Bullies' Dr. Tenpenny." *Drtenpenny. com.* Accessed July 12. http://drtenpenny.com/boycott-pediatrician-bullies/.

Thinking Moms' Revolution. 2014. "Home | The Thinking Moms' Revolution." Accessed April 30. http://thinkingmomsrevolution.com/.

Thompson, L., and D. Nuell. 1982. "DPT: Vaccine Roulette." WRC-TV (NBC), April.

Tuana, Nancy. 2006. "The Speculum of Ignorance: The Women's Health Movement and Epistemologies of Ignorance." *Hypatia* 21(3): 1–19.

Wagner, Marsden. 2008. *Born in the USA: How a Broken Maternity System Must Be Fixed to Put Mothers and Infants First.* University of California Press.

Wakefield, Andrew J. 2011. *Callous Disregard: Autisms and Vaccines: The Truth Behind a Tragedy.* Skyhorse Publishing.

Wakefield, Andrew J., S. H. Murch, A. Anthony, J. Linnell, D. M. Casson, M. Malik, M. Berelowitz, et al. 1998. "RETRACTED: Ileal-Lymphoid-Nodular Hyperplasia, Non-Specific Colitis, and Pervasive Developmental Disorder in Children." *The Lancet* 351(9103): 637–641.

Wazana, Ashley. 2000. "Physicians and the Pharmaceutical Industry: Is a Gift Ever Just a Gift?" *JAMA: The Journal of the American Medical Association* 283(3): 373–380.

Weiner, Lynn Y. 1994. "Reconstructing Motherhood: The La Leche League in Postwar America." *The Journal of American History* 80(4): 1357–1381.

Wiessinger, Diane, Diana West, and Teresa Pitman. 2010. *The Womanly Art of Breastfeeding.* 8th Ed. Rev. Upd. Ballantine Books.

Williams, Mary Elizabeth. 2014. "Alicia Silverstone's Clueless Vaccine Advice." April 23. www.salon.com/2014/04/23/alicia_silverstones_clueless_vaccine_advice/.

Wolf, Jacqueline H. 2003. "Low Breastfeeding Rates and Public Health in the United States." *American Journal of Public Health* 93(12): 2000–2010. doi:10.2105/AJPH.93.12.2000.

Women Chairs of the Association of Medical School Pediatric Department Chairs. 2007. "Women in Pediatrics: Recommendations for the Future." *Pediatrics* 119(5): 1000–1005. doi:10.1542/peds.2006-2909.

Young, Iris Marion. 1990. "The Five Faces of Oppression." In *Justice and the Politics of Difference*, 39–65. Princeton University Press.

Zagzebski, Linda Trinkaus. 1996. *Virtues of the Mind: An Inquiry into the Nature of Virtue and the Ethical Foundations of Knowledge*. Cambridge University Press.

2 Bias and the 'irrationality' of vaccine denialism

"Our findings show a strong presence of omission bias in our respondents: participants would accept a higher risk of their child catching a disease than they would of their child reacting to a vaccine."
(Brown, Kroll, Hudson, Ramsay, Green, Vincent, et al. 2010, 4183)

In the last chapter I argued that parents, and especially mothers, have reasons to be skeptical about the testimony of pediatricians and to form resistant epistemic communities. In this chapter, I continue to argue that vaccine denialism need not result from especially blameworthy forms of parental ignorance or irrationality. In particular, I resist the common charge that vaccine denialists are uniquely vulnerable to 'biased' thinking about the risks and benefits of vaccines.

Vaccination choices involve judgments of probability under conditions of uncertainty. When people make these sorts of judgments about topics outside their areas of expertise, they often use a set of cognitive shortcuts, or *heuristics*. Parents are not usually experts about vaccine science. So, we may conclude that when they arrive at false beliefs about vaccines, i.e. when they become vaccine denialists, it is because their cognitive shortcuts have failed to deliver true beliefs. I think this is largely true. Common cognitive heuristics likely contribute to vaccine denialism. However, I object to the way that this (naïve) narrative of bias-based vaccine denialism focuses our attention on the epistemic failures of individual parents.

First, parents who become vaccine denialists do not rely on cognitive heuristics more than parents who vaccinate their children do. The same forms of automatic reasoning that lead some parents to reject vaccines lead other parents to embrace them. Also, pediatricians are not immune to the influence of common cognitive shortcuts.[1] Therefore, instead of focusing on the fact that vaccine denialists use cognitive shortcuts, we should ask why automatic reasoning processes incline only some parents towards vaccine denialism. We should ask how we might help restructure the conditions in which parents make choices about vaccines, so that more parents will be led by their automatic reasoning processes towards true beliefs.

Second, vaccine denialists are vulnerable to cognitive biases, but not because they are unintelligent or unwilling to engage in effortful reasoning. On the contrary, vaccine denialists are intelligent and educated, and they deliberate about vaccines more than parents who vaccinate do. But their intelligence and confidence lead them astray. (Unfortunately, excessive self-confidence in areas outside our expertise will often lead us astray.) Furthermore, vaccine denialists' resistant epistemic communities usually do not practice forms of adversariality and epistemic accountability that challenge the results of parents' automatic reasoning processes.

Third, what appear to be cases of bias-based vaccine denialism may be something else entirely. In particular, people can believe vaccines are unsafe without rejecting the scientific consensus about the likelihood of vaccine complications. In this case, a disagreement about the safety of vaccines may be caused by a disagreement about non-epistemic values, rather than a disagreement about scientific research.[2]

Automatic reasoning and vaccine denialism

People who talk and write about vaccine denialism – in both popular media and academic research – often point to the (supposed) cognitive failures of vaccine denialists. We hear the following: Parents are overwhelmed by their emotions. They focus too much on high-profile cases of vaccine complications. They do not know anyone who had polio, but they know children with autism spectrum disorders. They are easily convinced by simple narratives about vaccine dangers, for example that 'mercury causes autism'. In short, vaccine denialists are supposed to give free rein to their immediate responses to vaccines, and they fail to correct these intuitions with the evidence of medical science. In contrast, pediatricians and parents who vaccinate are supposed to be less susceptible to biased thinking. Either they do not have anti-vaccine gut responses or, if they do, they successfully block these negative automatic reactions.

Many academic journal articles point to cognitive biases as a cause of vaccine denialism (D. A. Asch et al. 1994; Ball, Evans, and Bostrom 1998; Betsch et al. 2011; Betsch, Renkewitz, and Haase 2013; Brown, Kroll, Hudson, Ramsay, Green, Long, et al. 2010; Brown, Kroll, Hudson, Ramsay, Green, Vincent, et al. 2010; Connolly and Reb 2003; Gong et al. 2013; Larson et al. 2011; Lewandowsky et al. 2012; Ritov and Baron 1990; Smith, Appleton, and MacDonald 2013).[3] Popular depictions of vaccine denialism also often explicitly invoke cognitive biases (see e.g. Allen 2007b). Even though many people who write about vaccine denialism do not refer to social psychology or cognitive science, insights from these disciplines may help to organize our thinking about the (supposed) cognitive failures of vaccine denialists.

It will be useful to summarize some of the main themes of the academic literature on cognitive biases: Over the last fifty years, work in cognitive science and social psychology has provided powerful evidence that we can best understand human reasoning in terms of a relationship between two kinds of thought processes (see e.g. Gilovich 2008; Haidt 2012; Kahneman 2011; Slovic 2000; Taleb 2010; Thaler and Sunstein 2009). Following Tversky and Kahneman, I use the terms 'System 1' and 'System 2' to mark this distinction, but what I say is consistent with similar distinctions marked by different terms, e.g. elephant/rider or automatic/reflective systems. System 1 is continually active and nearly impossible to turn off. It reaches conclusions in an automatic and cognitively easy manner, and it makes frequent use of cognitive shortcuts, or heuristics, to arrive at its conclusions.[4] When it is presented with a complicated question, System 1 identifies a similar and less complicated question and provides an answer to the less complicated question (Kahneman 2011, chap. 9). In particular, these kinds of reasoning processes are informed by our feelings (affect), by vivid associations, and by our tendency to construct plausible causal explanations from limited evidence. In many cases, these heuristics work well: They are the basis of the 'expert intuitions' of veteran firefighters, chess champions, and neonatal intensive care unit nurses (Klein 1999).[5] But the heuristics of System 1 can also lead to false beliefs, and in some domains of inquiry these cognitive shortcuts are prone to systematic errors. In these cases, System 1's heuristics become cognitive biases; a bias is a form of reasoning that systematically leads to errors (Ariely 2010).

In contrast, System 2 reaches conclusions through deliberate and effortful activity and, in principle, it should be able resist and correct the errors that System 1 makes.[6] It engages in the sorts of activities that commonsense psychology associates with thought: counting objects, measuring volumes, analyzing statistical data, and evaluating chains of inferences. However, System 2 is cognitively burdensome and we use it sparingly, usually only to affirm the results of System 1 processes. Depending on the domain of inquiry, it may take years of training and experience – along with robust self-control and institutional safeguards – to use System 2 to successfully block or redirect the conclusions of System 1.

Before moving on, I want to clarify that these two 'systems' are *models* for thinking about different kinds of reasoning. They do not refer to different regions of the brain or to other material objects. Instead, they are tools that reliably represent the evidence we have about how human beings reason. Here, I leave unaddressed the many metaphysical and epistemological questions that one may raise about the status of models in science (see e.g. Weisberg 2013).

In this section of the chapter I discuss some ways in which forms of automatic (System 1) reasoning may lead to vaccine denialism. This is a speculative discussion. My aim is to present what I take to be a simplified (though generally accurate) view of the etiology of many cases of vaccine denialism. My arguments take the following form:

1   Human reasoning is often subject to automatic process X.
2   If people have beliefs/feelings/experiences of kind Y, then automatic process X may lead them to vaccine denialism.
3   Vaccine denialists often have beliefs/feelings/experiences of kind Y.
4   Therefore, automatic process X may lead people to vaccine denialism.

Of course, (4) is not a radical conclusion. But it should be sufficient for me to explain a popular account of how vaccine denialism is supposed to result from cognitive biases.

In the next four subsections I discuss the possible influence of the following System 1 cognitive processes upon vaccination decisions: affect, availability, causal narratives, and groupishness.

Affect

Much of our thinking begins with our feelings. We experience the world 'flavored' by affect (Damasio 1994; Haidt 2012). Our affective responses play an essential role in decision making, so much so that people who experience a restricted scope of emotions, for example as a result of brain injuries, often struggle to make everyday choices. Why are emotions so important for our decisions? This is a bigger question than I will try to answer. For now, it is enough to observe that our minds often automatically replace factual questions about an object of inquiry with questions about our feelings towards that object. When we ask 'Does X work?' or 'Is X safe?', we often provide an answer to a different question: 'How do I *feel* about X?' (Zajonc 1980).[7] The affect heuristic also inclines us to endorse a tidy view of our decision-space, according to which the objects or acts we like have no downsides and those we dislike have no benefits. Kahneman says that the affect heuristic leads us to believe that "[g]ood technologies have few costs [and] bad technologies have no benefits" (Kahneman 2011, 140). Of course, affect is usually not sufficient for belief. We often disbelieve things that we would like to be true. However, the affect heuristic can incline Systems 1 and 2 to seek out (or to generate) 'permission' for us to believe what we want to believe.

The affect heuristic can contribute to vaccine denialism when our minds replace the question, 'Are vaccines safe and effective?' with the question, 'Do I like vaccines?' When this heuristic is operating, it may lead parents who have negative feelings about vaccines to become less likely to believe that vaccines are safe and effective.

People may have negative feelings about vaccines for different reasons, but I want to start by resisting an account that I think is clearly false. Some writers have tried to explain diverse forms of science denialism, e.g. the rejection of climate change, evolution, vaccines, and GMO science, in terms of a broad aversion to science. On such a view, all of these phenomena of science denialism result from the same anti-science sentiment

(Mooney and Kirshenbaum 2010; Otto 2011; Otto 2012; Prothero, Linse, and Shermer 2013).[8] But there is no evidence for the existence of a coherent constituency of science-denialists. For example, there is no significant overlap between vaccine denialists and people who reject climate change or evolution (Kahan 2014).[9] Furthermore, vaccine denialists claim to embrace science. They do not display a generalized hatred of the methods and results of science, biomedical or otherwise (National Vaccine Information Center 2015; Wakefield 2011).

If affect contributes to vaccine denialism, then the relevant feelings are likely to be focused on targets that are narrower than 'science'. In particular, affect-based vaccine denialism will result from negative feelings about vaccines or phenomena that are directly related to vaccination. Perhaps a mother recalls the discomfort or anxiety she experienced when she received shots. Maybe she felt awful when she restrained her flailing and screaming child while the nurse inserted the needles.[10] A mother may develop negative feelings about vaccines indirectly, for example from media reports about (real or supposed) vaccine complications. Also, vaccine denialism may result from an affect bias even if the negative feelings are not directed at objects or activities that are directly associated with vaccination.[11] One might dislike pharmaceutical companies or the way that government is involved in health care. Alternatively, one might be averse to performing medical interventions on healthy persons' bodies.[12] Recall that another manifestation of the affect heuristic is that we have a tendency to believe things we dislike have no upside, while things we like have no downside. So, one consequence of the affect heuristic is that it will lead people who dislike *something* associated with vaccines to form negative opinions about *everything* associated with vaccines.

I am not primarily interested in the nearly trivial fact that cognitive biases can contribute to vaccine denialism. Instead, I want to resist the conclusion that vaccine denialists are cognitively deficient, relative to both pediatricians and parents who vaccinate. Even if cognitive biases contribute to vaccine denialism, vaccine denialists are no more biased than either parents who vaccinate or mainstream pediatricians.

First, we ought not to valorize the rational capacities of parents who decide to vaccinate. These people are just as likely to depend on cognitive shortcuts as vaccine denialists do. (An overarching theme of the cognitive bias literature is that everyone relies on automatic forms of reasoning.) Instead, the cognitive heuristics of vaccine denialists incline them towards (or do not much to disincline them from) false beliefs about vaccine science, while the cognitive heuristics of vaccinating parents incline them towards (or do not much disincline them from) true beliefs about vaccine science. Let's return to the affect heuristic. Parents who vaccinate generally have good relationships with their pediatricians. The existence of a strong parent-pediatrician relationship correlates strongly with parents fully vaccinating their children. Parents with good relationships with pediatricians generally like their pediatricians. And since we all rely on cognitive short-cuts, it follows that parents who vaccinate may have done so (at least in part) because they like the people and objects associated with vaccination. Recall, also, our tendency to have 'tidy beliefs', that is, to think that what we like is entirely good, and that what we dislike is entirely bad. Parents who like their pediatricians will tend to like their pediatricians' testimony on behalf of vaccines. Parental assent to this testimony may result less from rational reflection on research science than from a fortunate spillover of positive parental feelings.[13]

What about the ways pediatricians reason? We should not think that pediatricians are immune to cognitive biases. Indeed, they may be as vulnerable to the distorting influence of various heuristics – such as affect – as are members of the general public (Gilovich 2008; McNeil et al. 1982; Tversky and Kahneman 1971). Furthermore, clinicians are some-times *worse* at diagnosing disorders than are civilians who are armed with simple algorithms for matching symptoms to diseases.[14] I do not mean to criticize physicians. It is not their fault that they are vulnerable to the same cognitive biases that burden us all. Instead, I want to emphasize that the epistemic authority of physicians does not rest on their superior ability to overcome the sorts of cognitive biases that may lead some parents to become vaccine denialists. Rather, one ought to defer to the medical exper-tise of physicians because they are usually reliable conduits for biomedical knowledge. Pediatricians are not usually active scientific researchers. But they are members of institutions that are committed (albeit imperfectly) to acquiring and distributing medical knowledge. There is good reason to trust what pediatricians say about vaccines because they are generally faithful in reporting the results of biomedical research (or at least the state of the research when they received their medical training). Why? It's not because they have deliberated and reflected on all the information they distribute to their patients. Pediatricians usually lack both the time and the training for that. Instead, it is because they believe what they have been taught. This is likely for many reasons, but we should not be surprised to find that the affect heuristic plays a role. The comfort and familiarity physicians have with the institutions of medical science likely contribute to their endorsement of these institutions' results.

The affect bias likely plays only a positive role when it comes to the ways physicians form beliefs about vaccines. But this heuristic may lead physicians into error in other domains. In particular, we ought to worry that physicians are often 'educated' by pharmaceutical sales repre-sentatives at resort-vacation continuing medical education conferences. Many people and organizations have worried about the epistemic and ethical issues surrounding this practice (Campbell et al. 2007; de Melo-Martín and Intemann 2009; Grande, Shea, and Armstrong 2012; Steinman, Landefeld, and Baron 2012). My worry is that physicians are likely to form good feelings about pharmaceutical companies as a result of the 'gifts' they receive. Since physicians are just as susceptible to the affect heuristic as everyone else, the fact that they like pharmaceutical company representatives means that they will be more likely to believe what these people say about the value of prescribing their drugs. Also, some parents may be aware that physicians are vulnerable to cognitive biases, and they may know that these biases can reasonably lead physicians astray in some domains. Accordingly, some parents may decide to grant less credibility to the testimony of physicians than they otherwise would, as I discussed in the last chapter.

Availability

We have a greater tendency to endorse beliefs when we can recall information that is consistent with those beliefs. We rely on the availability heuristic when we answer questions by reflecting on our ability to recall dramatic events and personal experiences that are related to the phenomena under consideration (Kahneman 2011, 130). This heuristic often works well. For example, we are less willing to trust someone with a secret if we remember an occasion when he betrayed our trust. However, our personal experiences and vivid memories are often poor guides to phenomena that are best understood through statistical analysis. For example, people believe that highly publicized crimes (such as child abductions) and natural disasters (such as tornadoes) are both more common and more dangerous than less-publicized events, such as acquaintance rape and automobile accidents.[15] And the mere fact that an idea is familiar – it is easily accessible in our memory – makes it more likely that we will endorse it (Kahneman 2011, 62). We believe what we remember, even if we do not understand it (Begg, Armour, and Kerr 1985; Zajonc 1968). Furthermore, when a familiar idea is conjoined with an unfamiliar idea, the conjunction becomes familiar, and more likely to receive our assent.

The availability heuristic may contribute to vaccine denialism when someone's most vivid and accessible ideas about vaccines are consistent with the belief that vaccines are unsafe or ineffective (Ball, Evans, and Bostrom 1998). And information that is consistent with the conclusions of vaccine denialism may be easy to remember and recall. Smith, Appleton, and MacDonald report that "negative vaccine anecdotes are much more likely to be recalled than evidence [in favor of vaccines]" (Smith, Appleton, and MacDonald 2013, 88).[16] Lewandowsky et al. add that emotional anti-vaccine narratives are more likely to be shared and distributed than less-emotional narratives (Lewandowsky et al. 2012). Also, the news media and social media prominently feature stories about vaccine complications, both of the real and of the fake variety. For example, a 2013 episode of Katie Couric's television show (*Katie*) focused on a mother who claimed her daughter died after receiving the HPV vaccine, but the episode did not mention that multiple studies have found no link between HPV vaccine and either short- or long-term negative health consequences (Arnheim-Dahlström et al. 2013; Centers for Disease Control and Prevention 2014; McDonough 2013). Even when media reports include expert opinions favorable to vaccination, cold and considered presentations by experts usually pale in contrast with the impassioned narratives of vaccine denialists. Dry discussions of data do not make for the formation of vivid memories. Finally, when someone watches a debate between vaccine denialists and vaccine advocates, the loudest message the media may communicate is that 'vaccination is controversial'.

In previous generations, I suspect that the availability heuristic more frequently inclined people to believe that vaccines were safe and effective. People had more personal memories of the horrors of the childhood diseases against which vaccines offer protection. They had nightmares about iron lungs. Their childhood friends went blind from measles. Their mothers gave birth to babies who were deaf from congenital rubella syndrome. Earlier generations of parents were often relieved to realize that new vaccines could save their babies from diseases that had harmed so many people who they knew. Even if today's parents know this history, their thinking about vaccines is less likely to be colored by these sorts of feelings of relief.[17] Instead, the most *available* thoughts that some of today's parents may have about vaccines likely include worries about (supposed) vaccine complications, including autism spectrum disorders.[18]

Recall that when familiar ideas are combined with unfamiliar ideas, this can make us more likely to endorse the truth of the conjunction of these ideas. Vaccine denialism is often associated with familiar (and attractive) ideas, such as the avoidance of industrial toxins, 'natural' parenting, the self-healing body, resistance to over-medication, the protection of vulnerable children, and the exercise of parental responsibilities and prerogatives. When these familiar and likeable ideas get associated with the idea that vaccines are not as safe as pediatricians say they are, people may be more likely to reject the scientific consensus about the safety of vaccines.[19]

I have suggested some ways in which the availability heuristic may contribute to vaccine denialism. But the same heuristic may lead other parents to believe vaccines are safe, and it may lead pediatricians to be more confident in their testimony on behalf of vaccination. Consider that many parents think of vaccines as a routine part of children's health care. When they think of vaccines, they likely think of healthy children, of well-baby visits, and of normal care for one's child. These good thoughts about vaccines do not result from extensive parental research about the science or history of vaccines. In fact, the overwhelming majority of parents do not think about vaccines at all until their children are vaccinated (Glanz et al. 2013). Instead, it is a fortunate accident if the availability heuristic leads some parents to endorse the scientific consensus about the safety and efficacy of vaccines.

Consider, also, how the availability heuristic may influence pediatricians.[20] Many pediatricians likely have easily recallable memories of treating children who suffered from vaccine-preventable diseases. At the very least, pediatricians are more likely than your average parent to have seen children suffering from these diseases. When pediatricians think about vaccines, they likely think about how they can help prevent other children from experiencing this sort of suffering.

Causal narratives

We are natural storytellers. Our minds automatically create narratives to explain phenomena that puzzle us. Thomas Gilovich argues that this is because of a combination of two tendencies of our automatic reasoning: (1) we 'see' (nonexistent) patterns in random data, which call out for explanation, and (2) we fabricate causal narratives to explain these patterns (Gilovich 2008). We do this even when we have very little evidence about the phenomena our narratives aim to explain. In fact, we create more convincing stories when we have less evidence, since in those cases our stories need to account for only a small number of factors. But when we know more, our stories have to be more complicated to account for additional details, and more complicated stories tend to be less satisfying (Taleb 2010). Finally, even people who are experts at resisting naïve narratives in one domain of activity, e.g. scientists in the lab, will rely on unjustified causal narratives in other domains of activity, e.g. in interpersonal relationships.[21]

When we and our loved ones suffer, we want to know why. Friedrich Nietzsche, a 19th-century philosopher, described the human tendency to make up stories about the origins of our pain:

> The sufferers ... enjoy being mistrustful and dwelling on wrongs and imagined slights: they rummage through the bowels of their past and present for obscure, questionable stories that will allow them to wallow in tortured suspicion, and intoxicate themselves with their own poisonous wickedness ... 'I suffer: someone or other must be guilty' – and every sick sheep thinks the same.
>
> (Nietzsche 2006, 94)

Nietzsche thought that most people cannot help but make up stories to lay the blame for their suffering on others (and sometimes on themselves). Nietzsche criticized this tendency, but he was clear that it was all too common.

Parents who are aware of the immense burdens of caring for an autistic child may want to blame someone. They may know that some vaccines have contained mercury, and that the symptoms of mercury poisoning somewhat resemble some of the symptoms of autism spectrum disorders.

Parents may also know that autistic children sometimes have gastro-intestinal disorders, and they may believe that vaccines can change the intestinal microbiome (as Wakefield's retracted research suggested). When some children develop (what appear to be) symptoms of autism in the months after receiving a vaccine, this may be enough further evidence for parents to endorse the quick narrative that vaccines cause autism.

Consider another tidy causal narrative. This one, from Jennifer Margulis (who wrote *The Business of Baby*), is even less complicated than stories about mercury or gastrointestinal disorders. Margulis observes that societies with more coercive vaccination policies have higher rates of infant mortality. For example, the United States has more coercive vaccination policies than Denmark, and the United States also has higher rates of infant mortality than Denmark. Margulis concludes that this correlation shows that "our current vaccine schedule … is not in the best interests of our babies' health" (Margulis 2013, 222). In her view, mandatory vacci-nation policies contribute to infant mortality, and societies could achieve lower levels of infant mortality if they relaxed their mandatory vaccination policies.

Some parents who are exposed to these sorts of anti-vaccine narratives become less likely to vaccinate their children (Betsch et al. 2011; Betsch, Renkewitz, and Haase 2013). In particular, parents who are exposed to anti-vaccine narratives (e.g. 'vaccines cause autism') are more likely to refuse vaccines than are parents who are exposed only to raw statistics about the risks of vaccine complications. However, once someone has been exposed to anti-vaccine narratives, being provided with statistical information about vaccine risks makes them even more likely to refuse vaccines.[22] Emotionally powerful narratives have an even greater impact (Betsch et al. 2011).

Recall that we are more confident about our causal narratives when they account for all of our existing beliefs about the objects of our nar-ratives. The less we know about vaccines, the more likely we are to be confident in our (relatively simple) narratives. But someone who knows a good deal about vaccine science, or who trusts mainstream pediatricians, or who has vivid positive associations with vaccines is going to struggle to integrate all of this information into a coherent and persuasive vaccine denialist narrative. For example, people who know something about mercury poisoning and autism may know that the symptoms of mercury poisoning are not at all identical to the symptoms of autism. They may also know that rates of autism have continued to increase long after mercury had been removed from vaccines. Also, parents may know that there is no evidence of links between vaccines and the gastrointestinal disorders that are common for people with autism. Furthermore, people who know something about public health may realize that societies with the most coercive vaccination programs also tend to have relatively high poverty rates, and they may know that poverty correlates strongly with infant mortality.

Simple vaccine denialist causal narratives cannot easily incorporate these kinds of additional information.

To return to a frequent refrain: We should not valorize parents who vaccinate. It is unlikely that they rely on more *sophisticated* causal narratives when they reason about vaccines (Glanz et al. 2013). Parents who vaccinate don't know much about vaccines, and they don't spend much time thinking about vaccines. Instead, it's very likely that they rely on simple narratives, too. They may believe that 'vaccines keep children from getting sick'. But this is simplistic. Some children do not develop individual immunity from vaccines, individual immunity sometimes wears off over time, and much of the protection that vaccines provide comes from herd immunity. I am not criticizing parents who believe simple pro-vaccine narratives. Instead, I want to emphasize that these parents may rely just as much on simple causal narratives as do vaccine denialists. So, we should not try to explain vaccine denialism in terms of some parents' disproportionate susceptibility to the power of simple causal narratives.

What about pediatricians and simple narratives? On one hand, pediatricians' narratives about vaccines are likely to be more complicated. Physicians know more about vaccines. But I do not want to valorize physicians either. They sometimes rely on uninformed simple narratives about vaccine refusal and denialism. For example, I have heard physicians blame the increase in pertussis (whooping cough) infections on vaccine refusers. This can be a compelling narrative: People who are not vaccinated against pertussis are more vulnerable to infection, rates of pertussis vaccination refusal are up, and rates of pertussis have increased. But the story that results from this sort of thinking – 'vaccine refusal caused increased pertussis infections' – is false. Most of the increase in rates of pertussis can be attributed to the fact that the immunity generated by the newer pertussis vaccine is not as long-lasting as the individual immunity that the earlier pertussis vaccine generated (Centers for Disease Control and Prevention 2013).[23]

Groupishness

We are social reasoners. We have a tendency to believe what we believe others believe.[24] In a set of famous and much-replicated experiments from the 1950s, Solomon Asch showed that people will often endorse clearly false beliefs if they think there is a group consensus in favor of those false beliefs (S. Asch 1955). In one of his experiments, Asch found that subjects would agree that two sticks of obviously different lengths were actually the same size, as long as the subjects first heard their fellow putative research subjects (who were in fact part of the research team) announce that they thought the sticks were the same length.

Many questions are not as easy to answer as the ones Asch gave his subjects. When the answers to factual questions are less obvious, groupishness may have even more profound consequences. Of particular interest to me is that we have a tendency to endorse factual judgments that we believe are consistent with the beliefs – and the values – of those with whom we share cultural commitments.[25] This is not only a tendency to believe what 'people like us' already believe. It is also a proactive cognitive mechanism. We have an automatic tendency to endorse beliefs that we think are consistent with policies our group supports, and to reject beliefs that are consistent with policies that our group rejects, even if members of our group have not yet spoken out on the particular issue under consideration.[26]

Contemporary research on the impact cultural commitments may have on factual judgments began with the pioneering work of the anthropologist Mary Douglas. Along with the political scientist Aaron Wildavsky, Douglas argued that political conflicts surrounding the anticipated risks of proposed public policies can often be explained in terms of one's cultural values (M. Douglas and Wildavsky 1983).[27] For example, people who are committed to hierarchical and individualistic social ideals tend to believe that the environmental and safety risks of nuclear power are relatively low. According to Douglas and Wildavsky, these people refuse to believe that risks are higher, because if they believed that risks were higher they would have to support greater restrictions on the private economic activity of the owners of nuclear power plants (M. Douglas and Wildavsky 1983, 138–151). In contrast, people who are committed to egalitarian and solidaristic socio-political values tend to believe that nuclear power has greater environmental and safety risks. According to Douglas and Wildavsky, these people are more willing to believe that there are higher risks of nuclear power because their cultural commitments make them less averse to public regulation of the private economic activity of business owners.

Recent work on the 'cultural theory' of risk assessment – under the title of 'cultural cognition' – has generated robust empirical support for the claim that people often make factual judgments about risk on the basis of their cultural or political values.[28] Much of this work has been carried out by Dan Kahan at the 'Cultural Cognition Project' at Yale University. Kahan explains the thesis of 'cultural cognition' (or 'cultural cognition of public policy') with the following slogan: "cultural commitments are prior to factual beliefs on highly charged political issues."[29] This cultural cognition thesis has a set of component parts. First, we have a tendency to reject beliefs that would force us to renounce aspects of our cultural identity.[30] Second, violations of cultural values are laden with affect. It follows – from my earlier discussion of affect – that we will tend to reject beliefs when endorsing them would cause us to feel badly. Finally, most people – on most issues – rely on the opinions of experts to shape their beliefs.[31] But when we decide who is an expert, we tend to pick people who share our values (Cohen 2003; Kahan, Jenkins-Smith, and Braman 2011).[32]

At first glance, groupishness may seem irrelevant to vaccine denialism. After all, vaccine refusal and denialism do not correlate with particular religious identities or political orientations (Kahan 2014). No large religious denominations preach against vaccines, and no major political party endorses vaccine denialism or refusal. On the contrary, there is widespread support for vaccination among members of different religious groups, and among people with different political ideologies. To be clear: There are partisan disagreements about coercive vaccination programs, including exemption programs, but I leave these issues until chapters five and six. For now, it is enough to note that inasmuch as there are partisan disagreements about vaccination policies, the fights are over the use of state power and not the truth of vaccine science or the prudence of routine childhood vaccination.

Groupishness may contribute to vaccine denialism even though vaccine denialism does not correlate with religiosity or political ideology. First, the social and media prominence of vaccine denialism may lead people to mistakenly believe that vaccine denialism is prevalent in their social groups. False beliefs about consensus views can trigger groupishness, especially if vaccine refusers are geographically clustered (Lewandowsky et al. 2012).[33] The fact that vaccine denialists tend to be more vocal than advocates of vaccination makes it likely that people will believe vaccine denialism to be more common than it is.[34] (Here, the availability heuristic may contribute to groupishness.) Also, as I discuss above, public advocates of vaccine denialism are often sympathetic figures, for example concerned mothers. The fact that media discussions of vaccine safety often feature debates between vaccine denialist mothers and public health officials also tells in favor of the possibility that groupishness can lead parents to vaccine denialism. If mothers see debates about vaccine denialism as debates between mothers and doctors, it is unsurprising that some mothers will be inclined to side with their own. This can happen even though the overwhelming majority of mothers support vaccination, since the media's portrayal of factual disagreement about vaccines is often radically distorted.

Second, vaccine denialism may be common within some niche cultural groups, including communities organized around fundamentalist religion, libertarian politics, and natural ('purity-focused') parenting. These groups may be so small that their contribution to vaccine denialism/refusal can be difficult to detect in empirical research. Also, membership in these cultural affinity groups may cross political and religious lines and, therefore, be invisible to studies that track only religiosity and political ideology.

Finally, vaccine denialism is likely to be common in groups that have emerged in response to (perceived and actual) abuses of mainstream medicine. In the previous chapter, I discussed ways in which parents (usually mothers) have formed in-person and online communities of mutual support in response to what they believe to be the shortcomings of mainstream obstetric and pediatric medical practices. These resistant epistemic communities position themselves in opposition to a collection of mainstream practices, including prenatal testing, hospital births, caesarean sections, childbirth analgesia, regular well-baby visits, and childhood antibiotics. The affective flavor of these communities is of righteous anger at the tendency of mainstream medical authorities to undermine the power and autonomy of parents, and to act for profit rather than for the well-being of children.[35] In such communities, groupishness may lead to vaccine denialism in a straightforward manner: The identity of these groups consists in active resistance to medical interventions to which they object (Luyten et al. 2013).

To return to the recurring theme of this section of the chapter: Pediatricians and parents who vaccinate are also likely to be influenced by automatic reasoning processes when they reason about vaccines. But, in their case, groupishness likely inclines them towards vaccine science. First, most parents who vaccinate are members of social, political, religious, and cultural groups whose members overwhelmingly believe that vaccines are safe. At a more basic level, 'vaccinating your kids' is just something that most members of most social groups do. Questions about vaccine safety – and questions about whether concerns about vaccine safety warrant vaccine denialism and refusal – are unlikely to arise for many parents. Most parents do what most people like them are doing, and they do it because most people like them are doing it. But as vaccine denialists sometimes observe, following the herd is not usually an epistemically or morally virtuous strategy. I am glad that groupishness inclines many parents to believe that vaccines are safe. But the fact that groupishness leads some parents to endorse true beliefs about vaccines does not mean that these parents have acted more rationally than vaccine denialists.

We may say something similar about groupishness and pediatricians. Pediatricians are members of the medical establishment. The medical establishment endorses the safety and efficacy of vaccines. So, groupishness likely inclines pediatricians to embrace the safety and efficacy of vaccines. To be clear: I do not mean to say that pediatricians are wrong to defer to the expert opinion of mainstream medical authorities and research science. But inasmuch as groupishness – an automatic reasoning process – inclines pediatricians towards embracing vaccine science, we have reason to resist the conclusion that vaccine denialists are uniquely reliant upon automatic reasoning when it comes to thinking about the safety and efficacy of vaccines.

Why does unconscious reasoning incline only some parents towards vaccine denialism?

I have argued that automatic reasoning processes are unlikely to play a larger role in the reasoning of vaccine denialists than they play in the reasoning of pediatricians and parents who vaccinate. So, we should not conclude that vaccine denialism is a consequence of the putative fact that vaccine denialists are relatively more reliant on their 'gut feelings', emotions, easily recallable memories, simple stories, or cultural affiliations. Instead, we ought to wonder why some parents are led by their automatic reasoning processes towards vaccine denialism, while most parents are not.

First, some parents have beliefs and memories that prime their automatic reasoning processes to incline them towards vaccine denialism, while others do not. For example, some parents are predisposed to be skeptical about the claims and practices of mainstream medicine and pharmaceutical companies, for the reasons I discussed in chapter one. Others are political libertarians, and are skeptical about public (health) programs. Some have had direct experience with autistic children or with people who they believe have suffered from vaccine complications.

I want to focus most of my attention, here, on another reason why only some parents are led by their automatic reasoning processes to embrace vaccine denialism: When parents do independent research about vaccines, they may prime their automatic reasoning processes to lead them towards vaccine denialist conclusions. (This may seem counterintuitive, since it's common to think that reading and thinking about a topic can help people to resist the force of their emotions and gut feelings.)

People who end up becoming vaccine denialists frequently turn to the Internet to get advice about vaccines (Einsiedel 2011; Healy and Pickering 2011; Omer et al. 2009). And parents who turn to the Internet to learn about vaccines are much more likely to become vaccine denialists than those who do not (Jones et al. 2012). This is understandable, when we reflect on how much bad information about vaccines the Internet contains, and how easy it is to find it.[36] In particular, less than 20% of parents who did Internet research about vaccines spent time reading official medical information websites (Downs, Bruine de Bruin, and Fischhoff 2008). Other studies found that 52% of parents generally trust the information about vaccines that they find online, and that 70% of the parents who found information about vaccines online used that information when deciding whether to vaccinate (Berman and Dees 2013; Tafuri et al. 2014).

One problem with Internet research about vaccine safety is that it leads people to false information. Another is that people are sometimes more likely to believe things they read online than things they are told in person (Sperber et al. 2010). But even the *true* information people find online can incline them to embrace vaccine denialist conclusions. For example, popular vaccine denialist websites often tell heartbreaking stories about children who supposedly experienced vaccine complications. Some of these stories may be false, but at least some of them are likely to be true. A person who reads these stories may develop bad feelings about vaccines and vaccination policy. These feelings may prime affect-based automatic reasoning towards vaccine denialism. Furthermore, vaccine denialist websites often focus on compelling narratives about the ways in which vaccines can harm children (Healy and Pickering 2011). When vaccine-hesitant parents go online to learn about vaccines, they will find emotionally evocative narratives that will incline them to believe that vaccines are unsafe (Betsch et al. 2012). Finally, online spaces are perfect places for cultivating resistant epistemic communities in which vaccine denialism is a core practice.

Conscious reasoning and vaccine denialism

Recall the two different kinds of reasoning processes: System 1 is automatic and System 2 is effortful. It is a paradigm of good thinking when System 2 evaluates the results of System 1 (Kahneman 2011).[37] When the automatic reasoning of System 1 inclines people towards vaccine denialism, we may hope that effortful deliberation by System 2 will redirect them towards true beliefs about vaccines. And it seems natural to conclude that people who become firmly committed to vaccine denialism have failed to make appropriate use of the effortful reasoning processes of System 2. I think this account is inaccurate and unfair.

First, vaccine denialists deliberate about vaccines. Earlier in this chapter (and in the Introduction), I provided evidence that vaccine denialists actually do *more* reading, thinking, and talking about vaccines than parents who vaccinate do. So, we ought not to conclude that vaccine denialists lack the ability or the will to engage in effortful reasoning about vaccines, or that these supposed cognitive deficits explain vaccine denialism. It's true that vaccine denialists fail to use effortful reasoning to reject vaccine denialist beliefs, but it's false to say that they have failed to use effortful reasoning all together.

Second, vaccine refusers are not uniquely bad at effortful reasoning. Their System 2 reasoning functions as well as the System 2 reasoning of parents who vaccinate, even though vaccine denialists have failed to use their effortful reasoning to reject the vaccine denialist beliefs towards which their automatic reasoning has inclined them. Most people (most of the time) use System 2 reasoning to give assent to (and create rationalizations for) the intuitive judgments that System 1 generates. The primary use of System 2 is to immunize our gut reactions against the critical attention that we might otherwise direct their way.[38] For example, we resist changing our minds.[39] In particular, we have a lower standard of evidence for maintaining our beliefs than for changing our beliefs.[40] When we want to believe something, we ask only whether we can believe it, i.e. whether there is any evidence at all. If there is, we hold onto our existing belief and we "stop thinking" (Haidt 2012, 84). In contrast, when we don't want to believe something, we ask whether we must believe it. Then we search for contrary evidence, and, if we find any at all, we reject the belief we do not want to accept. This is *confirmation bias*, and there is ample evidence that it affects us all.[41]

Like everyone else, vaccine denialists are resistant to revising their beliefs in the face of contradictory evidence (Betsch and Sachse 2013; Lewandowsky et al. 2012). They continue to believe what they want to believe, until there is no longer any evidence for their views.[42] Recall the claim that vaccines cause autism.[43] According to one narrative (which traces itself to the famous Wakefield paper), the MMR vaccine causes a bowel disorder ('autistic enterocolitis') that is (supposedly) linked to behavioral regression and autism (Wakefield et al. 1998). According to another narrative, mercury (i.e. thimerosal/thiomersal) in vaccines causes autism (Kennedy 2005; Kirby 2006).[44] The case for either of these etiologies of autism was always weak. But, for some years, the evidence against these hypotheses was not yet overwhelming. Parents could still find some reason to worry about a vaccine-autism link. For example, Anna Kirkland argues (persuasively, I think) that there were reasonable questions about MMR-autism and thimerosal-autism links from about 1998 to 2003 (Kirkland 2012, 73–74). During these years vaccine denialists had *permission* to believe there was a causal link between MMR and autism (or between thimerosal and autism), even if that conclusion was not well supported by the evidence. It was only after the little evidence in favor of MMR-autism and mercury-autism links evaporated (after a flurry of papers was published in 2003–2004) that the more thoughtful vaccine denialists abandoned these specific narratives. (Of course, some vaccine denialists still endorse these narratives.) Today, it is more common for vaccine denialists to claim that other vaccine ingredients contribute to autism, such as formaldehyde or aluminum (Fombonne 2008; Frompovich 2011; Gerber and Offit 2009; Palevsky 2012). Even though there is almost no evidence that these vaccine ingredients are harmful, thoughtful vaccine denialists may hold out as long as their causal narratives about vaccine harms retain some plausibility, i.e. as long as the medical community has not completely demolished the plausibility of these links. And vaccine denialists have kept researchers busy. Indeed, a common complaint about vaccine denialists is that they have forced a great deal of otherwise unnecessary research to be conducted, in order to entirely demolish the plausibility of vaccine denialist narratives.

Another example of a System 2 bias that may contribute to vaccine denialism is *motivated reasoning*. Like confirmation bias, motivated reasoning directs our cognitive capacities to defend what we already believe to be true. While confirmation bias inclines us to grant disproportionate weight to facts that count in favor of our existing beliefs, motivated reasoning affects our judgments about what the facts are in the first place. It leads us to believe 'facts' that lend support to our non-epistemic goals (Kahan, Jenkins-Smith, and Braman 2011; Kunda 1990). For example, our judgments about how to solve arithmetic problems can depend upon whether potential solutions are consistent with the views that we are otherwise (i.e. non-epistemically) motivated to adopt.

Unfortunately, intelligence and education do not make it easier for people to resist confirmation bias and motivated reasoning. The opposite is true. Being more intelligent can sometimes make it harder to overcome the conclusions of System 1 reasoning. For example, Perkins, Faraday, and Bushey found that more intelligent people are better at coming up with arguments for their side of an argument, but they are no better at coming up with arguments for the opposing side (Perkins, Faraday, and Bushey 1991). The first aspect of their finding is unsurprising. We expect more intelligent people to be able to identify additional arguments for what they believe. But we should worry about the second part: More intelligent people are no better at anticipating objections to their views than less intelligent people are. Accordingly, more intelligent people may be more vulnerable to confirmation bias, since they will have an easier time identifying reasons to continue believing what they already believe, but will be no better at identifying reasons to revise their beliefs. The reasoning of more intelligent people may be more distorted by motivated reasoning, too. Indeed, there is evidence that smarter people are more likely to make up 'facts' to support their position (Kahan et al. 2013; Lodge and Taber 2013). So, the fact that vaccine denialism may result from (or at least be reinforced by) confirmation bias and motivated reasoning is not evidence that vaccine denialists are less intelligent than parents who vaccinate. (If anything, it is evidence that vaccine denialists are smarter, which we have independent reason to believe is true.) I would like to agree with Poland and Spier that we can resist vaccine denialism with "better scientific and public education," but I doubt such efforts would address the main causes of the problem (Poland and Spier 2010, 2361).

The fact that vaccine denialists have not overcome their System 2 biases is not evidence that they are especially blameworthy for failing to resist their biases, since System 2 biases are very difficult to resist. Even with great effort and training, individuals are often able to make only small progress towards resisting confirmation bias or motivated reasoning (Camerer and Hogarth 1999; Sperber et al. 2010; Willingham 2008). It follows that we cannot blame vaccine denialists much for their failure to resist the ways System 2 biases contribute to vaccine denialism. Furthermore, we have no reason to think that parents who vaccinate have resisted either confirmation bias or motivated reasoning about vaccines. Vaccine denialism is an epistemic failure, but it does not follow that parents who vaccinate their children have reached true beliefs about vaccines through epistemically commendable reasoning practices. On the contrary, parents who vaccinate have likely been inclined by System 1 reasoning to accept the medical consensus about vaccines, and their System 2 biases have likely rationalized the results of their automatic reasoning processes. Neither vaccine denialists nor parents who vaccinate are more likely to have successfully resisted confirmation bias or motivated reasoning.

If we really want to understand vaccine denialism, we ought to focus on institutions, not individuals. I made some efforts towards institutional arguments in chapter one, where I focused on the resistant epistemic communities that vaccine denialists often participate in. These groups have various attributes that foster forms of System 2 reasoning that reinforce vaccine denialism. For one, these are often relatively homogenous groups. People join because they are already vaccine denialists or because they are sympathetic to vaccine denialism. But System 2 biases may be magnified when we deliberate only with people who agree with us (Kruglanski et al. 2006; Sunstein 2002; Tesser 1978). (This is one of the many reasons why diversity is so important in epistemic communities (Intemann 2011; Longino 2002).) It does not help that vaccine denialist communities often explicitly endorse epistemic norms that are not conducive to criticizing the results of System 1 reasoning processes. Members of these groups are often implored to 'trust your gut' or 'rely on your mommy instinct'. Furthermore, the continued existence of vaccine denialist groups depends upon their commitment to vaccine denialism. As Anna Kirkland observes, the "leadership [of vaccine denialist communities] must remain committed to these theories to hold the organizations together" (Kirkland 2012, 71). (Institutional self-preservation is a powerful force.) Finally, a primary purpose of vaccine denialist communities is to offer mutual support to parents who are making (or who believe themselves to be making) difficult decisions. Parents who are conflicted about their decision not to vaccinate are looking for others to affirm their choices. And parents with disabled children are looking for reassurance that vaccines are to blame for their burdens. It almost certainly violates the norms of these 'supportive' communities to expect others to engage in a critical give-and-take of reasons with you. (It took me far too long to realize that Socratic questioning can make me unwelcome in many social spaces.)

Contrast these attributes of vaccine denialist spaces with the corresponding attributes of well-functioning scientific communities. Membership in the scientific community is not marked primarily by scientists' beliefs about particular phenomena, but by their commitment to particular methods of inquiry and by their engagement with institutions that hold them accountable for their claims under (constructive) adversarial conditions, such as anonymous peer review and public criticism of one's methods and results. System 2 biases are difficult for individuals to resist, and this includes individual scientists, but *communities* can do a great deal to resist biased reasoning, when their members are committed to pursuing truth under conditions of accountability and adversariality. Communities of scientific inquiry are not support groups. A scientist does not transgress the norms of her professional community when she sharply criticizes the claims of a fellow researcher. Instead, she acts in accordance with some of the central norms of scientific practice when she expects other researchers to support their conclusions with good evidence and inferences. This is not to say that scientific communities always function well, or that adversarial argumentation is always appropriate.[45] Instead, the point is that the virtues of scientific institutions, rather than the virtues of individual scientists, allow scientific communities to (sometimes) resist powerful cognitive biases, such as confirmation bias and motivated reasoning.

Motivational biases

So far, I have discussed ways in which cognitive biases may incline people towards vaccine denialism. A combination of both automatic reasoning processes and distortions in our effortful reasoning can lead people to endorse false beliefs about vaccines. Now I want to discuss some ways in which cognitive biases can lead people to become vaccine refusers, without making them vaccine denialists. Automatic reasoning processes and distortions in effortful reasoning may incline a parent to refuse vaccines, even if they do not incline her to reject the scientific consensus about vaccines.

A *framing bias* is a tendency for our judgments about how to act to be influenced by differences in how we receive information about possible outcomes. In particular, we are more likely to choose an option when our information about it focuses on positive potential outcomes, and we are less likely to choose an option when our information about it focuses on negative possible outcomes. In one famous study, two groups of physicians at Harvard Medical School were presented with a cancer case study (McNeil et al. 1982). Members of each group were asked to recommend either surgery or radiation. Each group received only one of the following messages about the short-term mortality rates for surgery:

1   The one-month survival rate is 90%.
2   There is a 10% mortality rate in the first month.

These statements contain statistically identical information. But the two groups of physicians made different recommendations. Of the physicians who received statement (1), 84% recommended surgery, but only 50% of the physicians who received statement (2) recommended surgery. This kind of study has been repeated many times, with similar results. Our responses to risk can be influenced by the ways in which we receive information about the likelihood of positive and negative outcomes.

A framing bias could contribute to vaccine refusal if vaccine refusers were more likely than vaccinating parents to reflect on information about vaccine safety that emphasized the possible negative outcomes of vaccination (Ball, Evans, and Bostrom 1998; Gong et al. 2013). The fact that vaccine refusers often find evocative information about vaccines online – and are attentive to the possibility of vaccine complications – provides evidence that the framing bias sometimes plays a role in vaccine refusal. Consider the following example of two different ways parents might encounter information about serious vaccine complications:

1 Every year, children around the world receive hundreds of millions of vaccines, and over 99.999% of them have no serious complications.
2 Every year, hundreds of children around the world experience serious vaccine complications, out of the hundreds of millions who are vaccinated.[46]

These two statements contain statistically identical information. A person who endorses (1) believes neither more nor less about the rates of vaccine complications than does a person who endorses (2). But given what we know about framing bias, parents who receive information about vaccine risks framed like (2) may be more likely to refuse vaccines than parents who receive information about vaccine risks framed like (1). Statement (2) foregrounds the negative potential consequences of vaccination; statement (1) does not. Statement (2) may also encourage what Slovic et al. call *denominator neglect* (Slovic et al. 2004). This occurs when people's judgments about risk focus on the number of good or bad outcomes and ignore the magnitude of the pool from which those outcomes are drawn. Hundreds of serious vaccine complications may sound like a lot, even when we know that those hundreds were drawn from a pool of hundreds of millions of immunizations.

Another example of how a cognitive bias can have motivational rather than epistemic consequences is the *omission bias*. This is a tendency to think that it would be worse for a bad outcome to result from one's action (commission) than for the same bad outcome to result from one's inaction (omission) (Spranca, Minsk, and Baron 1991). Kahneman says that "people expect to have stronger emotional reactions (including regret) to an outcome that is produced by action than to the same outcome when it is produced by inaction" (Kahneman 2011, 348).[47] A tendency to prefer bad outcomes that arise from omission, over bad outcomes that arise from commission, is supposed to be a bias since what really matters is (supposed to be) whether the world becomes a better or worse place, and not whether *it is our actions* that bring about better or worse states of the world. Many studies have pointed to this (supposed) bias as a cause of vaccine refusal (D. A. Asch et al. 1994; Ball, Evans, and Bostrom 1998; Brown, Kroll, Hudson, Ramsay, Green, Vincent, et al. 2010; Downs, Bruine de Bruin, and Fischhoff 2008; Dubé et al. 2013; Meszaros et al. 1996; Sadaf et al. 2013; Wroe et al. 2005). As in the case of framing bias, the omission bias does not lead people to endorse false beliefs about vaccines. Instead, it affects their judgments about how to prioritize different potential outcomes.

The risks of vaccine complications are lower than the risks of contracting vaccine-preventable diseases. However, the omission bias may explain why some vaccine refusers prefer to face the risks of vaccine-preventable diseases. Brown et al. found that:

> participants would accept a higher risk of their child catching a disease than they would of their child reacting to a vaccine, would consider a number of symptoms/signs as less serious if they were caused by a disease than if they were caused by a vaccine reaction, and would regard as acceptable a longer duration of symptoms/signs as a consequence of disease than as a consequence of vaccine reaction. It follows that vaccine reactions which objectively appear less unpleasant than or equally unpleasant to disease outcomes may be perceived by parents to be sufficient to warrant vaccine refusal.
>
> (Brown, Kroll, Hudson, Ramsay, Green, Vincent, et al. 2010, 4183)

Brown et al. conclude that omission bias seems to play a role in the reasoning of many vaccine refusers.

In preparing for this book project, I often came across declarations from parents to the effect that they would rather have their child risk getting measles, etc., than risk vaccine complications, even though the evidence is clear that the risks of vaccine complications are much lower than the risks of vaccine-preventable diseases. Omission bias may explain why some parents prefer to risk the potential negative outcomes of vaccine refusal (e.g. a disease contraction), even though the expected outcome of vaccination is "objectively ... less unpleasant" than the expected outcome of vaccine refusal.

We should not conclude that parents who vaccinate are immune to the omission bias. Instead, they may also prefer negative outcomes from omissions over negative outcomes from commissions, but they may disagree with vaccine refusers about how to sort different vaccine-related choices into the 'commission' and 'omission' categories. For instance, parents who vaccinate may think that it is an *omission* to allow one's child to get vaccinated, since this is a choice not to deviate from a default medical practice. In contrast, they may think that it is a *commission* to refuse vaccines, since this choice involves the performance of various actions aimed at deviating from default pediatric health care, e.g. rejecting a pediatrician's treatment schedule and requesting exemptions from mandatory school vaccination laws.

This may seem to be an odd conclusion, since it suggests that there isn't an a priori truth about whether choices to vaccinate are omissions or commissions. If I'm right, then how we resolve this question depends on our understanding of normal childhood health and health care. If it is normal to get vaccinated, then vaccine refusal is a commission. But if it is normal for children to be vulnerable to vaccine-preventable diseases, then vaccination is a commission. That is, the omission bias is a bias relative to *baseline expectations*, and people with different values may have different baselines.

I agree with Tim Dare that it would be a mistake to think that decisions about the *normalcy* of diseases or vaccine complication risks depends only on individuals' beliefs about what is 'natural';

> It might seem that the threat posed by vaccine preventable diseases is natural – 'any harm done by nonimmunisation is done by the disease' – and therefore part of our normal baselines. Anything done to reduce that threat would be to move the beneficiaries above the baseline and so to benefit them ... But I propose that we should not so link 'normal' to 'natural' so closely. The positioning of normal baselines should be seen in part at least as a function of community decisions and expectations which impose demands, distribute risks, and set standards.
>
> (Dare 1998, 139)

I think Dare is right to emphasize that our baseline expectations for public health depend upon community decisions, and cannot be resolved by reflecting on what seems 'natural' to individuals. For example, the fact that chicken pox was common thirty years ago meant that chicken pox infection was a baseline expectation at that time. But the community's introduction of widespread chicken pox vaccination has transformed baseline expectations. It is now abnormal for children to get chicken pox.

In the next chapter, I argue that some parents are committed to ideals about 'pure' or 'natural' parenting, and that these ideals pick out different baseline expectations for children's health and health care than the baselines to which statistically normal parents are committed. For now, though, I want to say some more about vaccine refusal and the omission bias, on the assumption that vaccine refusers' ways of categorizing of omissions and commissions is uncontroversial.

Even if it were clear which choices were omissions and which were commissions, which I doubt, we might still wonder whether the omission bias is really a *bias*.[48] Some people seem to think that the distinction between doing and allowing sometimes makes a moral difference, for example when the choice is between killing and letting die. They think it is worse to act to bring about someone's death than it is to allow them to perish, even though the expected outcome of one's choice would be the same in either case. This kind of ethical conviction may help to explain widespread legal prohibitions on 'active euthanasia' and equally widespread legal toleration of 'passive euthanasia' in palliative end-of-life care.

But perhaps the widespread intuitive appeal of the doing/allowing distinction, e.g. in the case of killing and letting die, is merely evidence that a common cognitive bias has colonized our moral thinking? In a famous (for philosophy) article, James Rachels argues that the doing/allowing (commission/omission) distinction does *not* make an important moral difference, at least in life-and-death scenarios (Rachels 1975). Rachels asks us to consider two cases. In the first case, Smith drowns his nephew in a bathtub with the intent to kill him and collect an inheritance. In the second case, Jones allows his nephew to drown in a bathtub, with the intent to let him die (though he could have saved him) and collect an inheritance. We are supposed to agree (with Rachels) that Jones's inaction is just as morally wrong as Smith's action. Passive euthanasia is supposed to be no better than active euthanasia and, more generally, bad outcomes that result from omission are supposed to be no better than bad outcomes that result from commission.

Even if we share Rachels's intuition about Jones and Smith, this is not a sufficient reason to either reject the doing/allowing distinction or to agree that the phenomena which are categorized as instances of 'omission bias' involve faulty reasoning. A distinction can be meaningful even if it does not make a difference in every case, and there may be cases in which the doing/allowing distinction does make a difference. Consider one of the 'trolley cases' introduced by Philippa Foot and Judith Thomson (Foot 1978; Thomson 1985). In what Thomson calls *Fat Man*, you are a bystander to an out-of-control trolley that is about to kill five innocent people by running them over. You may intervene by pushing one person off a bridge. He will land on the tracks and his body will slow down the train enough to prevent the five people from being killed. The consensus view is that it would be wrong for you to push the man.[49] Most people think it would be better for you to *allow* five people to die, than for you to *do* something (in this case, push someone) to kill one person.

Our intuitions about *Fat Man* cannot vindicate the doing/allowing distinction by themselves. But they may undermine an argument for the 'omission bias' that is based only on our intuitions about the Jones and Smith cases. (An argument based on intuitions can be defeated by contrary intuitions.) However, even if many more of our intuitions supported the moral significance of the doing/allowing distinction, this may not be enough to defend the distinction against the charge of bias. For example, Joshua Greene acknowledges that the doing/allowing distinction has popular support, but he nonetheless thinks that support for it is irrational. Greene has studied fMRI images of the brains of people who are in the process of deciding not to push the fat man onto the tracks. The parts of their brains that are associated with automatic reactions and emotions are much more active than the parts of their brains that are associated with calculation and deliberate thinking. The opposite is true of the brain activity of the people who ultimately decide to push the fat man (Greene 2013; Greene et al. 2001). Greene argues that his studies show that people who embrace the doing/allowing distinction are basing their judgments on automatic and emotion-driven forms of reasoning. They are victims of cognitive bias.

Rather than let myself get carried off into the details of contemporary 'trolleyology', I want to draw this discussion to a close with a few take-away points. First, it is not obvious that a commitment to the doing/ allowing distinction reflects biased thinking. Many moral philosophers (and many more non-philosophers) think that respecting this distinction is a core part of the moral life. When vaccine refusal results from the sort of thinking some have characterized as 'omission bias', it may not follow that vaccine refusal results from biased thinking.

However, even if we can defend the doing/allowing distinction against the charge of bias, it may not be morally permissible to choose to allow harms, when allowing harms would cause *much worse* outcomes than doing harm would cause. For example, it may be immoral to refuse to push one person to his death if you could save a billion people by doing so, even if it is morally permissible to refuse to kill one to save five. I lack the space to defend this sort of 'threshold deontology'. But if something like this view is correct, it follows that whether it is morally permissible to refuse vaccines because of the doing/allowing distinction depends on the relative risks of vaccination and vaccine refusal.[50] Suppose that the risk of serious vaccine complications is 1/10,000,000 and the risk of disease contraction for non-vaccinated people is 1/10,000. Suppose, too, that serious vaccine complications are as bad as contracting vaccine-preventable diseases (though this is not generally true). Then, there would be a 1000:1 ratio between the expected badness of vaccine refusal and the expected badness of vaccination. Is this enough of a difference to cross the threshold? Would it be unreasonable to refuse to push one person onto the tracks to save a thousand people? I don't know, but this case is less clear to me than is the case of pushing one to save five.

Finally, we may question whether the 'omission bias' makes more than a trivial contribution to most instances of vaccine refusal (Connolly and Reb 2003; Tanner and Medin 2004). Omission bias is supposed to be widespread, but there are few vaccine refusers. This may be because vaccine refusers suffer from an extreme version of omission bias, but we lack evidence for that claim. Indeed, no study has shown that there is any cognitive bias to which vaccine refusers are disproportionately vulnerable.

Cognitive bias or value conflicts?

Public health advocates sometimes seem to take it for granted that rational reflection on medical facts leads to particular health care decisions. This conception of health care decision making can cause people to think that those who disagree with them about health care choices must disagree with them about the relevant medical facts. For example, if it were true that everyone who knew the facts about vaccines supported vaccination, then vaccine *refusal* could be caused only by vaccine *denialism*. Of course, it's true that disagreements about medical facts can cause disagreements about health care choices. I spent the first half of this chapter focused on some ways in which cognitive biases can contribute to vaccine denialism (and, thereby, to vaccine refusal). But not everyone who endorses the same medical facts will make the same health care decisions. This is because *values* play a necessary role in deliberations about medical interventions, since our values inform how we prioritize the potential outcomes of our medical choices. Accordingly, rational health care decision making is underdetermined by facts. This is not a novel claim, and there is an immense literature on the relationship between science and non-epistemic values (see e.g. H. E. Douglas 2009; Kitcher 1993; Longino 1990). But rather than engage in a systematic summary, I will instead draw on a single paper that is relevant for my purposes. I hope that this will promote accessibility and relevance, even at a cost to comprehensiveness.

Inmaculada de Melo-Martín and Kristen Intemann have written about parental deliberations surrounding birthing practices (de Melo-Martín and Intemann 2012). They argue that physicians and public health officials are mistaken if they believe that disagreements about homebirth result from disagreements about the statistical risks of birthing in the hospital and the home environment (de Melo-Martín and Intemann 2012, 60). Instead, de Melo-Martín and Intemann argue that opponents in debates about homebirth often agree about the medical research regarding the relative risks of various birthing options. But parties to these disputes "disagree about how particular risks should be weighed, how much risk is acceptable when adopting public policies that involve pregnancy and delivery, and how competing goods should be balanced in light of existing limitations in the available evidence" (de Melo-Martín and Intemann 2012, 64). These are disagreements about values, not facts.

One of the main disagreements concerns how much weight to give worst-case scenarios. Proponents of homebirth are willing to bear a higher risk of their new baby being injured or dying, in order to realize various goods associated with homebirth. These include avoiding undesirable aspects of hospital births, e.g. fetal heart monitoring, episiotomy, epidural analgesia, caesarean section; and having access to goods made available by homebirth, e.g. greater comfort and control of the birthing space, easy involvement of family and friends in caring for mother and baby (de Melo-Martín and Intemann 2012, 64). Advocates of hospital births disagree with homebirth advocates about the relative (un)desirability of these aspects of birthing in hospital and at home.

Furthermore, advocates of homebirth and hospital births often have "different views about the nature of pregnancy and childbirth" (de Melo-Martín and Intemann 2012, 65). Opponents of homebirth see pregnancy and childbirth as "intrinsically risky activities," and therefore believe that these activities should take place only in a hospital setting (de Melo-Martín and Intemann 2012, 65).[51] In contrast, proponents of homebirth see "pregnancy, labor, and delivery for low-risk women as generally safe activities that can at times be risky" (de Melo-Martín and Intemann 2012, 66). For homebirth proponents, complications from a homebirth are like falling down the stairs or getting into a car accident. The fact that there are possible negative outcomes of these routine activities is not a reason to be risk averse in ways that compromise goods associated with those activities. Most people do not wear safety equipment to climb stairs or refuse to live in multi-story homes. They do not hire professionals to drive their cars, even when they drive their new baby home from the hospital. Some people think childbirth is a similarly routine experience, and they don't want their birthing experiences to be structured around the demands of hospital protocols that may make birth only marginally safer.

De Melo-Martín and Intemann argue that a failure to recognize the influence of values on homebirth choices may lead to three kinds of problems (de Melo-Martín and Intemann 2012, 67). (All three kinds of problems can also result from a failure to recognize the ways values influence vaccine choices.) First, an excessive focus on medical facts (rather than values) may impede communication, since it may redirect conversations away from the features of homebirth (or vaccination) that are relevant to the disagreement. In the case of vaccine refusal, we would do well not to focus exclusively on vaccine denialism, which is an instance of epistemic failure, if we want to understand and properly respond to vaccine refusal.[52] Second, focusing on nonexistent factual disputes may lead to unfruitful (and wasteful) calls for 'more research', when the medical research is not in question. For example, I will argue in the next chapter that parental worries about 'toxins' in vaccines may reflect a parental embrace of 'natural' health, rather than a rejection of vaccine science. We are unlikely to alleviate concerns about 'toxins' with more studies. Finally, obscuring the roles played by values in disputes about health care choices may lead to unsound public policy. If public health care policy promotes particular health care choices (e.g. hospital births and childhood vaccination), and if arguments for these choices are informed by disputed values, then public policy that pretends to be value neutral is a lie. What is worse, this deceptive sort of public policy will leave important questions about disputed values unaddressed, and may lead advocates of homebirth and vaccine refusal to suspect the motives of health care policymakers. At the very least, democratic public health policy must be transparent about its underlying values.

Conclusion

The arguments in this chapter should generate a sense of urgency about the breakdown in trust I discussed in the previous chapter. Recall that most parents believe vaccines are safe and effective. Vaccine denialists are a small minority. But parents who vaccinate their children do not usually read scientific studies or analyze the confidence intervals of the statistical predictions of vaccine science. Instead, they believe that vaccines are safe and effective because they trust and like their children's pediatricians, and because they have constructed various pro-vaccine causal narratives on the basis of that trust. Vaccine denialists are not cognitively deficient compared to parents who vaccinate. Their minds work just as well (or as poorly). Instead, the breakdown in parental trust in pediatricians – which may occur for good reasons – leaves otherwise truth-oriented parents vulnerable to cognitive biases that impede their efforts to arrive at true beliefs about the risks of vaccination. And these biases can have consequences for parents' choices, even when they do not distort parents' beliefs about vaccine science. Even when cognitive biases do not lead parents to become vaccine *denialists*, they can sometimes lead parents to become vaccine *refusers*. Finally, some cases of apparent bias-based vaccine refusal are better understood as cases of disagreement about the values that ought to inform parental decisions about routine childhood vaccines.

Notes

1 For some examples of the overwhelming literature documenting the ways cognitive biases distort physicians' judgments, see Baumann, Deber and Thompson (1991); Berner and Graber (2008); Eva and Norman (2005); Sibbald and Cavalcanti (2011); and Swindell, McGuire, and Halpern (2010).
2 If biases were implicated in our value commitments, then biases would be relevant to these forms of vaccine denialism. I take up worries about bias-based values towards the end of the next chapter, where I discuss whether there are reasons to reject the values of 'purity' and 'sanctity'.
3 There has been almost no philosophical engagement with the role that cognitive heuristics may play in vaccination choices. A notable exception is Dare (1998).
4 Thaler and Sunstein: "The Automatic System is rapid and feels instinctive, and it does not involve what we usually associate with the word 'thinking'... [t]he Automatic System is your gut reaction and the Reflective System is your conscious thought" (Thaler and Sunstein 2009, 19, 21).
5 I leave it to epistemologists to determine whether true beliefs that are formed through reliable forms of automatic reasoning count as knowledge. That question is beyond the scope of my work here.
6 Thaler and Sunstein: "The Reflective System is more deliberate and self-conscious" (Thaler and Sunstein 2009, 20).
7 Zajonc writes that "[in] practice affective reactions are so fast and compelling that they act like blinders on a horse: they 'reduce the universe of alternatives' available to later thinking" (Zajonc 1980, 171, quoted in Haidt 2012, 56).
8 By 'anti-science', I mean a large-scale rejection of the methods and results of science. See Holton (1993).
9 Furthermore, there is little reason to think that 'anti-scientific' attitudes are driving these other forms of science rejection. Instead, a higher level of scientific literacy correlates with a stronger denial of some kinds of scientific consensus, among members of groups who are more likely to reject that science (Kahan et al. 2012).
10 On the role of fear (e.g. of needles) and pain in vaccine denialism/refusal, see Smith, Appleton, and MacDonald (2013, 93).

11 For example, a parent may distrust and dislike her child's pediatrician. Recall that, in the last chapter, I argued that parents sometimes have good reasons to refuse to grant quick assent to the testimony of pediatricians and to form resistant epistemic communities. Here, I make a different (though related) claim: Parents may develop negative feelings about their child's pediatrician, even if they do not have a good reason for doing so. There is a strong correlation between parental trust of pediatricians and vaccination (Benin et al. 2006; Wei et al. 2009; Williams and Swan 2014).

12 Seth Mnookin provides a helpful summary of some aspects of vaccination that may lead a person to have negative feelings about vaccines: "Vaccines contain viruses, viruses are dangerous, infants' immune systems aren't fully developed, drug companies are interested only in profit, and the government can't always be trusted" (Mnookin 2011, 18).

13 Among other reasons, this is because parents who vaccinate do not do much thinking about vaccination.

14 Paul Meehl (1954) showed that the subjective impressions of trained clinical psychologists were less accurate at predicting the behavior of their patients/ clients than were statistical predictions based on a few inputs for each client/patient. Even the expert intuitions of medical practitioners can be less accurate than judgments that result from statistical algorithms and minimal data inputs.

15 "[E]stimates of causes of death are warped by media coverage … Unusual events (such as botulism) attract disproportionate attention and are consequently perceived as less unusual than they really are" (Kahneman 2011, 138).

16 The fact that negative emotionally charged anecdotes have such power is a reason for vaccine advocates to support efforts to widely distribute stories about people who have been harmed by vaccine-preventable diseases, such as the "Story Gallery" at ShotByShot (2014).

17 In this way, the availability bias may help to explain some of the transitions in what Robert Chen et al. call the Life-cycle of an Immunization Program (Chen et al. 1994). For example, Chen et al. argue that once a vaccine becomes so widely used that few people have experienced the disease, then people will start to worry more about vaccine complications. One reason for this change is that information about vaccine-preventable diseases becomes less available to memory when people have fewer direct experiences of the disease.

18 Brown et al. (2012) have shown that *direct* experience with an autistic child correlates with vaccine denialism/refusal.

19 In the next chapters I often highlight how vaccine refusal is connected to moral and non-moral values: In chapter three, I focus on the values of purity and sanctity (and the feeling of disgust). In chapter four, I focus on parental moral rights. In chapter five, I focus on the claim that medical interventions ought always to be voluntary. And, in chapter six, I focus on the idea that individual citizens have a liberty right to be exempted from forms of government coercion which they find (morally) objectionable.

20 For evidence of the distorting impact of the availability heuristic on physicians' diagnostic practice, see Eva and Norman (2005).

21 Some residents of suburban neighborhoods with relatively high numbers of cancer diagnoses have claimed that their so-called 'cancer clusters' had environmental causes, e.g. high-voltage power lines. However, the distribution of the proximities of cancer patients to the supposed causes of these 'cancer clusters' is random (Thaler and Sunstein 2009, 31). Another evocative example of this phenomenon is that some WWII Londoners believed that some areas of London were hit by relatively fewer German bombs because German spies lived in those areas (Gilovich 2008).

22 Betsch, Renkewitz, and Haase (2013) provided study participants with both statistical and narrative information about vaccines and adverse vaccination events. They found that "[w]hen the relative frequency [of vaccine complications] was communicated in the form of statistical information, 35.7% of the reported sample must have experienced adverse events for participants to shift their intentions from vaccinating to not vaccinating. When communicated in the form of narratives, the relative frequency need only be 25.5% for participants to change their intentions (i.e. roughly 10% fewer cases than when using statistical information)" (22).

23 It is notable that vaccine safety worries in the 1980s – fueled by a previous generation of vaccine denialists – influenced the change to the newer (and less effective) pertussis vaccine. So, 'vaccine refusal caused pertussis increase' is true, but not in the straightforward way many suppose.

24 See Robert Shiller (2005) on the psychological factors which explain market prices in boom-and-bust cycles.

25 People believe what supports their 'team', not only (or even primarily) when it is in their interest to do so. Political opinions are not primarily strategies of instrumental rationality, but are markers of group membership. They are like "the array of bumper stickers people put on their cars showing the political causes, universities, and sports teams they support" (Haidt 2012, 86).

26 For an evolutionary explanation of our tendency to endorse the beliefs (we believe) the majority of our community endorses, see Boyd and Richerson (1988).

27 In 1970, Mary Douglas published *Natural Symbols*, which introduced a two-axis model for sorting cultural values. She argued that one could categorize cultural commitments according to whether they scored higher or lower on the axes of *group* and *grid*. Someone with low-group values prioritizes individual liberty when thinking about public policies, while someone with high-group values prioritizes collective political projects. Someone with low-grid values is more likely to believe that social goods – including opportunities, positions of power/privilege, wealth, and income – ought to be distributed equally or in accordance with egalitarian values (e.g. merit), while someone with high-grid values is more likely to think that such goods ought to be distributed according to physical or social facts such as race, gender, religion, class, or family wealth.

28 A mark of this new research is that it rejects (or does not emphasize) the 'functionalist' explanations offered by Douglas, Wildavsky, and others for the tendency of one's values to influence one's factual beliefs. Douglas and Wildavsky argued that we believe unjust or immoral actions are also dangerous because doing so may lend support to our conceptions of morality and justice. On Douglas and Wildavsky's 'functionalism', see M. Douglas (2002) and Thompson, Ellis, and Wildavsky (1990). For Kahan's criticism of the earlier functionalism of 'cultural theory', see Kahan and Braman (2006, 154–155).

29 Kahan and Braman continue: "Culture is prior to facts, moreover, not just in the evaluative sense that citizens might care more about how gun control, the death penalty, environmental regulation and the like cohere with their cultural values than they care about the consequences of those policies. Rather, culture is prior to facts in the cognitive sense that what citizens believe about the empirical consequences of those policies derives from their cultural worldviews. Based on a variety of overlapping psychological mechanisms, individuals accept or reject empirical claims about the consequences of controversial polices based on their vision of a good society" (Kahan and Braman 2006, 150).

30 The term 'cognitive dissonance' was coined by Leon Festinger. See Festinger, Riecken, and Schachter (1956). Also see Akerlof and Dickens (1982) and Sherman and Cohen (2002).

31 On the general idea of the importance of expert testimony in belief formation, see Coady (1995), Goldberg (2010), and Goldman (2001).

32 Kahan, Jenkins-Smith, and Braman argue that the factual judgments of experts are also affected by their values (Kahan, Jenkins-Smith, and Braman 2011, 156n26). On this point, Kahan, Jenkins-Smith, and Braman cite Paul Slovic (2000, at 406–409). In this way, judgments based on expert opinion may be influenced by cultural cognition at two levels: first, in the selection of the expert; second, in the judgment of the expert. On a related note, Elizabeth Anderson argues that there are easy-to-use methods to accurately identify true experts, but she acknowledges that it may take a massive democratization of politics, culture, and the media for people to reliably use those methods (Anderson 2011).

33 On geographic clustering and opinion formation about vaccines, see Omer et al. (2008) and Salathé and Bonhoeffer (2008).

34 Jacobson, Targonski, and Poland (2007) argue that mass media communication about vaccination gives an "exaggerated impression of social support" for vaccine denialism/refusal (3150).

35 Consider some of the chapter titles of Margulis's book, *The Business of Baby*: Chapter 4, "CUTTING COSTS: The Business of Cesarean Birth;" Chapter 5, "PERINATAL PRICES: Profit-Mongering After the Baby is Born;" Chapter 6, "FORESKINS FOR SALE: The Business of Circumcision;" and Chapter 9, "BOOST YOUR BOTTOM LINE: Vaccinating for Health or Profit?" (Margulis 2013).

36 It may also reflect the fact that people who do Internet research are already questioning. We should not be too surprised that people who refuse to 'go with the flow' are more likely to refuse vaccines.

37 Brownstein and Madva (2012a; 2012b) disagree that System 2 processes *always* ought to test the results of System 1 processes. They think we need to have a good reason for System 1 to face potential revision. But this should be easy enough in the case of vaccine denialism, since there are good reasons to subject one's automatic judgments to criticism when they lead to the rejection of widely endorsed scientific claims.

38 System 2 is more often "an apologist for the emotions of System 1 than a critic of those emotions – an endorser rather than an enforcer. Its search for information and arguments is mostly constrained to information that is consistent with existing beliefs, and not with an intention to examine them" (Kahneman 2011, 103–104).

39 As Abelson has said, 'beliefs are like possessions' – we do not want to give them up once we have them (and once we have found some use for them) (Abelson 1986).

40 Gilovich writes that "we tend to use different criteria to evaluate propositions or conclusions we desire, and those we abhor. For propositions we want to believe, we ask only that the evidence not force us to believe otherwise – a rather easy standard to meet, given the equivocal nature of much information. For propositions we want to resist, however, we ask whether the evidence *compels* such a distasteful conclusion – a much more difficult standard to achieve" (Gilovich 2008, 83–84). Also see Kunda (1990) and Zajonc (1980).

41 For a review of the literature, see Nickerson (1998). See also Ditto, Pizarro, and Tannenbaum (2009), Mercier and Sperber (2011), and Wason (1960).

42 This tendency was noted among the early vaccine denialists. In 1910, Dr. Jay Frank Schamberg wrote for the *Ladies' Home Journal* that "[t]he opponents of

vaccine ... accept as true every alleged accident after vaccination as resulting therefrom, but assiduously shut their eyes to the evidence offered of the efficacy of vaccination" (Allen 2007a, 106–107).

43 For a review of the different narratives, see Baker (2008).

44 CDC and the American Academy of Pediatrics (AAP) did not help matters when they issued a joint statement requesting that vaccine manufacturers remove thimerosal from vaccines, absent any evidence that ingredient was harmful (Centers for Disease Control and Prevention 1999; Centers for Disease Control and Prevention 2001). Jason Schwartz discusses how a similar commitment to maintain public trust in vaccines led to the withdrawal of the RotaShield rotavirus vaccine in 1999, and how that decision resulted in similar kinds of unintended consequences as did CDC and AAP advocacy for the removal of thimerosal (Schwartz 2012).

45 Adversarial argumentation can be more or less conducive to truth-oriented inquiry, depending on how it is conducted (Moulton 1983; Rooney 2010).

46 Kahneman discusses an example like this (Kahneman 2011, 329).

47 I have so far taken for granted that the metaphysical distinction between action and inaction, or commission and omission, has some intuitive force. If we cannot sensibly make these distinctions, then we cannot make sense of the omission bias.

48 My discussion in this paragraph benefited from Howard-Snyder (2011).

49 For summary and discussion of much of the empirical work on trolley problems, see Edmonds (2013).

50 On 'threshold deontology', see Moore (2008).

51 In particular, "in risk assessments related to pregnancy, often the assumption at work is that any risk to the fetus, however small or theoretical, outweighs considerations that may be of substantial importance to the woman herself" (de Melo-Martín and Intemann 2012, 65). See also Lyerly et al. (2007; 2009).

52 Here, I am reminded of Mark Largent's claim that debates about whether vaccines cause autism are unhelpful proxy fights over a complex set of value-laden concerns surrounding contemporary vaccine policy (Largent 2012).

Bibliography

Abelson, Robert P. 1986. "Beliefs Are Like Possessions." *Journal for the Theory of Social Behaviour* 16(3): 223–250.

Akerlof, G. A., and W. T. Dickens. 1982. "The Economic Consequences of Cognitive Dissonance." *The American Economic Review* 72(3): 307–319.

Allen, Arthur. 2007a. *Vaccine: The Controversial Story of Medicine's Greatest Lifesaver.* W. W. Norton & Company.

Allen, Arthur 2007b. "True Believers: Why There's No Dispelling the Myth That Vaccines Cause Autism." *Slate.com.* June 29. www.slate.com/articles/health_and_science/medical_examiner/2007/06/true_believers.html.

Anderson, Elizabeth. 2011. "Democracy, Public Policy, and Lay Assessments of Scientific Testimony." *Episteme* 8(2): 144–164.

Ariely, Dan. 2010. *Predictably Irrational, Revised and Expanded Edition: The Hidden Forces That Shape Our Decisions.* Rev. ed. Harper Perennial.

Arnheim-Dahlström, Lisen, Björn Pasternak, Henrik Svanström, Pär Sparén, and Anders Hviid. 2013. "Autoimmune, Neurological, and Venous Thromboembolic Adverse Events after Immunisation of Adolescent Girls with Quadrivalent Human Papillomavirus Vaccine in Denmark and Sweden: Cohort Study." *British Medical Journal* 347(October): f5906. doi:10.1136/bmj.f5906.

Asch, David A., Jonathan Baron, John C. Hershey, Howard Kunreuther, Jacqueline Meszaros, Ilana Ritov, and Mark Spranca. 1994. "Omission Bias and Pertussis Vaccination." *Medical Decision Making* 14(2): 118–123.

Asch, Solomon E. 1955. "Opinions and Social Pressure." *Scientific American* 193(5): 31–35.

Baker, Jeffrey P. 2008. "Mercury, Vaccines, and Autism: One Controversy, Three Histories." *American Journal of Public Health* 98(2): 244–253.

Ball, Leslie K., Geoffrey Evans, and Ann Bostrom. 1998. "Risky Business: Challenges in Vaccine Risk Communication." *Pediatrics* 101(3): 453–458.

Baumann, Andrea O., Raisa B. Deber, and Gail G. Thompson. 1991. "Overconfidence among Physicians and Nurses: The 'Micro-Certainty, Macro-Uncertainty' Phenomenon." *Social Science & Medicine* 32(2): 167–174.

Begg, Ian, Victoria Armour, and Therese Kerr. 1985. "On Believing What We Remember." *Canadian Journal of Behavioural Science/Revue canadienne des sciences du comportement* 17(3): 199.

Benin, A. L., D. J. Wisler-Scher, E. Colson, E. D. Shapiro, and E. S. Holmboe. 2006. "Qualitative Analysis of Mothers' Decision-Making about Vaccines for Infants: The Importance of Trust." *Pediatrics* 117(5): 1532–1541.

Berman, David M., and Paola Dees. 2013. "Vaccines and the Internet." In *Vaccinophobia and Vaccine Controversies of the 21st Century*, edited by Archana Chatterjee, 399–418. Springer.

Berner, Eta S., and Mark L. Graber. 2008. "Overconfidence as a Cause of Diagnostic Error in Medicine." *The American Journal of Medicine* 121(5): S2–23.

Betsch, Cornelia, Noel T. Brewer, Pauline Brocard, Patrick Davies, Wolfgang Gaissmaier, Niels Haase, Julie Leask, Frank Renkewitz, Britta Renner, and Valerie F. Reyna. 2012. "Opportunities and Challenges of Web 2.0 for Vaccination Decisions." *Vaccine* 30(25): 3727–3733.

Betsch, Cornelia, Frank Renkewitz, and Niels Haase. 2013. "Effect of Narrative Reports about Vaccine Adverse Events and Bias-Awareness Disclaimers on Vaccine Decisions: A Simulation of an Online Patient Social Network." *Medical Decision Making* 33(1): 14–25.

Betsch, Cornelia, and Katharina Sachse. 2013. "Debunking Vaccination Myths: Strong Risk Negations Can Increase Perceived Vaccination Risks." *Health Psychology* 32(2): 146.

Betsch, Cornelia, Corina Ulshöfer, Frank Renkewitz, and Tilmann Betsch. 2011. "The Influence of Narrative v. Statistical Information on Perceiving Vaccination Risks." *Medical Decision Making* 31(5): 742–753.

Boyd, Robert, and Peter J. Richerson. 1988. *Culture and the Evolutionary Process.* University of Chicago Press.

Brown, Katrina. F., J. S. Kroll, M. J. Hudson, M. Ramsay, J. Green, S. J. Long, C. A. Vincent, G. Fraser, and N. Sevdalis. 2010. "Factors Underlying Parental Decisions about Combination Childhood Vaccinations Including MMR: A Systematic Review." *Vaccine* 28(26): 4235–4248.

Brown, Katrina F., J. Simon Kroll, Michael J. Hudson, Mary Ramsay, John Green, Charles A. Vincent, Graham Fraser, and Nick Sevdalis. 2010. "Omission Bias and Vaccine Rejection by Parents of Healthy Children: Implications for the Influenza A/H1N1 Vaccination Programme." *Vaccine* 28(25): 4181–4185.

Brown, Katrina F., Susannah J. Long, Mary Ramsay, Michael J. Hudson, John Green, Charles A. Vincent, J. Simon Kroll, Graham Fraser, and Nick Sevdalis.

2012. "UK Parents' Decision-Making about Measles–Mumps–Rubella (MMR) Vaccine 10 Years after the MMR-Autism Controversy: A Qualitative Analysis." *Vaccine* 30(10): 1855–1864.

Brownstein, Michael, and Alex Madva. 2012a. "Ethical Automaticity." *Philosophy of the Social Sciences* 42(1): 68–98.

Brownstein, Michael, and Alex Madva. 2012b. "The Normativity of Automaticity." *Mind & Language* 27(4): 410–434.

Camerer, Colin F., and Robin M. Hogarth. 1999. "The Effects of Financial Incentives in Experiments: A Review and Capital-Labor-Production Framework." *Journal of Risk and Uncertainty* 19(1–3): 7–42.

Campbell, Eric G., Russell L. Gruen, James Mountford, Lawrence G. Miller, Paul D. Cleary, and David Blumenthal. 2007. "A National Survey of Physician–Industry Relationships." *New England Journal of Medicine* 356(17): 1742–1750.

Centers for Disease Control and Prevention. 1999. "Thimerosal in Vaccines: A Joint Statement of the American Academy of Pediatrics and the Public Health Service." July 9. www.cdc.gov/mmwr/preview/mmwrhtml/mm4826a3.htm.

Centers for Disease Control and Prevention. 2001. "Impact of the 1999 AAP/USPHS Joint Statement on Thimerosal in Vaccines on Infant Hepatitis B Vaccination Practices." *Morbidity and Mortality Weekly Report (MMWR)* 50(6): 94.

Centers for Disease Control and Prevention. 2013. "CDC – Pertussis: Frequently Asked Questions." *Pertussis (Whooping Cough)*. December 19. www.cdc.gov/pertussis/about/faqs.html#increasing.

Centers for Disease Control and Prevention. 2014. "Human Papillomavirus Vaccination: Recommendations of the Advisory Committee on Immunization Practices (ACIP)." *Morbidity and Mortality Weekly Report (MMWR)*. August 29. www.cdc.gov/mmwr/preview/mmwrhtml/rr6305a1.htm.

Chen, Robert T., Suresh C. Rastogi, John R. Mullen, Scott W. Hayes, Stephen L. Cochi, Jerome A. Donlon, and Steven G. Wassilak. 1994. "The Vaccine Adverse Event Reporting System (VAERS)." *Vaccine* 12(6): 542–550.

Coady, C. A. J. 1995. *Testimony: A Philosophical Study*. Oxford University Press.

Cohen, G. L. 2003. "Party over Policy: The Dominating Impact of Group Influence on Political Beliefs." *Journal of Personality and Social Psychology* 85(5): 808.

Connolly, Terry, and Jochen Reb. 2003. "Omission Bias in Vaccination Decisions: Where's the 'Omission'? Where's the 'Bias'?" *Organizational Behavior and Human Decision Processes* 91(2): 186–202.

Damasio, A. R. 1994. *Descartes' Error*. Putnam.

Dare, Tim. 1998. "Mass Immunisation Programmes: Some Philosophical Issues." *Bioethics* 12(2): 125–149.

De Melo-Martín, Inmaculada, and Kristen Intemann. 2009. "How Do Disclosure Policies Fail? Let Us Count the Ways." *The FASEB Journal* 23(6): 1638–1642.

De Melo-Martín, Inmaculada, and Kristen Intemann. 2012. "Interpreting Evidence: Why Values Can Matter as Much as Science." *Perspectives in Biology and Medicine* 55(1): 59–70.

Ditto, Peter H., David A. Pizarro, and David Tannenbaum. 2009. "Motivated Moral Reasoning." *Psychology of Learning and Motivation* 50: 307–338.

Douglas, Heather E. 2009. *Science, Policy, and the Value-Free Ideal*. University of Pittsburgh Press.

Douglas, Mary. 2002. *Purity and Danger: An Analysis of the Concepts of Pollution and Taboo*. Routledge.

Douglas, M., and A. Wildavsky. 1983. *Risk and Culture: An Essay on the Selection of Technological and Environmental Dangers.* University of California Press.

Downs, Julie S., Wändi Bruine de Bruin, and Baruch Fischhoff. 2008. "Parents' Vaccination Comprehension and Decisions." *Vaccine* 26(12): 1595–1607.

Dubé, Eve, Caroline Laberge, Maryse Guay, Paul Bramadat, Réal Roy, and Julie A. Bettinger. 2013. "Vaccine Hesitancy: An Overview." *Human Vaccines & Immunotherapeutics* 9(8): 1763–1773.

Edmonds, David. 2013. *Would You Kill the Fat Man? The Trolley Problem and What Your Answer Tells Us about Right and Wrong.* Princeton University Press.

Einsiedel, E. F. 2011. "Publics and Vaccinomics: Beyond Public Understanding of Science." *OMICS: A Journal of Integrative Biology* 15(9): 607–614.

Eva, Kevin W., and Geoffrey R. Norman. 2005. "Heuristics and Biases – a Biased Perspective on Clinical Reasoning." *Medical Education* 39(9): 870–872.

Festinger, Leon, Henry W. Riecken, and Stanley Schachter. 1956. *When Prophecy Fails.* Harper-Torchbooks.

Fombonne, E. 2008. "Thimerosal Disappears but Autism Remains." *Archives of General Psychiatry* 65(1): 15–16.

Foot, Philippa. 1978. "The Problem of Abortion and the Problem of Double Effect." In *Virtues and Vices and Other Essays*, 19–32. University of California Press.

Frompovich, Catherine. 2011. "Formaldehyde in Vaccines | Vactruth.com." *Vactruth.com.* June 14. http://vactruth.com/2011/06/14/formaldehyde-in-vaccines/.

Gerber, Jeffrey S., and Paul A. Offit. 2009. "Vaccines and Autism: A Tale of Shifting Hypotheses." *Clinical Infectious Diseases: An Official Publication of the Infectious Diseases Society of America* 48(4): 456–461.

Gilovich, Thomas. 2008. *How We Know What Isn't So.* Simon and Schuster.

Glanz, Jason M., Nicole M. Wagner, Komal J. Narwaney, Jo Ann Shoup, David L. McClure, Emily V. McCormick, and Matthew F. Daley. 2013. "A Mixed Methods Study of Parental Vaccine Decision Making and Parent–Provider Trust." *Academic Pediatrics* 13(5): 481–488.

Goldberg, Sanford C. 2010. *Relying on Others: An Essay in Epistemology.* Oxford University Press.

Goldman, A. I. 2001. "Experts: Which Ones Should You Trust?" *Philosophy and Phenomenological Research* 63(1): 85–110.

Gong, Jingjing, Yan Zhang, Zheng Yang, Yonghua Huang, Jun Feng, and Weiwei Zhang. 2013. "The Framing Effect in Medical Decision-Making: A Review of the Literature." *Psychology, Health & Medicine* 18(6): 645–653.

Grande, David, Judy A. Shea, and Katrina Armstrong. 2012. "Pharmaceutical Industry Gifts to Physicians: Patient Beliefs and Trust in Physicians and the Health Care System." *Journal of General Internal Medicine* 27(3): 274–279.

Greene, Joshua. 2013. *Moral Tribes: Emotion, Reason and the Gap between Us and Them.* Atlantic Books.

Greene, Joshua, R. Brian Sommerville, Leigh E. Nystrom, John M. Darley, and Jonathan D. Cohen. 2001. "An fMRI Investigation of Emotional Engagement in Moral Judgment." *Science* 293(5537): 2105–2108.

Haidt, Jonathan. 2012. *The Righteous Mind: Why Good People Are Divided by Politics and Religion.* Penguin.

Healy, C. Mary, and Larry K. Pickering. 2011. "How to Communicate with Vaccine-Hesitant Parents." *Pediatrics* 127 (Supplement 1): S127–133.

Holton, Gerald James. 1993. *Science and Anti-Science.* Harvard University Press.

Howard-Snyder, Frances. 2011. "Doing vs. Allowing Harm." In *The Stanford Encyclopedia of Philosophy*, edited by Edward N. Zalta,Winter. http://plato.stanford.edu/archives/win2011/entries/doing-allowing/.

Intemann, Kristen. 2011. "Diversity and Dissent in Science: Does Democracy Always Serve Feminist Aims?" In *Feminist Epistemology and Philosophy of Science: Power in Knowledge*, edited by Heidi E. Grasswick, 111–132. Springer.

Jacobson, R. M., P. V. Targonski, and G. A. Poland. 2007. "A Taxonomy of Reasoning Flaws in the Anti-Vaccine Movement." *Vaccine* 25(16): 3146–3152.

Jones, Abbey M., Saad B. Omer, Robert A. Bednarczyk, Neal A. Halsey, Lawrence H. Moulton, and Daniel A. Salmon. 2012. "Parents' Source of Vaccine Information and Impact on Vaccine Attitudes, Beliefs, and Nonmedical Exemptions." *Advances in Preventive Medicine* 2012: 1–8.

Kahan, Dan M. 2014. *Vaccine Risk Perceptions and Ad Hoc Risk Communication: An Empirical Assessment.* SSRN Scholarly Paper ID 2386034. Social Science Research Network. Accessed June 11, 2015. http://papers.ssrn.com/abstract=2386034.

Kahan, Dan M., and D. Braman. 2006. "Cultural Cognition and Public Policy." *Yale Law & Policy Review* 24: 149.

Kahan, Dan M., H. Jenkins-Smith, and D. Braman. 2011. "Cultural Cognition of Scientific Consensus." *Journal of Risk Research* 14(2): 147–174.

Kahan, Dan M., Ellen Peters, Erica Cantrell Dawson, and Paul Slovic. 2013. *Motivated Numeracy and Enlightened Self-Government.* SSRN Scholarly Paper ID 2319992. Social Science Research Network. Accessed June 11, 2015. http://papers.ssrn.com/abstract=2319992.

Kahan, Dan M., Ellen Peters, Maggie Wittlin, Paul Slovic, Lisa Larrimore Ouellette, Donald Braman, and Gregory Mandel. 2012. "The Polarizing Impact of Science Literacy and Numeracy on Perceived Climate Change Risks." *Nature Climate Change* 2(10): 732–735.

Kahneman, D. 2011. *Thinking, Fast and Slow.* Farrar, Straus and Giroux.

Kennedy, Robert F. 2005. "Deadly Immunity." *Rolling Stone*, July 14.

Kirby, David. 2006. *Evidence of Harm: Mercury in Vaccines and the Autism Epidemic: A Medical Controversy.* St. Martin's Griffin.

Kirkland, Anna. 2012. "The Legitimacy of Vaccine Critics: What Is Left After the Autism Hypothesis?" *Journal of Health Politics, Policy and Law* 37(1): 69–97.

Kitcher, P. 1993. *The Advancement of Science: Science without Legend, Objectivity without Illusions.* Oxford University Press.

Klein, Gary A. 1999. *Sources of Power: How People Make Decisions.* MIT Press.

Kruglanski, Arie W., Antonio Pierro, Lucia Mannetti, and Eraldo De Grada. 2006. "Groups as Epistemic Providers: Need for Closure and the Unfolding of Group-Centrism." *Psychological Review* 113(1): 84–100.

Kunda, Ziva. 1990. "The Case for Motivated Reasoning." *Psychological Bulletin* 108(3): 480.

Largent, M. A. 2012. *Vaccine: The Debate in Modern America.* Johns Hopkins University Press.

Larson, H. J., L. Z. Cooper, J. Eskola, S. L. Katz, and S. Ratzan. 2011. "Addressing the Vaccine Confidence Gap." *The Lancet* 378(9790): 526–535.

Lewandowsky, Stephan, Ullrich K. H. Ecker, Colleen M. Seifert, Norbert Schwarz, and John Cook. 2012. "Misinformation and Its Correction: Continued Influence and Successful Debiasing." *Psychological Science in the Public Interest* 13(3): 106–131.

Lodge, Milton, and Charles S. Taber. 2013. *The Rationalizing Voter.* Cambridge University Press.

Longino, Helen E. 1990. *Science as Social Knowledge: Values and Objectivity in Scientific Inquiry.* Princeton University Press.

Longino, Helen E. 2002. *The Fate of Knowledge.* Princeton University Press.

Luyten, Jeroen, Pieter Desmet, Veronica Dorgali, Niel Hens, and Philippe Beutels. 2013. "Kicking Against the Pricks: Vaccine Sceptics Have a Different Social Orientation." *The European Journal of Public Health* 24(2): 310–314.

Lyerly, Anne Drapkin, Lisa M. Mitchell, Elizabeth M. Armstrong, Lisa H. Harris, Rebecca Kukla, Miriam Kuppermann, and Margaret Olivia Little. 2007. "Risks, Values, and Decision Making Surrounding Pregnancy." *Obstetrics & Gynecology* 109(4): 979–984.

Lyerly, Anne Drapkin, Lisa M. Mitchell, Elizabeth Mitchell Armstrong, Lisa H. Harris, Rebecca Kukla, Miriam Kuppermann, and Margaret Olivia Little. 2009. "Risk and the Pregnant Body." *Hastings Center Report* 39(6): 34–42.

Margulis, Jennifer. 2013. *Business of Baby: What Doctors Don't Tell You, What Corporations Try to Sell You, and How to Put Your Pregnancy, Childbirth, and Baby Before Their Bottom Line.* Scribner.

McDonough, Katie. 2013. "Katie Couric Gets Called out for Promoting Bogus Science on HPV Vaccine." December 4. www.salon.com/2013/12/04/katie_couric_gets_called_out_for_promoting_bogus_science_on_hpv_vaccine/.

McNeil, Barbara J., Stephen G. Pauker, Harold C. SoxJr., and Amos Tversky. 1982. "On the Elicitation of Preferences for Alternative Therapies." *New England Journal of Medicine* 306(21): 1259–1262.

Meehl, Paul E. 1954. *Clinical Versus Statistical Prediction: A Theoretical Analysis and a Review of the Evidence.* University of Minnesota Press.

Mercier, Hugo, and Dan Sperber. 2011. "Why Do Humans Reason? Arguments for an Argumentative Theory." *Behavioral and Brain Sciences* 34(2): 57.

Meszaros, Jacqueline R., David A. Asch, Jonathan Baron, John C. Hershey, Howard Kunreuther, and Joanne Schwartz-Buzaglo. 1996. "Cognitive Processes and the Decisions of Some Parents to Forego Pertussis Vaccination for Their Children." *Journal of Clinical Epidemiology* 49(6): 697–703.

Mnookin, Seth. 2011. *The Panic Virus: A True Story of Medicine, Science, and Fear.* Simon & Schuster.

Mooney, Chris, and Sheril Kirshenbaum. 2010. *Unscientific America: How Scientific Illiteracy Threatens Our Future.* Basic Books.

Moore, Michael S. 2008. "Patrolling the Borders of Consequentialist Justifications: The Scope of Agent-Relative Restrictions." *Law and Philosophy* 27(1): 35–96.

Moulton, Janice. 1983. "A Paradigm of Philosophy: The Adversary Method." In *Discovering Reality*, edited by Sandra Harding and Merrill Hintikka, 149–164. Springer.

National Vaccine Information Center. 2015. "About Us." Accessed February 23. www.nvic.org/about.aspx.

Nickerson, Raymond S. 1998. "Confirmation Bias: A Ubiquitous Phenomenon in Many Guises." *Review of General Psychology* 2(2): 175.

Nietzsche, Friedrich. 2006. *"On the Genealogy of Morality" and Other Writings.* Edited by Keith Ansell-Pearson. Translated by Carol Diethe. 2nd ed. Cambridge University Press.

Omer, S. B., K. S. Enger, L. H. Moulton, N. A. Halsey, S. Stokley, and D. A. Salmon. 2008. "Geographic Clustering of Nonmedical Exemptions to School

Immunization Requirements and Associations with Geographic Clustering of Pertussis." *American Journal of Epidemiology* 168(12): 1389–1396.

Omer, S. B., D. A. Salmon, W. A. Orenstein, M. P. deHart, and N. Halsey. 2009. "Vaccine Refusal, Mandatory Immunization, and the Risks of Vaccine-Preventable Diseases." *New England Journal of Medicine* 360(19): 1981–1988.

Otto, Shawn Lawrence. 2011. *Fool Me Twice: Fighting the Assault on Science in America.* Rodale.

Otto, Shawn Lawrence. 2012. "Antiscience Beliefs Jeopardize US Democracy." *Scientific American* 307(5): 62–71.

Palevsky, Lawrence. 2012. "Aluminum and Vaccine Ingredients – National Vaccine Information Center." *National Vaccine Information Center.* Accessed June 14. www.nvic.org/Doctors-Corner/Aluminum-and-Vaccine-Ingredients.aspx.

Perkins, David N., M. Faraday, and B. Bushey. 1991. "Everyday Reasoning and the Roots of Intelligence." In *Informal Reasoning and Education*, edited by J. F. Voss, David N. Perkins, and J. W. Segal, 83–105. Lawrence Erlbaum Associates.

Poland, Gregory A., and Ray Spier. 2010. "Fear, Misinformation, and Innumerates: How the Wakefield Paper, the Press, and Advocacy Groups Damaged the Public Health." *Vaccine* 28(12): 2361–2362. doi:10.1016/j.vaccine.2010.02.052.

Prothero, Donald R., Pat Linse, and Michael Shermer. 2013. *Reality Check: How Science Deniers Threaten Our Future.* Indiana University Press.

Rachels, James. 1975. "Active and Passive Euthanasia." *New England Journal of Medicine* 292(2): 78–80.

Ritov, Ilana, and Jonathan Baron. 1990. "Reluctance to Vaccinate: Omission Bias and Ambiguity." *Journal of Behavioral Decision Making* 3(4): 263–277.

Rooney, Phyllis. 2010. "Philosophy, Adversarial Argumentation, and Embattled Reason." *Informal Logic* 30(3): 203–234.

Sadaf, Alina, Jennifer L. Richards, Jason Glanz, Daniel A. Salmon, and Saad B. Omer. 2013. "A Systematic Review of Interventions for Reducing Parental Vaccine Refusal and Vaccine Hesitancy." *Vaccine* 31(40): 4293–4304.

Salathé, Marcel, and Sebastian Bonhoeffer. 2008. "The Effect of Opinion Clustering on Disease Outbreaks." *Journal of the Royal Society Interface* 5(29): 1505–1508.

Schwartz, Jason L. 2012. "The First Rotavirus Vaccine and the Politics of Acceptable Risk." *Milbank Quarterly* 90(2): 278–310. doi:10.1111/j.1468-0009.2012.00664.x.

Sherman, D. K., and G. L. Cohen. 2002. "Accepting Threatening Information: Self-Affirmation and the Reduction of Defensive Biases." *Current Directions in Psychological Science* 11(4): 119.

Shiller, Robert J. 2005. *Irrational Exuberance.* Random House.

ShotByShot. 2014. "Story Gallery." *ShotByShot.org.* Accessed July 13. http://shotbyshot.org/story-gallery/.

Sibbald, Matthew, and Rodrigo B. Cavalcanti. 2011. "The Biasing Effect of Clinical History on Physical Examination Diagnostic Accuracy." *Medical Education* 45(8): 827–834.

Slovic, Paul. 2000. "Trust, Emotion, Sex, Politics and Science: Surveying the Risk-Assessment Battlefield." In *The Perception of Risk*, 390–412. Routledge.

Slovic, Paul, Melissa L. Finucane, Ellen Peters, and Donald G. MacGregor. 2004. "Risk as Analysis and Risk as Feelings: Some Thoughts about Affect, Reason, Risk, and Rationality." *Risk Analysis* 24(2): 311–322.

Smith, Jennifer C., Mary Appleton, and Noni E. MacDonald. 2013. "Building Confidence in Vaccines." In *Hot Topics in Infection and Immunity in Children IX*, edited by Nigel Curtis, Adam Finn, and Andrew J. Pollard, 81–98. Springer.

Sperber, Dan, Fabrice Clément, Christophe Heintz, Olivier Mascaro, Hugo Mercier, Gloria Origgi, and Deirdre Wilson. 2010. "Epistemic Vigilance." *Mind & Language* 25(4): 359–393.

Spranca, Mark, Elisa Minsk, and Jonathan Baron. 1991. "Omission and Commission in Judgment and Choice." *Journal of Experimental Social Psychology* 27(1): 76–105.

Steinman, Michael A., C. Seth Landefeld, and Robert B. Baron. 2012. "Industry Support of CME – Are We at the Tipping Point?" *New England Journal of Medicine* 366(12): 1069–1071.

Sunstein, Cass R. 2002. "The Law of Group Polarization." *Journal of Political Philosophy* 10(2): 175–195.

Swindell, J. S., Amy L. McGuire, and Scott D. Halpern. 2010. "Beneficent Persuasion: Techniques and Ethical Guidelines to Improve Patients' Decisions." *The Annals of Family Medicine* 8(3): 260–264.

Tafuri, S., M. S. Gallone, M. G. Cappelli, D. Martinelli, R. Prato, and C. Germinario. 2014. "Addressing the Anti-Vaccination Movement and the Role of HCWs." *Vaccine* 32(38): 4860–4865.

Taleb, Nassim Nicholas. 2010. *The Black Swan: The Impact of the Highly Improbable Fragility*. Random House.

Tanner, Carmen, and Douglas L. Medin. 2004. "Protected Values: No Omission Bias and No Framing Effects." *Psychonomic Bulletin & Review* 11(1): 185–191.

Tesser, Abraham. 1978. "Self-Generated Attitude Change." In *Advances in Experimental Social Psychology*, edited by L. Berkowitz, 289–338. Academic.

Thaler, Richard H., and Cass R. Sunstein. 2009. *Nudge: Improving Decisions about Health, Wealth, and Happiness*. Penguin Books.

Thompson, Michael, Richard Ellis, and Aaron Wildavsky. 1990. *Cultural Theory*. Vol. xvi. Political Cultures. Westview Press.

Thomson, Judith Jarvis. 1985. "The Trolley Problem." *The Yale Law Review* 94(6): 1395–1415.

Tversky, Amos, and Daniel Kahneman. 1971. "Belief in the Law of Small Numbers." *Psychological Bulletin* 76(2): 105.

Wakefield, Andrew J. 2011. *Callous Disregard: Autisms and Vaccines: The Truth Behind a Tragedy*. Skyhorse Publishing.

Wakefield, Andrew J., S. H. Murch, A. Anthony, J. Linnell, D. M. Casson, M. Malik, M. Berelowitz, et al. 1998. "RETRACTED: Ileal-Lymphoid-Nodular Hyperplasia, Non-Specific Colitis, and Pervasive Developmental Disorder in Children." *The Lancet* 351(9103): 637–641.

Wason, P. C. 1960. "On the Failure to Eliminate Hypotheses in a Conceptual Task." *Quarterly Journal of Experimental Psychology* 12(3): 129–140. doi:10.1080/17470216008416717.

Wei, F., J. Mullooly, M. Goodman, M. McCarty, A. Hanson, B. Crane, and J. Nordin. 2009. "Identification and Characteristics of Vaccine Refusers." *BMC Pediatrics* 9(1): 18.

Weisberg, Michael. 2013. *Simulation and Similarity: Using Models to Understand the World*. Oxford University Press.

Williams, S. Elizabeth, and Rebecca Swan. 2014. "Formal Training in Vaccine Safety to Address Parental Concerns Not Routinely Conducted in US Pediatric Residency Programs." *Vaccine* 32(26): 3175–3178.

Willingham, Daniel T. 2008. "Critical Thinking: Why Is It so Hard to Teach?" *Arts Education Policy Review* 109(4): 21–32.

Wroe, Abigail L., Angela Bhan, Paul Salkovskis, and Helen Bedford. 2005. "Feeling Bad about Immunising Our Children." *Vaccine* 23(12): 1428–1433.

Zajonc, Robert B. 1968. "Attitudinal Effects of Mere Exposure." *Journal of Personality and Social Psychology* 9 (2p2): 1.

Zajonc, Robert B. 1980. "Feeling and Thinking: Preferences Need No Inferences." *American Psychologist* 35(2): 151.

3 Purity, disgust, and 'unsafe' vaccines

> "[V]accines are metaphors ... for capitalist corruption, cultural decadence, and environmental pollution."
>
> (Biss 2013, 33)

Vaccine refusers often say that vaccines are unsafe. This is by far the most common reason parents give for refusing routine childhood vaccines (see e.g. Brown et al. 2010; Downs, Bruine de Bruin, and Fischhoff 2008; Dubé et al. 2013; Glanz et al. 2013; Gust et al. 2008; Healy and Pickering 2011; Leask et al. 2012; Parrella et al. 2013; Sadaf et al. 2013; Tafuri et al. 2014; Wei et al. 2009). Sometimes parents identify specific worries, e.g. that vaccines cause autism, but they often express indeterminate concerns. Mark Largent and Elena Conis have argued that sometimes parents endorse particular narratives about vaccine harms because that is often easier than explaining their true motivations, which may be opaque even to them (Conis 2015; Largent 2012). In this chapter I identify the source and content of some of these more general worries about vaccine safety.

Some parents with vaccine anxieties do not contest the factual claims of vaccine science. Instead, they think vaccines are unsafe because they disagree with vaccine advocates about the *values* that ought to inform vaccination choices. In particular, some parents seem inclined to refuse vaccines because they are especially committed to a cluster of ideals, including 'purity', 'cleanliness', 'sanctity', and 'the natural'. Jonathan Haidt groups these values under the banner of the 'ethics of sanctity/purity', though for convenience I will speak generally about an 'ethics of purity', even though I mean to include these other values (Haidt 2012). What makes an ethics of purity distinct is the importance it attaches to protecting one's metaphysical status (the sort of being that one is). On such a view, we must be on guard to avoid contact with objects or activities that could degrade our status through 'taint' or 'contamination'. For example, to preserve spiritual purity, we must not touch objects or perform acts that are spiritually impure. To live naturally, we must avoid contact with what is unnatural. To preserve our humanity, we must avoid behaviors that could brutalize our nature. And so on. An ethics of purity also often includes the expression of both moralized and non-moralized forms of *disgust*. This emotion motivates people to resist or to otherwise reject potential contamination.[1]

I think purity-motivated vaccine refusers are sometimes committed to ideals of naturalness, sanctity, purity, etc. that are practically unrealizable or morally objectionable. At the end of this chapter, I will criticize the purity ideals that seem to motivate some vaccine refusers. But my arguments about purity and disgust are circumscribed: I sidestep ongoing debates about whether disgust (including its associated ideals) can ever be an 'admissible social tool'.[2] For context, some people defend a limited role for disgust in law and society (Kahan 1999; Kass 1997; W. I. Miller 1997), while others are much less sanguine about the political usefulness of disgust and purity (Kelly 2011; Kelly and Morar 2014; Nussbaum 2004; Nussbaum 2010; Plakias 2013). Even though I will ultimately criticize the sorts of purity ideals that seem to motivate some vaccine refusers, I am at least open to the possibility that purity and disgust could play valuable roles in public policy debates.

There are three reasons to focus on the role that an ethics of purity may play in vaccine refusal. First, an ethics of purity may help to explain the relative historical invariability of vaccine refusal.[3] Vaccine refusers have been making many of the same objections for two hundred years, even though vaccine complications are now much lower (and vaccine effectiveness much higher) than ever before (Allen 2007, 333–337; Durbach 2005; Kitta 2012, 11; Offit 2010, 105; Oshinsky 2006; Salmon et al. 2006; Wolfe and Sharp 2002). If people are worried that vaccines transgress boundaries between the sacred and the profane, then facts about complication rates are not going to change their minds.

Second, if some vaccine refusers are motivated by an ethics of purity, then this would explain why vaccine refusers tend to be more educated, even though there is overwhelming scientific evidence that complication rates are low (Healy and Pickering 2011; Largent 2012, 32; Mnookin 2011a, 12; Omer et al. 2009; Wei et al. 2009). More educated people may know more (and be able to learn more) about vaccines and vaccine policy. Their knowledge may trigger disgust or other adverse purity-based responses.

Third, an ethics of purity may help to explain why vaccine refusal does not correlate with broad forms of political and social identity. Vaccine refusal is equally (un)common among liberals and conservatives, and among the religious and the non-religious (Kahan 2014; Kirby 2006, xiv; Mooney 2011). But vaccines contain (or are believed to contain) ingredients that are among the core objects of disgust across human populations (and across political divides): the decaying parts of animal and human bodies. Also, when the scope of disgust extends beyond these core objects, it is informed by diverse social, political, and religious ideals, that is, ideals that participants in various political and religious communities embrace.

I begin this chapter's discussion by showing how vaccine refusal may emerge from a commitment to relatively universal ideals of bodily purity.

Then, I turn my attention to ways that socially contingent sanctity norms may inform the conclusion that vaccines contain disgusting objects (or are associated with disgusting activities). In particular, I take up the following claims: vaccines violate spiritual purity, vaccines contain industrial 'toxins', vaccination violates childhood innocence, and vaccines objectify human persons. Later, I explain how the conviction that vaccines are unnecessary or inappropriate may emerge from a belief that 'pure' or 'natural' ways of living are sufficient for good health. Finally, I explain how the belief that diseases sanctify individuals and communities may incline people to refuse vaccines. I conclude by discussing some objections to the particular purity ideals to which some vaccine refusers seem committed.

Bodily purity, vaccines, and the core objects of disgust

Almost all human beings share some ideas about purity. We are disgusted by a common core group of objects, including bodily waste, spoiled foods, corpses, and animal body parts. The scope of purity varies between cultures, but these core objects attract near-universal aversion (Curtis and Biran 2001; Haidt 2012; W. I. Miller 1997; Schaller and Park 2011). Our disgust at these objects is not merely an emotional response, but it also has cognitive content. It includes the underlying belief that we can become contaminated and degraded if decaying matter (e.g. from dead animals or human beings) enters our bodies (Rozin and Fallan 1987; Rozin, Haidt, and McCauley 2000). Becoming contaminated by this material is supposed to undermine our humanity by compromising our purity, our nonanimality, and our lives.[4]

In *Yuck! The Nature and Moral Significance of Disgust*, Daniel Kelly develops an instructive account of the nature of disgust, by drawing on the extensive empirical and interpretive work that has been done on this topic (Kelly 2011). Kelly argues that we best understand the nature of disgust in terms of a conjunction of two claims, which he calls the *Entanglement Thesis* and the *Co-opt Thesis*. The Entanglement Thesis claims that the human disgust response combines two adaptations that, individually, are common among other animals: a strategy for avoiding poisons and a strategy for avoiding parasites. Therefore, we best understand disgust as part of our evolved extended immune system. The Co-opt Thesis claims that the disgust response is flexible and susceptible to learning, and can be coopted to serve social and political purposes. For instance, disgust can be 'moralized' and deployed to defend moral, religious, and political norms.

The conjunction of Kelly's Entanglement and Co-opt theses (what he calls 'the E & C view') helps us to distinguish between two different forms of disgust (and purity ideals). First, one form of disgust focuses on protecting the body against poisons and parasites, by directing us to avoid ingesting or otherwise having intimate contact with decaying animal and human tissues. This primitive form of disgust is motivated by an ideal of bodily non-contamination, and it is not responsive to ideas about interpersonal wrongs or measurable harms. Jonathan Haidt illustrates this idea when he reflects on the near-universal human aversion to bestiality: "Even if it does no harm and violates nobody's rights when a man has sex with a chicken carcass, [people believe that] he still shouldn't do it because it degrades him" (Haidt 2012, 100).[5] As Haidt implies, the beliefs that underlie bodily disgust are not likely to be responsive to measurable evidence about harms and benefits. This is because our primitive disgust response is informed by our thoughts about the metaphysical status of the human person, and not by scientific evidence or naturalized moral arguments. As Martha Nussbaum puts it, the cognitive content of disgust "is typically unreasonable, embodying magical ideas of contamination, and impossible aspirations to purity, immortality, and nonanimality" (Nussbaum 2004, 14).[6]

The second form of disgust is *moralized*. This form of disgust focuses on activities and objects of moral or political concern. I will say more about moralized disgust at the beginning of the next section. For now, though, I turn to the role that bodily disgust may play in vaccine refusal.

In 1798, Edward Jenner first publicized his success in immunizing people against smallpox (Jenner 1798).[7] To vaccinate against smallpox, he extracted pus from the blisters of a person infected with cowpox. Then, he made an incision on a healthy person's body and he inserted the cowpox pus into the wound. The vaccinated person later experienced a non-life-threatening infection, but was thereafter immune to smallpox. This procedure was much safer than the then-prevalent method for artificially generating immunity against smallpox (called 'variolation'), which involved deliberately infecting people with a less virulent strain of smallpox (*Variola minor*). Using cowpox was just as effective, but it caused far fewer complications and deaths.

Pus is disgusting. The pus from *animal disease blisters* is even worse. It was predictable that people would respond to Jenner's methods with revulsion, and that they would object to vaccination on the grounds that it contaminated children's bodies with cowpox pus. Recall that there is a near-universal human aversion to incorporating decaying animal material into our bodies. In 1806, Benjamin Moseley wrote a book-length criticism of Jenner's methods, titled *Commentaries on the Lues Bovilla; or Cow Pox* (Moseley 1806). Moseley objected to the fact that Jenner's immunizations involved "the injection of the morbific matter of a diseased animal into a healthy child" (Moseley 1806). Moseley thought it beyond belief "[t]hat a people would be found to contaminate their offspring with a poison taken from the brute creation" (Moseley 1806). (Of course, the immediate source of Jenner's vaccine was cowpox blisters on the bodies of *human beings*, but the original source of the disease was a *cow*.) Moseley did not claim Jenner's methods were ineffective at preventing smallpox, nor did he claim that smallpox vaccination caused an unacceptably large amount of measurable harms. Instead, he thought there was something intrinsically damaging about putting decaying animal material into the bodies of healthy children. This sentiment was pervasive among members of early anti-vaccine movements, who worried that vaccination placed one's humanity at risk, and who feared that "a beast be put into their children" (Durbach 2005, 125).[8] Great Britain's Anti-Vaccination Society published an evocative engraving in 1802. This work, entitled "The Cow-Pock – or – the Wonderful Effects of the New Inoculation!", shows Jenner vaccinating a room full of patients (Gillray 1802). They sprout cows (and parts of cow bodies) from their heads, torsos and appendages.

Doctors today do not spread cowpox pus into wounds they have opened on children's bodies. We have moved vaccination away from the filth of the barnyard into the sterility of a pediatrician's office. There, a syringe conceals the contents of vaccines from patients (and from their parents). For these reasons, Seth Mnookin observes that "[r]eceiving a shot in a doctor's office might not activate the disgust response in the way that early inoculation methods did" (Mnookin 2011a, 195). Even so, contemporary vaccine refusers continue to claim that vaccination contaminates healthy persons by introducing decaying animal (and now human) body parts into their bodies. The common core objects of bodily impurity still seem to play a role in the thinking of some of today's vaccine refusers.

Consider Neil Miller, the author of many best-selling anti-vaccine books. He writes that one reason not to vaccinate is that vaccines contain "[m]onkey kidney, calf serum, and chick embryo [which] are foreign proteins – biological matter composed of animal cells" (N. Z. Miller 1996, 48). Miller does not present scientific evidence to support his claims. Instead, Miller adds a contemporary twist to the age-old claim that animal materials will contaminate our bodies. He worries that these foreign substances will "change our genetic structure," by introducing animal genes into the human genome (N. Z. Miller 1996, 48).[9] For a similar example, consider the title of a 2012 article from *Vactruth.com*: "The Ultimate Gamble: Do Childhood Vaccines Result in Genetic Hybridization from Alien Human and Animal DNA Contents?" (Buttram 2012). (The author's answer to his titular question is 'yes'.) The idea that vaccines transfer harmful animal genes to human beings is pervasive among some vaccine refusers, and also among a broader community of conspiracy theorists. For example, Edward Hooper wrote a book entitled *The River*, in which he argued that HIV transferred from chimpanzees to human beings when HIV-infected chimp kidney was used in the oral polio vaccine (Hooper 1999). This claim has been definitively refuted (Blancou et al. 2001; Poinar, Kuch, and Paabo 2001). But research science can do little to block the worry that decaying and diseased animal tissues will contaminate human bodies.

To be clear: Gene transfer is a real phenomenon. My point is that there is no evidence that vaccination contributes to a harmful transfer of genes from animals to humans. Instead, I suspect that Miller and others like him are driven by a traditional aversion to animal contamination, rather than by a scientific hypothesis about measurable outcomes. In this way, contemporary vaccine refusers who express worries about animal contamination may have a lot in common with early vaccine refusers. Even though Miller expresses his concerns using the rhetoric of contemporary genetics, he seems motivated by an age-old aversion to the contamination of the human body.

Some of today's vaccines include (or, more accurately, are made from) one of the core objects of disgust that was *not* associated with Jenner's smallpox vaccine. Contemporary vaccine refusers sometimes express disgust that vaccines contain "aborted fetal tissue" (Kirby 2006, 97).[10] They object that many vaccines contain viruses that were grown in human cell cultures, and that these human cell cultures were cultivated from tissues harvested from aborted fetuses. For example, the human cell line WI-38 is used to make rubella vaccine, the human cell line MRC-5 is used to make hepatitis A vaccine, and the human cell line PER. C6 is now being used in vaccine research. All of these cell lines originated from the tissues of aborted fetuses (Plotkin 2011; Wong 2010).[11] Consider the concerns of Shelley Reynolds, a mother who spoke before the US House Government Reform Committee about vaccine safety. Reynolds claimed that it was foolish to think that one could inject material grown from aborted fetal tissue into children "and not expect [that] ... it will not [sic] alter their minds and bodies" (Kirby 2006, 97). The implication is that it is damaging to children to inject them with these materials. Why?

An anti-abortion group – "Physicians for Life" – may fill in the blanks. According to them, "more than 23 vaccines are *contaminated* by the use of aborted fetal cells," and this contamination causes genetic damage which leads to diseases including lupus, multiple sclerosis, and autism (Deisher 2009, emphasis added). Like Miller, the members of "Physicians for Life" frame their objection in the rhetoric of science, and like Miller, they invoke the possibility of harmful gene transfer between vaccines and the genomes of vaccinated children. But these worries are not based on scientific evidence. Instead, the members of this group seem primarily motivated by the worry that decaying human body parts will contaminate our bodies.

People who believe that abortion consists in the murder of a human person may believe that they have moral reasons to resist methods of producing vaccines that make use of aborted fetal tissues. The Roman Catholic Church, for example, has advocated the development of vaccines that do not rely on cell lines derived from fetal tissues, though it teaches that it is morally permissible to receive current vaccines (Luño 2006). Furthermore, the Church claims that people who choose not to vaccinate are morally responsible for any harms they cause to vulnerable people (including fetuses). However, the worry I focus on here is different from concerns about participation in moral evil. Instead, I am interested in the idea that vaccines containing materials derived from aborted fetal tissues may *contaminate* one's body. This concern is not reducible to the worry that vaccination involves cooperation (licit or not) with moral evil, since its focus is bodily purity, rather than the moral rightness of one's actions.[12]

Impure vaccines and socially contingent objects of (moralized) disgust

In this section, I look at ways that vaccine refusal emerges from culturally specific purity ideals. In particular, I explore how one might come to believe vaccines violate spiritual purity, contain industrial 'toxins', violate childhood innocence, or objectify human persons.

My work in this section is more speculative than my work in the previous section. This is because I will discuss forms of disgust that focus not only on *bodily* purity, but also on *moralized* forms of purity.[13] While the former is relatively straightforward, the latter raises a number of empirical and interpretive issues (see e.g. Chapman and Anderson 2013; de Melo-Martín and Salles 2011). For example, bodily disgust can be relatively easily identified. It focuses on avoiding the core objects – vectors for poisons and parasites – which include the decaying tissues of animal and human bodies. But it is not always so clear when a particular negative emotional response is an instance of *moralized* disgust, rather than an instance of another negative emotion, such as moral anger. The concept is clear enough: Moralized disgust is an adverse emotional response to (potential) contamination or diminishment through involvement with moral impurity, i.e. violations of moral norms. But we may manifest many different kinds of negative emotional responses to violations of moral norms, and some of them (including anger) may resemble disgust.

Russell and Giner-Sorolla argue that we can identify moralized disgust by its context insensitivity (Russell and Giner-Sorolla 2013). You become tainted by doing what is (morally) disgusting, regardless of the circumstances in which you violate the relevant moral norm (Russell and Giner-Sorolla 2011; Liane Young and Saxe 2011). For example, incest is morally disgusting even if it is accidental. In contrast, moral anger is context dependent. Suppose that you act in a way that harms me. I will become angry with you if I believe you intended to harm me, but I will become less angry if I think you harmed me as the result of an accident. Because moral disgust is less sensitive to your intentions, it is in principle possible to distinguish moralized disgust from other negative emotions about moral norm violations. The problem for my work is that I have incomplete information about the negative emotional responses of vaccine refusers.

Therefore, my claims about the ways in which moralized disgust (and moralized purity) may contribute to vaccine refusal are more speculative than I would like.

Spiritual purity and contamination

Early vaccine refusers often claimed that vaccines contaminated the body in ways that compromised a person's spiritual status. In particular, they invoked biblical commands against making cuts upon the body (Allen 2007, 56). For example, Leviticus 19:28 commands the Israelites: "Do not cut your bodies for the dead or put tattoo marks on yourselves." Many of the other Levitical edicts also focus on practices of bodily purity and holiness, with the ultimate goal of maintaining the privileged relationship between the Israelite community and God.[14] Even the parts of Leviticus that discuss procedures for priestly sacrifices also focus on purity, for example the prohibitions on physical defects among both priests and sacrificial animals in chapters 21 and 22. In this context of bodily/spiritual purity, deliberately marking one's body – such as with the wounds from smallpox vaccination – could constitute defilement and could jeopardize one's link to God. Such a transgressive act might have dire consequences for one's metaphysical status.

Some early vaccine refusers also relied on 'purity' texts from the Christian New Testament to justify their refusal of vaccines. They claimed that scars from smallpox vaccination were "the mark of the beast," i.e. outward signs of a person's rejection of God and of their commitment to follow Satan (Durbach 2005, 118). For example, Revelation 13:16 says: "It [the beast from the earth] also forced all people, great and small, rich and poor, free and slave, to receive a mark on their right hands or on their foreheads." (Of course, smallpox vaccination was not performed on one's hand or forehead, but never mind about that.) For these vaccine refusers, becoming vaccinated was "unchristian" and a form of "devil worship," and some went so far as to say that vaccination turned a child into an "anti-Christ" (Durbach 2005, 118, 121).

I think that an ethics of purity likely played a role in these early religious forms of vaccine refusal. These vaccine refusers did not (merely) think vaccination was immoral or that God would punish them if they vaccinated. They (also) believed that vaccination would diminish or degrade them. It would make them impure and their impurity would cut them off from a relationship with God and the Christian community.[15] The ultimate authority was God's command, but what God commanded was that people maintain a particular metaphysical status. And vaccination put that status in jeopardy.

It is much less common for today's vaccine refusers to invoke religious reasons for their refusal. Very few contemporary religions publicly support vaccine refusal; many endorse vaccination as a moral duty (Grabenstein

2013).[16] Accordingly, Mark Largent argues that public health officials make a serious error if they conclude that religious convictions contribute much to contemporary vaccine refusal (Largent 2012, 25–26). Many people claim to object to vaccines for religious reasons. But these people are usually lying in order to take advantage of vaccine waiver programs that prioritize religious objections (Reiss 2014). (I address questions about vaccine waivers in chapter six.)

Some of today's vaccine refusers are linked to religious communities. Recent outbreaks of measles in the 'Bible Belt' of the Netherlands have been tied to forms of conservative Protestant Christianity that are prevalent in that region (Mintz 2013). Also, there was a recent outbreak of measles in Texas among members of the same megachurch (Szabo 2013). But the objections that members of these religious groups have are different from those I discussed earlier. In some cases, including in the Netherlands measles outbreaks, religious believers were worried that vaccination expressed an unwillingness to trust in God's providence. The Dutch vaccine refusers were not concerned about vaccination violating their spiritual purity. Instead, they thought their health status ought to be left up to God. Also, some cases of vaccine refusal may emerge in church communities, but not be motivated by religious commitments. Indeed, the leaders of the Texas megachurch promoted secular reasons for vaccine refusal, for example that vaccines contain harmful industrial toxins. I take up these sorts of secular purity concerns below.

Industrial 'toxins'

Sarah Pope, who blogs as *The Healthy Home Economist* (and claims to have 46,000 subscribers) says, "these vaccines are loaded with toxins and I'm not gonna inject them into my kids, period" (Abrams 2014). It is common for contemporary vaccine refusers to worry about one or more of the following scary-sounding ingredients that have been in vaccines: thimerosal/thiomersal, aluminum, formaldehyde, and anti-bacterial agents such as Neomycin, Polymyxin B, and Streptomycin. Vaccine refusers often direct people to read the 'package inserts' that come with vaccines, as if an ingredient list were enough to conclude that vaccines were unsafe. But there is no evidence that these ingredients are harmful to people in the formulations and quantities that are present in vaccines. For example, the toxicity of *ethyl* mercury (which is one of the metabolites of the thimerosal/thiomersal that used to be included in some vaccines) is much lower than the toxicity of *methyl* mercury (for which the EPA mercury standards are written). Also, worries about 'toxins' in vaccines seem indifferent to the fact that 'the dose makes the poison' (as Paracelsus said).[17] Almost anything can be toxic, in a high enough dose (even water and chocolate), and almost anything can be harmless in a low enough dose. In particular, there is overwhelming evidence that the 'toxins' in vaccines appear in such low doses that they are very unlikely to cause adverse health effects.

I think an ethics of purity helps to explain why the presence of scary-sounding ingredients in vaccines (albeit in safe formulations and quantities) leads some people to believe vaccines are unsafe. Of course, none of these ingredients is among the core objects of disgust. For example, most people do not hesitate to wrap food in aluminum foil. And for many generations, parents placed mercury thermometers in the mouths of sick children without worry (though perhaps they should have been concerned, since the mercury in thermometers could have become a harmful vapor if those thermometers broke). So, the idea that the presence of 'toxins' in vaccines renders them impure must emerge from a particular cultural context.

I think that vaccine refusers sometimes associate the 'toxic' ingredients in vaccines with industrial pollution. We live in a polluted world and pollution harms our health. Industrial wastes emitted into the air cause respiratory problems and contribute to climate change. Chemicals used in hydraulic fracturing ('fracking') may make groundwater undrinkable for centuries. Eating crops grown in urban agricultural soil may lead to poisoning with lead, cadmium, and arsenic. And consumer products contain harmful ingredients, too. There are hormones in meat and milk, pesticides in produce, BPA in plastics, and VOCs in paints. The effects of these ingredients either are known to be harmful or are not known not to be harmful.

There are good reasons to resist harmful forms of pollution. We ought to refuse to ingest or otherwise expose ourselves to products that can harm our bodies. But it is important for these choices to be informed by scientific evidence about measurable harms. Unfortunately, I suspect that some consumer and environmental activism is motivated by a reverential attitude towards the natural world, and by a characterization of human industrial activity as a force that contaminates the sacred. According to the view I have in mind, we should avoid contact with consumer products that have become 'dirty' or 'impure' as a result of their connection to industrial processes. Instead, we should use only 'natural' and 'pure' products, which are marked by the absence of the 'toxins' we need to avoid. Accordingly, a purity-focused consumer aims to keep her family safe by seeking out 'alternative' products, i.e. those that don't contain the 'toxins' that might cause contamination.[18]

Some vaccine refusers seem to be acting out of a commitment to this kind of purity-focused consumerism. Consider Jenny McCarthy's message to pharmaceutical companies: 'Green Our Vaccines'. McCarthy says that she and her fellow vaccine refusers "are not an anti-vaccine group. We are demanding safe vaccines. We want to reduce ... the toxins" (Kluger 2009). But, of course, vaccines cause very low rates of complications. And when vaccines do lead to these predictable and measurable bad health outcomes, it is not because of the 'toxic' ingredients that worry McCarthy and others like her. But if McCarthy's judgments about safety are informed by ideals of purity, then facts about the causes of vaccine complications may do little to prevent her from concluding that vaccines are unsafe.

At the same time, it is not entirely unreasonable for parents to rely on an anti-toxin ('purity') heuristic when they make health and consumer decisions. Parents are not chemists or toxicologists, and they may have difficulty making decisions about the safety of particular consumer products. Furthermore, parents who live in societies that allow dangerous products to be sold must be vigilant consumers. History shows that authorities (medical, political, and otherwise) will often vouch for the safety of products that are anything but safe. So, parents may have good reason to be unwilling to accept the assurance that vaccine 'toxins' are not dangerous. Here, then, we return to themes from my discussion in chapter one, where I focused on the ways that historical and social dynamics can reasonably undermine the trust parents place in the testimony of pediatricians and other officials.

Childhood innocence

Some vaccine refusers seem fixated on the idea that vaccines jeopardize childhood innocence. They express anxiety about perceived violations of the protective bubble in which (they imagine) previous generations of children were allowed to develop. On this view, vaccines are contaminated because they are tainted by 'adult' behaviors, including sexual activity and intravenous drug use.

Vaccine refusers commonly complain that some routine vaccines protect against diseases that are unlikely to affect children. For example, Jennifer Margulis says the following about the vaccine for hepatitis B:

> When my daughter was born in 1999, the nurse bustled in with her tray and said, "OK, it's time for your hepatitis B vaccine." And I looked at my daughter and I looked at the nurse and I said, "Isn't hepatitis B a sexually transmitted disease?" And I said, "Why am I supposed to vaccinate my newborn baby against a sexually transmitted disease?" And the nurse got really mad.
>
> (Palfreman 2010)

What distresses Margulis is that a nurse has presumed to vaccinate her child against a disease that is often transmitted sexually (or through intravenous needles associated with illegal drug use). But why does this distress her?

The facts are clear. There are many good (and easily accessible) reasons for the universal vaccination of newborns against hepatitis B. CDC says:

administering a birth dose to infants ... serves as a "safety net" to prevent perinatal infection among infants born to HBsAg-positive mothers who are not identified because of errors in maternal HBsAg testing or failures in reporting of test results.

(Centers for Disease Control and Prevention 2005)[19]

Early detection of hepatitis B can be difficult, and this disease can cause serious liver damage and death if left untreated. Infected mothers are likely to transmit hepatitis B to newborns during childbirth, unless their newborns receive the vaccine. Unfortunately, selective vaccination is not effective, since errors in testing or in reporting mothers' hepatitis B status are relatively common.

I don't know what motivates Margulis' spirited rejection of the hepatitis B vaccine.[20] But I wonder whether purity and disgust may play a role.[21] Perhaps Margulis has a visceral negative reaction to the idea of performing sexually related interventions on the body of an infant. She asks, "Why am I supposed to vaccinate my newborn baby against a sexually transmitted disease?" and the (implied) response to her (rhetorical) question is: "There is obviously no good reason to vaccinate a newborn against a sexually transmitted disease." Why is this? After all, there are good reasons to vaccinate infants against hepatitis B. Perhaps Margulis has a deep aversion to associating babies with adult sexuality (and with its consequences).[22]

The idea of childhood innocence may also contribute to vaccine refusal in a different way. I suspect that vaccination is sometimes associated with disruptions in social practices concerning the care of children. In particular, I think vaccine refusal is sometimes based on cultural anxieties about recent changes in motherhood and childhood. Contamination legends often emerge in times of great social upheaval, where they serve to focus general anxieties towards concrete objects (Kitta 2012, 80). In recent years, developed societies have experienced a rapid increase in (middle-class) women's participation in the formal workforce. This change has been accompanied by women's transition away from traditional forms of housewife mothering, and towards a greater reliance on mass-produced foods and alternative childcare relationships. Cultural anxieties about the changing practices of motherhood have contributed to contamination legends (often 'urban legends') about mass-produced convenience foods. These stories feature children who find fingers in hamburgers, rats in french fries, and semen in ketchup (Kapferer 1990). Andrea Kitta has argued that similar anxieties inform some instances of vaccine refusal (Kitta 2012).

I admit it may seem like a stretch to think that worries about contamination sometimes express underlying anxieties about broader cultural changes. So, I want to take a bit of time to defend the plausibility of this view by starting with a discussion about anxieties surrounding food safety. Our food is safer than it has ever been. Pasteurization prevents children from developing cholera or listeria after drinking tainted milk. Refrigeration allows consumers to purchase produce unspoiled by harmful bacteria. Contra the claims of some contemporary 'raw milk' advocates, pasteurization and refrigeration have saved many lives; raw milk is often dangerous (Centers for Disease Control and Prevention 2014b; Oliver et al. 2009). Furthermore, various regulations and inspection protocols now prevent unhealthy ingredients – such as lead, arsenic, and gypsum – from being added to food products. However, only 30% of Americans believe that technology has made their food safer (Matchar 2013). My point is not that people are now eating healthier foods (or have healthier eating habits) than they did in previous generations (though I suspect that 'grandma's homemade meals' were less healthy than we imagine them to have been). Instead, my point is that our food is much *safer* than it was in the past – it is less likely to cause discrete health harms – yet many people don't accept this obvious fact.

Some people have argued that contemporary food products and practices are tainted by their association with the demise of mythological middle-class motherhood. Cultural anxieties about the fact that fewer mothers now spend their days preparing home-cooked meals may contribute to a feeling that contemporary food is unsafe, even in the face of contradictory evidence. And public advocates for 'healthier' foods often explicitly blame feminist transformations of the family for the (supposed) decrease in the safety and health of food. Michael Pollan writes that cooking healthy foods was "a bit of wisdom that some American feminists thoughtlessly trampled in their rush to get women out of the kitchen" (Pollan 2009). Caitlin Flanagan, a regular contributor to *The Atlantic*, says that feminists in the 1970s thought that "[c]ooking nourishing dinners was an oppressive act" (Flanagan 2007, 175). British celebrity cookbook author Rose Prince writes that "it's feminism we have to thank for the spread of fast-food chains and an epidemic of childhood obesity" (Prince 2010).[23]

I think similar anxieties may lurk in the background of many of the 'contamination legends' told by vaccine refusers. 'Contaminated vaccines' may be a way to focus cultural anxieties about changes in mothering practices, for example the increased presence of small children in daycare (Kitta 2012). Accordingly, saying that 'vaccines are contaminated' may be a way of expressing otherwise inscrutable worries about whether children are well cared for, and whether there isn't *something more* mothers might do for their children.[24] In this light, it is no coincidence that vaccine refusers sometimes promote labor-intensive alternatives to vaccination (e.g. ongoing chiropractic care, home-cooked organic and gluten-free meals, chelation, and enemas). Vaccine refusers also often participate in intensive birthing and mothering activities, including homebirths, attachment parenting, baby-wearing, extended breastfeeding, elimination communication, and homeschooling.[25] It is also no coincidence that vaccine advocates have promoted some vaccines by pointing to the ways they could improve the lives of working parents. For example, media campaigns aimed at increasing rates of chicken pox vaccination have sometimes noted that parents should vaccinate to prevent their children from missing a week of school (and to prevent parents from missing a week of work). If every child had a mother waiting at home for him, then parents of healthy children would not have to worry as much about this consequence of the chicken pox. But those days are over (and never existed for many), and times of great social disruption can cause deep but inscrutable worries, including concerns about contamination.

Doctors, corporations and the objectification of patients

Earlier generations of vaccine refusers sometimes focused on the degrading ways they believed physicians treated patients. Some people claimed that physicians treated people's bodies as mere objects on which to work their craft. Even though young people might enter the medical profession with noble motives, they would soon become part of an inhuman machine. After time, their skills would be directed towards the accumulation of wealth and power, rather than human health and well-being.[26] An early 20th-century vaccine refuser worried that "[e]very doctor there [in the city] has become a cog in the medical machine. And once the machine gets its grip on you, you cannot escape, you are drawn in and ground through the mill" (Mnookin 2011a, 34–35). On this view, individual patients were raw materials for the medical machine, and vaccination was just one sign of this machine's inhumanity. Its unholy apparatus would cut open the bodies of innocent children and inject them with dangerous poisons. Here, the culture of modern professionalized medicine is degrading, and vaccination is just an instance of a broader problem.

The medical profession is the most-trusted profession in both the United Kingdom and the United States (Gallup 2012; Mludzinski 2011). Even so, some of today's vaccine refusers voice similar concerns about the profession of medicine as did earlier vaccine refusers. For example, Robert Mendelsohn, a prominent vaccine critic, locates his criticism of routine childhood vaccination within a broader criticism of mainstream medicine. On his view:

> There is never enough blood in the hospital temples of Modern Medicine to satisfy the surgeon's desire as he seduces his victims – primarily women – virgin and otherwise – to mount the holy altar so he can carry out his ritual mutilations. The wild blood-lust, starting with animal vivisection and proceeding to human mutilation, stamps Modern Medicine as the most primitive weapon this world has ever seen.
>
> (Mendelsohn 2003, cited at Offit 2010, 48)

These comments express an extremely cynical view of modern medicine, one that is certainly not widely shared, but which is contiguous with a more 'moderate' criticism that contemporary vaccine refusers often endorse (and which I discussed in chapter one). For example, David Kirby reports that many vaccine refusers think of pediatricians as sadists who "poked and prodded" children "like some pet science project" (Kirby 2006, 23). Barbara Loe Fisher, the founder of the National Vaccine Information Center (NVIC), claims that physicians are so interested in preserving their power that they are unwilling to listen to parents (Offit 2010, 81; Specter 2009, 7, 60). These sorts of accusations are commonplace among contemporary vaccine refusers, who locate their refusal of vaccines within a broader rejection of (what they take to be) the deceptive and dehumanizing practices of the medical profession. Here, vaccines are tainted by association with the abuses of modern medicine, and not only by the fact that they contain the core objects of disgust. Parents who reject vaccines because they associate vaccines with (what they believe to be) the degradations of modern medicine may think vaccines are 'unsafe', but their worries about vaccine safety will not be assuaged by CDC's efforts to better publicize vaccine science.

The idea that there is something *degrading* about contemporary medical practice is echoed by vaccine refusers who chafe at the profit-seeking behavior of pharmaceutical companies. They argue that corporations necessarily degrade the environment, poison people, and corrupt social and political institutions. Vaccine refusers who engage in this sort of rhetoric echo a classic leftist criticism of capitalist modes of production: Capitalism transforms people into mere instruments of production, and it turns all forms of social and political life into economic relationships; it leaves nothing sacred.

The fact that vaccines are manufactured by profit-seeking corporations also informs a broader worry: Industry has corrupted the practice of medicine and public health. Eula Biss discusses an example of this charge: The chair of the Council of Europe's health committee accused the World Health Organization (WHO) of faking the 2009 H1N1 pandemic in order to sell more vaccines (Biss 2012).[27] The idea that government officials and physicians have been bought off by pharmaceutical companies – and that they are now 'pushing' Big Pharma's drugs – is prevalent among vaccine refusers. One vaccine refuser writes that public vaccination programs are the same as "the federal government giving every kid a carton of cigarettes and saying, 'Get to work'" (Mnookin 2011a, 196). Another vaccine refuser says that doctors and governments "turn the pharmaceutical spigot on children" to make money for drug companies (Converse 2011, 106–107). On this view, vaccines are contaminated, not (only) by the presence of the core objects of disgust, but by their association with the corruptions of industrial capitalism.

Of course, there are many good reasons to object to the distorting influence of the profit motive in the practice of medicine, and vaccination programs are not immune to these objections. For example, we may reasonably worry that powerful pharmaceutical corporations overstate the benefits of their vaccines, while understating the potential harms. And we may be concerned that corporations use their economic and political power to sidestep (and supplement) the approval and recommendation procedures undertaken by public health authorities. The troubled rollout of the HPV vaccine is an example of how the impatience of pharmaceutical companies undermined public trust in vaccine safety (Charo 2007; Udesky 2007). But these concerns can be overblown. And when they are overblown, I suspect that disgust at the (supposed) impurities and degradations of profit-driven pharmaceutical companies is often a contributing factor.

Health through pure living

In the previous section I argued that the idea that vaccines are contaminated need not emerge only from reflection on the fact that vaccines contain the core objects of disgust. People may also be disgusted by the fact that vaccines are entangled with broader forms of social, political, and spiritual defilement and impurity. In this section I turn my attention to the idea that vaccines are unnecessary or ineffective, because disease results primarily from dirty or unnatural living, rather than from exposure to pathogens.[28] Accordingly, vaccines might not be impure, but they are unnecessary for people who pursue pure living.

Health from holiness and disease as divine judgment

The original vaccine refusers often claimed that disease was a divine punishment for humanity's sins (Allen 2007, 25).[29] From this point of view, "vaccination interfered with God's plans or cast doubt upon his omnipotence" (Allen 2007, 56). People who accepted vaccines were attempting to usurp God's providence; they were trying to redeem themselves from their 'fallen' condition through their own efforts, rather than by trusting in divine grace (Minardi 2004). (As I discussed above, some residents of the Dutch Bible Belt have similar ideas today.) The idea that health and disease are grounded in deeper spiritual realities, and that vaccines deny the spiritual core of health and disease, motivated many early anti-vaccination efforts. Importantly, this claim about vaccination is distinct from the claim that vaccines contain the core objects of disgust or that they otherwise violate spiritual purity. For example, one need not think that there is anything impure about vaccines to think that vaccination is unnecessary for people who live spiritually pure lives.

Contemporary vaccine refusers sometimes claim that vaccines mistake the spiritual causes or the supernatural purposes of disease. For example, they may resist vaccines against sexually transmitted diseases because they believe these diseases are divine punishments for sexual impurity. One parent writes that the hepatitis B vaccine "supports the devil in his effort to encourage [my] daughter to engage in sex and intravenous drug use" (Allen 2007, 391). Another writes that "immunizing my children against hepatitis B gives the appearance that my children will be sexually promiscuous or drug users," in violation of God's commands (Allen 2007, 391). Mark Largent gives voice to these worries: "Instead of engaging in the arduous task of altering people's behaviors, [some believe that] these vaccines, with the ease of a few simple shots, would do away with what moralists consider the natural consequences of problematic behaviors" (Largent 2012, 22). In this context, parental disgust may be directed at the behaviors for which it is imagined that diseases are the appropriate (super) natural punishment. Accordingly, people who manifest this sort of disgust may refuse vaccines, but they may do so without thinking vaccines are impure. Instead, they may believe vaccines are unnecessary (or counterproductive) for people who are living pure lives, while they prevent dirty people from receiving the punishments they deserve.

Natural health

The conditions of modernity provide new resources for characterizing the 'fallen' condition of mankind. Various aspects of life in industrialized societies prevent people from realizing 'natural' health. We no longer perform much manual labor, we wear constrictive clothing, we eat low-nutrient foods full of sugar and salt, and we live in filthy and overcrowded cities, where we breathe polluted air and are far removed from nature. The modern city is sometimes thought to illustrate humanity's degraded condition (Mnookin 2011a, 33). In the words of the famous naturalist Lord Alfred Russel Wallace, smallpox was a "filth disease" and it would go away on its own once cities got rid of "foul air and water, decaying organic matter, overcrowding and other unwholesome surroundings" (Wallace 1910, 267–268).[30] Vaccines would be unnecessary if people and their surroundings were less dirty. On a similar note, the president of the late 19th-century National Anti-Vaccination League (UK) wrote that "infection [by germs is] merely a theoretical bogey, worked to frighten laymen, and diverting attention from the real enemy of the human race: dirt" (Durbach 2005, 160). If cleanliness brings health, then vaccines are not the answer to disease outbreaks. Clean living is.

The theory that disease originates from, or is transmitted by, the sorts of dirt, decay, and corruption present in the modern city has had great staying power. For example, the records of mid-20th-century polio researchers indicate that "the most common misconceptions about how one contracted polio included bathing in polluted water ... and consuming lots of 'sugar drinks,' especially Coca-Cola" (Oshinsky 2006, 93n4). Albert Sabin, a lead polio researcher, received many letters from members of the public who wanted to share their ideas about the causes of (the transmission) of polio. Among the most popular ideas was that "polio came from ... the smoking habits of pregnant women" (Oshinsky 2006, 93). Lora Little, an early 20th-century advocate of 'natural health', claimed that we got sick from eating too much "white sugar" (Allen 2007, 104). Of course, it's bad for us to have a poor diet and an inactive lifestyle. But healthy eating and regular exercise will not prevent people from getting (or dying from) measles and polio. Lora Little's claims about the harms of refined sugar were prescient, but candy does not cause influenza. There is a large gap between the claim that good lifestyle choices can improve our health and the claim that good lifestyle choices are sufficient for our health. Scientific evidence supports the first claim, but an ethics of purity can convince you to endorse the second claim. And that's how I think some vaccine refusers – both past and present – have been able to convince themselves that they don't need vaccines. For a recent example, Annemarie Colbin writes that pathogens don't make children ill. Instead, they get sick from bottle-feeding, cow's milk, processed foods, snacks, and insufficient fruits and vegetables (Colbin 2011). According to Colbin, we do not need to vaccinate to be healthy, since we can achieve natural health through pure living.

People who advocate purity-based conceptions of health are unlikely to support vaccination, since they do not believe vaccines address the real causes of disease. Among other reasons, this is because vaccines presuppose a false 'germ theory of disease', according to which diseases are caused by the presence and growth of microorganisms. In contrast, advocates of 'natural' health embrace 'holistic' theories. They believe that proper care of the body, including maintenance of its inner purity, is the pathway to health. Of course, they may think that bacteria and viruses play an ancillary role in illness, but they deny that so-called pathogens are significant determinants of whether one becomes ill.

Anna Meigs has called these conceptions of health "religion[s] of the body" (Meigs 1984). Followers of religions of the body go to great effort to protect and restore vital bodily essences, and they follow strict diets and purification rituals. For example, an early 19th-century vaccine refuser argued that the best way to prevent smallpox was not vaccination, but keeping "the blood pure, the bowels regular, and the skin clean" (Durbach 2005, 121). Among the founders of the Anti-Vaccination League of America were homeopaths and naturopaths, and chiropractors. They were practitioners of forms of 'medicine' which celebrated the body's ability to heal itself, by removing it from 'toxic' environments (Allen 2007, 102–103). The early 20th-century American vaccine refusers also included some of the founders of bodybuilding and personal fitness. These leaders of the US 'physical culture' movement prescribed spa treatments, enemas, and weight-lifting, in addition to good nutrition. One prominent figure was Bernarr Macfadden, who was a predecessor of fitness gurus Charles Atlas and Jack LaLanne. Macfadden published over 100 fitness books, ran a fitness-focused publishing empire, and established many fitness resorts (Adams 2010). Bernarr – he changed his name from 'Bernard' because he wanted a more masculine and powerful moniker – even founded a religion based on his principles. 'Cosmotarianism' combined mainstream Protestant Christianity with regular exercise, vegetarian diet, fasting, and a rejection of both mainstream medicine and processed foods.

The 'natural health' practices of today's vaccine refusers are continuous with the 'physical culture' movement that earlier vaccine refusers embraced. Today's vaccine refusers buy 'pure' products in order to resist disease. They don't buy clothes from Walmart or Target that contain carcinogenic flame retardants, they don't buy carpets with nasty chemicals, and they are sure to protect their bodies by consuming vitamins and supplements (Francl 2013; Haelle 2014; Mnookin 2011a, 16). Today's vaccine refusers are particularly focused on diet. The mother of a child who caused a recent measles outbreak in California explained her decision not to vaccinate by appealing to the protection she believed good nutrition provided. On her view, "[c]hildren will do fine with these diseases [e.g. measles] in a developed country that has good nutrition" (Mnookin 2011a, 19). This sort of reasoning leads Judy Converse to write that "nutrition status is what drives a child's ability to fight infections," not vaccines (Converse 2011, 107). And Arthur Allen observes that vaccine refusers claim to be able to "withstand diseases like whooping cough because of the healthy lifestyles they lived" (Allen 2007, 364).

One example of the role that 'natural health' plays in contemporary vaccine refusal is the prominence of the myth that there are no autistic Amish.[31] The Amish are traditional Christians who engage in simple living and who avoid many modern technologies, such as automobiles, electricity, or telephones, in their homes. According to the myth I have in mind, the Amish do not vaccinate and, for that reason, their children do not have autism. And, on the whole, the Amish are supposed to be much healthier than members of the general public. This story is common in contemporary vaccine refusal literature (Colbin 2011, 206; Kirby 2006, 112; Olmsted 2005). But both component claims of this myth are false. The Amish vaccinate, although some communities have lower vaccination rates than the general public (Mnookin 2011b; Yoder and Dworkin 2006). And some Amish are autistic, though rates of autism in Amish communities are slightly lower than rates among the general public. But much of this difference is likely due to underreporting, especially in the case of 'mild' or 'high-functioning' autism. The tight-knit Amish often do a good job of integrating such people into the full life of their communities and do not label people with manageable forms of autism as 'disordered' (Robinson et al. 2010).

Why do some vaccine refusers cling to the myth that there are no autistic Amish, in the absence of any good supporting evidence? I don't think that ignorance is a sufficient explanation. Disconfirming evidence is ample and accessible, and the people who are propagating this myth are well-educated. Instead, some form of confirmation bias is likely in play. In particular, I suspect vaccine refusers hold onto the myth that there are no autistic Amish because they are committed to an ideal of 'natural health', and because they believe that the Amish realize this ideal (though they do so in ways that 21st-century vaccine refusers do not want to entirely emulate). The idea of Amish cultural purity is a story about how hard physical work, limited engagement with technology and modernity, economic self-sufficiency, plain foods, and a close relationship with both farm animals and the land protects the noble Amish from the problems of the modern world. If vaccine refusers are committed to a conception of 'natural health' grounded in this sort of ethic of purity, then it follows easily enough that vaccine refusers would want to believe that the Amish way of life is sufficient for robust health.

Disease and the impurity of the 'other'

There is political upshot to the idea of 'health as purity' – and to its partner idea of 'disease as impurity'. This is because the contents of *purity* are partially constituted by the ideas that bind together political communities (M. Douglas 2002). Correspondingly, the contents of *impurity* are partially constituted by the ideas which shape the community's understanding of those who are outside of it. To be pure is to live according to the ideals of my people; to be impure is to live like foreigners.[32] According to this sort of view, vaccines are not as necessary when the community is intact as they are when foreigners are present (Kitta 2012, 89).

The United States has a long history of blaming diseases on the presence of 'others' within its borders. David Oshinsky writes:

> In the 1840s, the Irish were accused of bringing cholera to New York City; fifty years later, the Jews were suspected of spreading tuberculosis, also known as 'the tailor's disease.' Each time an epidemic appeared, native New Yorkers looked reflexively toward the immigrant slums.
>
> (Oshinsky 2006, 20)

The same was true of polio outbreaks, which were often blamed on the poor sanitation conditions in the neighborhoods populated by immigrants, blacks, and Latinos (Oshinsky 2006, 2). This tendency to blame disease on 'disgusting' and 'dirty' foreigners is not supported by the evidence. For example, the most serious outbreaks of polio "occur[ed] in the advanced 'sanitary' nations of the West," and were often concentrated within areas of those countries that had "the lowest population density and the best sanitary conditions" (Oshinsky 2006, 9, 22).

The belief that disease comes from outsiders persists and it plays a role in contemporary political debates, e.g. about immigration. For example, consider the following quote, which was featured on *Lou Dobbs Tonight* (a CNN program in the United States):

> We have some enormous problems with horrendous diseases that are being brought into America by illegal aliens [including] diseases we have only rarely had here in America, such as Chagas Disease, leprosy, malaria.
>
> (Waldman et al. 2008)[33]

Pat Buchanan, a conservative commentator and former political candidate, adds that "a lot [of] diseases are coming back. And it's because these 12 million illegals are coming across the border" (Waldman et al. 2008). Here, the object of disgust is the 'diseased foreigner' and the relevant purity is that of the political community. While a commitment to xenophobic conceptions of disgust and purity need not lead directly to vaccine refusal, it may direct attention towards 'public health' programs that emphasize deportations and other restrictions on immigration, rather than on mass vaccination. And it may contribute towards the establishment of coercive vaccination programs that disproportionately focus on immigrants and minorities.

Purification through illness

Another way in which an ethics of purity may inform vaccine refusal is through the idea that diseases have a purifying effect, on either individuals or the community. If communicable diseases purify, then we have a good reason to refuse routine childhood vaccines. Here, the idea is that diseases provide valuable personal and social forms of purification, and that vaccines interfere with disease-generated forms of purity and sanctity.

Disease and childhood development

Some vaccine refusers seem to believe that suffering from disease sanctifies individuals (especially children), and that vaccines prevent people from reaping the (spiritual) benefits that come from fighting disease. One form of this idea is that regular exposure to communicable diseases strengthens children, and that vaccines weaken children. Some vaccine refusers seek out infections for their children by hosting 'measles parties', 'pox parties', and 'flu parties'. At these events a gaggle of healthy children play a series of 'games' with a sick child to facilitate disease transmission (Kitta 2012, 9; Ubelacker 2009; Leslie Young 2010). A recent book, entitled *Melanie's Marvelous Measles*, celebrates the supposed developmental benefits of childhood diseases (Messenger 2012). The author, a vaccine refuser and activist named Stephanie Messenger, aims to "educate children on the benefits of having measles and how you can heal from them naturally and successfully" (Amazon 2014). In this book we learn about two children who were vaccinated against measles, but who got sick with measles anyway (since vaccines supposedly do not work). Unfortunately, these children had very severe symptoms of measles, because becoming vaccinated (and eating junk food!) largely destroyed their immune systems.[34] In contrast, we meet some unvaccinated children who have very mild symptoms from measles. These children enjoy their 'sick days' home from school. I don't think that Messenger (or others like her) is speaking the language of science. Instead, this sort of vaccine refusal seems to emerge from an ethics of purity and, in particular, from the idea that diseases such as measles purify and sanctify children in ways that prepare them for 'naturally' healthy adulthoods, while vaccination prevents children from realizing these benefits, by contaminating and corrupting the immune system.[35]

I don't think that everyone who goes to a 'pox party' is motivated by the idea that getting sick is *good* for children. Many likely believe that diseases are bad for children, but they choose to infect their children under controlled conditions to try to manage (what they may believe to be) inevitable illnesses. Also, some parents may believe that the symptoms of a disease will be milder if a child becomes infected at an earlier age (as is the case for chicken pox) (Centers for Disease Control and Prevention 2014a). But I think that Messenger and others like her have a different conception of the value of childhood illness, according to which diseases can *strengthen* young people (physically and spiritually) and prepare them for robust and naturally healthy living in the future.

In *Vaccine*, Arthur Allen tells about his exposure to a different (and, one hopes, rarer) form of the idea that diseases sanctify children. He discusses a belief that was taught by Rudolf Steiner – the founder of anthroposophy and the Waldorf schools – according to which "children need to become quite ill with infectious diseases in order to develop into spiritually whole beings" (Allen 2007, 328).[36] Steiner taught that parents ought to refuse vaccines because they prevent children from experiencing spiritual growth.[37] On his view, vaccines *degrade* children, not because vaccines are contaminated, but because vaccines keep children from becoming the sorts of spiritual beings that they otherwise would have become. Vaccines, Steiner thought, were a "spiritual trick" (Allen 2007, 344). Parents of students who attend today's Waldorf schools echo Steiner's views. One parent says

> [T]here's a little bit of soulfulness with getting ill. ... Sometimes people say that after a fever you see a difference in a child's being. It really strengthens them. ... [People who vaccinate their children] never allow them the soulfulness of being ill.
>
> (Allen 2007, 351)

Views like these might not be worth addressing if Waldorf schools were not experiencing a surge of popularity and growth. In the last thirty years, the number of accredited Waldorf schools has gone from around two hundred to over a thousand (International Forum for Steiner/Waldorf-Education 2014, 157). If you count Waldorf kindergartens and special education centers, the numbers reach almost four thousand worldwide, and this does not count Waldorf-themed charter schools and homeschooling communities. It should come as no surprise that "Waldorf schools around the world are disproportionately unvaccinated, and these schools have often been epicenters of vaccine-preventable illnesses, particularly in the United States and Germany" (Allen 2007, 343–344). Indeed, Waldorf schools consistently have the highest exemption rates in communities around the United States (Jadrnak 2013; Krieger 2015; Smith, Daniel, and Murphy 2015). Given their commitment to the sanctifying power of childhood illnesses, participants in Waldorf school communities are likely to be especially difficult targets for public health campaigns aimed at increasing the rates of childhood vaccination.

Some people have claimed that disease outbreaks purify and protect the broader community. They think that diseases are valuable natural mechanisms for maintaining the size and the health of the population. The most famous proponent of this view was Thomas Malthus. In the early 19th century he argued that smallpox played a commendable role in regulating the population of Europe (Malthus 1806). Malthus was an Anglican minister and he framed his concerns about the health of the community in religious terms: God allowed disease outbreaks in order to preserve the overall health of the human community. Accordingly, Malthus thought that attempts to prevent disease-related deaths only expanded the population beyond sustainable levels and would lead to unnecessary suffering. Malthus's views – or something like them – have been embraced at various times by a wide variety of people.

The Social Darwinists (e.g. Herbert Spencer) sometimes echoed themes from Malthus, though it is clear that Darwin did not. I point this out because we live in a time in which all manner of false and evil views have been wrongly attributed to the father of modern biology. One might look at the following, from chapter 5 of *Descent of Man*, and conclude that Darwin opposed vaccination:

> There is reason to believe that vaccination has preserved thousands, who from a weak constitution would formerly have succumbed to small-pox. Thus the weak members of civilised societies propagate their kind. No one who has attended to the breeding of domestic animals will doubt that this must be highly injurious to the race of man. It is surprising how soon a want of care, or care wrongly directed, leads to the degeneration of a domestic race; but excepting

in the case of man himself, hardly any one is so ignorant as to allow his worst animals to breed.

(Darwin 2004, 159)

Some writers have taken claims like these as evidence that Darwin opposed vaccination. He did not. Instead, Darwin argued that our *sympathy*, which emerges from "the noblest part of our nature," prevents us from allowing people to die when we have the means to save them (Darwin 2004, 159). Charles Darwin did not endorse the idea that disease 'purifies' human communities, even while others sometimes have.

Responding to the possibility of purity-based vaccine refusal

How should the possibility that vaccine refusal sometimes results from a commitment to an ethics of purity affect how we think about vaccine refusal and public vaccination policies? In the most general sense, the arguments of this chapter support one of the main theses of this book: Vaccine refusers are not irrational or otherwise uniquely cognitively deficient. They respond to reasons and they act for values, and their decisions about vaccines are understandable responses to the contexts in which they find themselves. Recall that, in chapter one, I argued that vaccine denialism may result from a reasonable refusal to show epistemic deference towards pediatricians, and that the breakdown in trusting physician-patient relationships results primarily from social and political forces beyond an individual person's control. In chapter two, I argued that vaccine denialism may result from poor reasoning, but I insisted that the cognitive liabilities that contribute to vaccine denialism are not unique to vaccine denialists. On the contrary, vaccine denialism may result from ordinary ways of thinking, under unfortunate social circumstances. In a similar vein, I have argued in this chapter that vaccine refusal may result from a commitment to an alternative system of values. In particular, vaccine refusers may believe that *vaccines are impure* or that *health requires only natural living* or that *diseases purify individuals and communities*. In this way, vaccine refusers may have reasons to refuse vaccines and they may appeal to various forms of evidence about relevant forms of (im)purity to defend their refusal of vaccines.

Aside from the general thesis that vaccine refusers are not 'irrational', I think my work in this chapter also supports a set of more specific claims.

First, greater educational outreach, aimed at teaching people the facts about vaccines, is unlikely to change the minds of people who refuse vaccines because of their commitment to an ethics of purity. This is because purity-based vaccine refusal may emerge from a commitment to different values than those that motivate public health advocates. Statistics about the low rates of vaccine complications and the various benefits of individual immunity may not address the following concerns: vaccines are contaminated (by their ingredients or their association with broader corruptions), vaccines are not necessary for people who otherwise avoid contamination, and vaccines prevent the sanctifying benefits of disease. Additional facts about the rates of vaccine complications are unlikely to change the minds of people who have these concerns. Instead, the facts that are likely to change these people's minds are facts that are relevant to the *values* that motivate their decisions to refuse vaccines. For example, someone who believes there are dangerous 'toxins' in vaccines is unlikely to respond to evidence that vaccines contain very low quantities of these materials. But her worries about vaccine safety might be alleviated if she were provided with evidence that these materials were *no longer present* in vaccines. This kind of vaccine refuser is willing to respond to evidence, but it must be evidence that is germane to the values that caused her to become a vaccine refuser.

Here, I want to resist the idea that vaccine refusers are motivated by extra-scientific values, while science is somehow value-free. See, for example, Arthur Allen, who says that "[b]y invoking science while implying that government and industrial science are corrupted by power and money, [some vaccine refusers] gloss over the extent to which alternative philosophies, rather than science, shape their critique of vaccination" (Allen 2007, 336). Also, Allen claims that science "cannot alter the fact that we are a fallen civilization" (Allen 2007, 334). Science is informed by values, too (H. E. Douglas 2009; Kitcher 2011). But the values that motivate scientific research and science policy may be quite different from those that motivate some vaccine refusers.

Second, if an ethics of purity can lead to vaccine refusal in a number of different ways, then this has consequences for how public health advocates should respond. Consider that many vaccine refusers claim that vaccines are impure, but they do not all agree about why vaccines are impure. Therefore, efforts that could appease some of these purity-focused vaccine refusers may not appease others. For example, removing animal body parts from vaccines could satisfy someone who finds vaccines disgusting because they contain animal materials, but is unlikely to satisfy a vaccine refuser who thinks vaccines are impure because they contain industrial 'toxins' or materials derived from aborted fetuses. Also, some purity-based vaccine refusers may not be disgusted by vaccines, but by something else. People who embrace *health-as-sanctity* may think vaccines are unnecessary for people who lead pure lives, while people who embrace *disease-as-sanctification* may think vaccines are an impediment to sanctified living. Efforts to remove 'impurities' from vaccines would do little to undermine most of these forms of vaccine refusal. Accordingly, public health efforts that focus on resisting the idea that vaccines are contaminated will not persuade vaccine refusers who are motivated by other purity-based considerations.

Third, my work in this chapter helps to explain why vaccine refusal is not a distinctively liberal or conservative practice. As I discussed in the

Introduction, there is good empirical evidence that vaccine refusal does not correlate with particular political ideologies. In this chapter, I have provided some additional evidence for why that is the case: At least some instances of vaccine refusal seem to result from a commitment to diverse ideals of purity. And these different purity ideals do not correspond to any (one) political ideology or to particular levels of religiosity.

Fourth, and following closely on my previous point, I have provided evidence that purity ideals (and the related emotion of disgust) are not as ideologically aligned as some have claimed they are. The fact that vaccine refusers express forms of moralized disgust that do not correlate with either liberal or conservative political views undermines the claim that an ethics of purity is a predominately conservative ethical framework, as Jonathan Haidt (2012) has claimed.[38] Of course, the ethics of purity looms large in the rhetoric of some conservative political arguments. For example, those who oppose equality for gays and lesbians often manifest disgust at the sexual acts which (they believe) gay and lesbian people perform, and they invoke the 'sanctity' of opposite-sex marriage as a reason to deny marriage rights to gays and lesbians (Inbar et al. 2009; Inbar, Pizarro, and Bloom 2009). Also, some who defend the conservative 'culture of life' – as part of their criticism on stem cell research and abortion rights – invoke and defend an ethics of purity and the value of disgust. For example, Leon Kass (the head of President George W. Bush's Bioethics Commission) has argued that disgust communicates a "wisdom" about the boundaries that should not be transgressed (Kass and Wilson 1998, 19; see also Kass 1997).

But conservatives do not have a monopoly on the ethics of purity (Dworkin 1994; Kahan 1998; Kahan 1999). For example, Dan Kahan argues that disgust helps liberals condemn cruelty (Kahan 1998). And Michael Sandel has argued that the reason why some things should not be for sale – including organs, soldiers, and citizenship – is because selling these things corrupts their intrinsic worth (Sandel 2012). On Sandel's view, these goods are defiled or degraded when prices are attached to them.

Conclusion: purity and reasoning about underlying values

Some people argue that the moral emotion of disgust – including the ideals of purity and sanctity connected to it – is a poor basis for making judgments about how to live our lives (Kelly 2011; Kelly and Morar 2014; Nussbaum 2004; Nussbaum 2010; Plakias 2013). Martha Nussbaum says that "disgust both hooks us on an unrealizable romantic fantasy of social purity and turns our thoughts away from the real measures we can take to improve [society]" (Nussbaum 2004, 107). She thinks disgust is an anti-social emotion, grounded in a commitment to maintain personal purity (at the cost of social improvement). On her view, ideals of purity lead a person to "repudiate this ugly world as not part of me. I vomit at these stultifying institutions, and I refuse to let them become part of my (pure) being" (Nussbaum 2004, 105). But moral action and political reform require individuals to engage actively in a 'dirty' and 'fallen' world. Since purity and disgust may lead us away from this kind of activity, (it is supposed to follow that) we should reject an ethics of purity. Also, moralized disgust may be intrinsically dehumanizing, since it portrays the objects of disgust as defiled or degraded (Kelly and Morar 2014).

Let us return to the example of debates about the social and political status of LGBT persons. On Nussbaum's view, our ideas about purity (and our feeling of disgust) should not influence either our interpersonal interactions with LGBT persons, or our advocacy of laws that will affect their lives (Nussbaum 2010). Instead, what matters is that we act on the basis of legitimate moral and political values, including liberty, equality, and well-being. So, for example, our opinions about gay marriage should be informed by the fact that same-sex marriage (like opposite-sex marriage) promotes personal and social goods (e.g. relationships of mutual lifelong caring), and by our commitment both to equality under the law and to freedom of association (see e.g. Corvino and Gallagher 2012).

I agree with Nussbaum that some ideals of purity are unreasonable and anti-social. The emotion of disgust can sometimes lead us astray. This much follows from two claims that I have endorsed: (1) Vaccine refusal is generally misguided and (2) Vaccine refusal sometimes results from an ethics of purity (and from the emotion of disgust). But it does not follow from the fact that disgust and an ethics of purity lead people astray in one case – such as vaccine refusal – that they always do so. Indeed, as I mentioned earlier, some have argued that we might harness the power of moralized disgust for progressive social purposes (Kahan 1998; Kahan 1999). But I want to sidestep this debate about the admissibility of disgust in public policy. My goal in the remainder of this conclusion is only to highlight some ways in which *vaccine refusers* may rely on unreasonable and unrealizable purity ideals.

Vaccine refusers may rely on purity ideals that are radically unrealizable. Consider our aversion to ingesting animal or human waste in order to preserve bodily purity. We consume 'insect filth' and other 'foreign matter' (including rodent hair and feces) in almost all of the food that we eat. We inhale aromatic compounds from other people's colons when we smell their flatulence. Consider (moralized) disgust at industrial toxins: We are swimming in toxins wherever we go. So, a choice to refuse vaccines that is informed by a commitment not to ingest animal/human waste or industrial toxins seems motivated by an unreasonable ideal. There are amazingly trivial amounts of both of these kinds of objects in vaccines compared to what we consume in our everyday lives. Even if we would do well to avoid these 'toxins', it is unreasonable to insist that we avoid them entirely. But if we don't need to entirely avoid these 'toxins', then the trace amounts present in vaccines should not trouble us.

Vaccine refusers are also sometimes committed to purity ideals that are morally objectionable. For example, it is morally wrong to refuse to provide your child with routine and readily available protection against a harmful disease, even if doing so violates your ideas about 'sexual purity'. Disease, suffering, and death are not fair punishments for sexual activities that you abhor. Also, it is racist and xenophobic to think people from other countries are dirty or impure. Finally, anxieties about the changing social roles of (middle-class) mothers are often informed by reactionary (and sexist) ideas about gender and family life. We ought to criticize these sorts of purity ideals and, therefore, we have good reason to criticize forms of vaccine refusal that emerge from these objectionable conceptions of purity and contamination.

Notes

1 I assume that an ethics of purity has the ability to influence our beliefs and actions. There is wide support for the idea that disgust can influence our decisions about what we ought to do (Greene 2008; Kelly 2011; Nussbaum 2004; Plakias 2013; Prinz 2007). Importantly, there are ongoing debates about the precise scope and intensity of disgust's causal powers. For example, Greene (2008) and Prinz (2006; 2007) defend an expansive scope and robust causal powers, while May (2014) claims that the empirical evidence supports a more restricted scope and more modest powers for disgust. But the arguments in this chapter do not depend on the outcome of such debates, since there is wide agreement that disgust can influence decisions within the domain of 'purity' or 'sanctity', which is all that I presuppose.

2 The term 'admissible social tool' comes from Kelly and Morar (2014).

3 In *Deadly Choices*, Offit argues that contemporary vaccine refusers have similar concerns as their historical counterparts did (Offit 2010, chap. 7). Offit thinks this historical continuity is supposed to undermine the legitimacy of contemporary vaccine refusal: There is something wrong with today's vaccine refusers if they are rehashing 150-year-old worries about vaccines. (After all, one and a half centuries of scientific evidence about the safety and efficacy of vaccines has accumulated during that time.) But Offit may be drawing the wrong conclusion from the historical consistency of vaccine refusers' concerns. I suspect that a better conclusion is that scientists, politicians, and public health officials have consistently done a poor job understanding the fact that some parents disagree with them about what a good and healthy childhood requires.

4 Martha Nussbaum captures the idea of contamination in this way: "if you ingest what is base, it debases you" (Nussbaum 2004, 88).

5 This is part of Haidt's discussion of the 'ethic of divinity' of Richard Shweder. See Shweder (1990) and Shweder et al. (1997).

6 Nussbaum continues: "Its core idea is the belief that if we take in the animalness of animal secretions we will ourselves be reduced to the status of animals. Similarly, if we absorb or are mingled with the decaying, we will ourselves be mortal and decaying" (Nussbaum 2004, 89).

7 For more information on the pre-history of vaccination, including the traditions of variolation that emerged from Turkey, India, and elsewhere, see the Introduction.

8 The early vaccine refusers' fear of animal contamination extended beyond the bovine origins of cowpox pus. Some early vaccine refusers believed that

smallpox vaccine included "poison of adders, the blood, entrails, and excretions of bats, toads, and suckling whelps" (Durbach 2005, 114; cited at Offit 2010, p. 110).

9 Miller is relying here on James (1988, 14–15).

10 Kirby is quoting parental testimony from the hearing of the House Government Reform Committee on April 7, 2000: "Autism: Present Challenges, Future Needs – Why the Increasing Rates?" 106th Congress, 2nd Session, *Congressional Record*, serial no. 106–80 (April 2000): 1–7.

11 Those who object to the fact that vaccines include these materials may have moral reasons for objecting. But my focus here is on the idea that there is something harmful in itself about injecting into the human body materials that originated from aborted fetuses.

12 This may be an oversimplification, since conservative sexual morality, including prohibitions on abortion, may be rooted in a valorization of sexual purity and a worry about sexual contamination.

13 John Deigh describes cultural and political disgust and contamination in the following way: "With regard to disgust, the phenomenon manifests itself in shared revulsion at actions and people who betray the beliefs, norms, and ideals of a group to which its subjects belong and with which they strongly identify. When people who belong to a group thereby share beliefs, norms, and ideals, when they subscribe to the same faith and support the same practices, then members who break faith with them or subvert their practices, have, if only symbolically, weakened the group. They have compromised, as it were, the group's integrity, and such compromises of integrity are seen as corruption and even defilement" (Deigh 2008, 119–120).

14 Here, consider Leviticus 15:31, "You must keep the Israelites separate from things that make them unclean, so they will not die in their uncleanness for defiling my dwelling place, which is among them."

15 Perhaps they believed that the causal relationship between one's impurity and one's relationship with God went the other way, too, i.e. that being severed from a relationship with God would defile a person.

16 The denominations that preach against vaccination are often very small. They are sometimes single congregations. For example, consider the Faith Tabernacle Congregation and the First Century Gospel Church in Philadelphia, which were the epicenters of a measles outbreak in the early 1990s (Lewin 1991).

17 Of course, I do not mean to endorse the details of Paracelsus's views. He may have been the 'father of toxicology', but most of his views should be rejected, e.g. that diseases are caused by combinations of mercury, sulfur and salt.

18 For example, *Honest.com* promises that its products are free of toxins. And it defines toxins broadly: "We define 'non-toxic' as chemicals that are generally safer for humans and the environment. While most manufacturers' assessments of toxicity only take acute impacts into consideration, we also assess chronic impacts, exposure routes, unique windows of vulnerability, and a wide spectrum of potential health impacts including carcinogenicity, teratogenicity, allergenicity, neurotoxicity, and more" (Honest 2013).

19 For some discussion of the ethical issues surrounding this protocol, see Isaacs et al. (2011).

20 For a discussion of the history of the evolving arguments public health officials have made on behalf of hepatitis B vaccine, see Conis (2015, chap. 8).

21 Perhaps I don't need to go so far afield to explain parental refusal of hepatitis B. Mothers who have good health care and who do not use intravenous drugs almost certainly do not have hepatitis B, and they will not transmit the virus to their children. But the chief reason for vaccinating infants against hepatitis B is to prevent mother-to-child transmission. Infants and children are not

otherwise vulnerable to this infection. And the reason to have universal infant vaccination against hepatitis B is because we cannot have a public policy that coerces only poor suspected drug users into vaccinating their children, not because every infant is at equal risk. But parents need not concern themselves with these political worries about state coercion. From their point of view, refusing hepatitis B vaccine may be entirely reasonable, even if public policy is also reasonable.

22 See, also, Dr. Sears's incredulity about vaccinating newborns against hepatitis B (askdrsears 2014).

23 For a broader discussion, see Matchar (2013), which was my immediate source for the three preceding quotations.

24 Consider, also, the history of blaming mothers for autism (Mnookin 2011a, 76–77). For example, Bruno Bettelheim wrote that autism resulted from dysfunctional early attachment between mother and child (Bettelheim 1959). If vaccine contamination legends express anxieties about changing mothering norms, then it is understandable that these legends would also invoke worries about autism, given the history of blaming autism on poor mothering.

25 For example, Sahni, Lai, and MacDonald found that vaccine refusal correlates with homebirth and with a refusal of neonatal vitamin K prophylaxis (Sahni, Lai, and MacDonald 2014).

26 On 'medicalization' and dehumanization, see Foucault (2003), though Foucault apparently approved of mass vaccination programs (Dreyfus 1996).

27 In response, WHO convened a group of independent experts to investigate this charge, and they found no merit to the charge (Biss 2012).

28 Of course, an individual vaccine refuser may invoke an ethics of purity in both ways: She may refuse vaccines because they are contaminated *and* because they are unnecessary or ineffective for people with natural health. But these two ways of invoking an ethics of purity in defense of vaccine refusal are analytically distinct; neither implies the other.

29 "The pious response to a smallpox epidemic was to accept its divine judgment as an opportunity for repentance" (Allen 2007, 25).

30 For an extended discussion of Wallace's reasons for believing smallpox vaccine was unsafe and ineffective, see Fichman and Keelan (2007) and Wallace (1910).

31 Other versions of this myth include the claim that the Amish do not suffer from measles, polio, or other communicable diseases.

32 For example, consider the arguments of Christine Hayes (2002, chap. 2). Hayes argues that the biblical requirements of ritual purity (e.g. Leviticus 12–15) help to mark the unique covenant between God and the Israelite people. The fact that gentiles are not bound by ritual purity laws marks them as outside of this covenant.

33 More recently, prominent conservative politicians and political commentators have claimed that the thousands of unaccompanied minors present at the southern US border in 2013–2014 portended a public health crisis, even though most of the immigrants came from countries that have higher vaccination rates than the United States has (Bouie 2014).

34 I could not access this book from my library or through interlibrary loan (and I refuse to purchase it). My summary of the text relies on Skepticat (2013). The book has since been pulled from some Australian bookstores (Sheperd 2013).

35 Mark Largent observes: "Chiropractors' emphasis on natural methods to enhance their patients' health sometimes leads them to argue that childhood diseases ultimately serve a protective purpose and that the use of vaccines undermines that benefit" (Largent 2012, 47).

36 Consider the following from Nietzsche's *Human All Too Human*, section 224: "For instance, a sickly man in the midst of a warlike and restless race will perhaps have more chance of being alone and thereby growing quieter and wiser" (Nietzsche 1996).

37 For a different example of the idea that diseases sanctify, consider a story Martha Nussbaum tells about a conference she attended: "[A] French anthropologist now delivers her paper. She expresses regret that the introduction of smallpox vaccination to India by the British eradicated the cult of Sittala Devi, the goddess to whom one used to pray to avert smallpox" (Nussbaum 1998, 35). The idea here is that vaccination destroys forms of spiritual life that existed prior to the introduction of vaccines. The cult of Sittala Devi involved *variolation* against smallpox, i.e. self-infection with a mild form of smallpox that made a person ill (and contagious) but that made her immune to later (and more severe) smallpox infections.

38 It is sometimes difficult to pin down what Haidt means by 'conservative'. For example, Blum (2013) argues that Haidt equivocates on the distinction between 'conservatives' and 'liberals'. According to Blum, Haidt sometimes marks the distinction in terms of different philosophical ideas, but other times he relies on different policy preferences or the political self-identification of his research subjects.

Bibliography

Abrams, Lindsay. 2014. "'The Daily Show': Anti-Vaxxers Are the Climate-Denying 'Nutjobs' of the Left." June 3. www.salon.com/2014/06/03/the_daily_show_anti_vaxxers_are_the_climate_denying_nutjobs_of_the_left/.

Adams, Mark. 2010. *Mr. America: How Muscular Millionaire Bernarr Macfadden Transformed the Nation Through Sex, Salad, and the Ultimate Starvation Diet.* HarperCollins.

Allen, Arthur. 2007. *Vaccine: The Controversial Story of Medicine's Greatest Lifesaver.* W. W. Norton & Company.

Amazon. 2014. "About the Author." *Amazon.com*. Accessed July 14. www.amazon.com/Melanies-Marvelous-Measles-Stephanie-Messenger/dp/1466938897.

askdrsears. 2014. "Hepatitis B Vaccine and Disease: Do Newborns Need a Vaccine for a Sexually Transmitted Disease?| The Trusted Resource for Parents." *Ask Dr Sears® | The Trusted Resource for Parents*. Accessed June 11. www.askdrsears.com/topics/health-concerns/vaccines/hepatitis-b-vaccine-and-disease-do-newborns-need-vaccine-sexually-transmitted.

Bettelheim, Bruno. 1959. "Joey: A Mechanical Boy." *Scientific American* 200(3): 117–126.

Biss, Eula. 2012. "On Vampire Capitalism and the Fear of Inoculation." *Harper's Magazine: The Stream*. December 7. http://harpers.org/blog/2012/12/on-vampire-capitalism-and-the-fear-of-inoculation/.

Biss, Eula. 2013. "Sentimental Medicine." *Harper's Magazine*, January, 33–40.

Blancou, Philippe, Jean-Pierre Vartanian, Cindy Christopherson, Nicole Chenciner, Claudio Basilico, Shirley Kwok, and Simon Wain-Hobson. 2001. "Polio Vaccine Samples Not Linked to AIDS." *Nature* 410(6832): 1045–1046.

Blum, Lawrence. 2013. "Political Identity and Moral Education: A Response to Jonathan Haidt's *The Righteous Mind*." *Journal of Moral Education* 42(3): 298–315.

Bouie, Jamelle. 2014. "America's Long History of Immigrant Scaremongering." *Slate*, July 18. www.slate.com/articles/news_and_politics/politics/2014/07/imm igrant_scaremongering_and_hate_conservatives_stoke_fears_of_diseased.html.

Brown, Katrina F., J. S. Kroll, M. J. Hudson, M. Ramsay, J. Green, S. J. Long, C. A. Vincent, G. Fraser, and N. Sevdalis. 2010. "Factors Underlying Parental Decisions about Combination Childhood Vaccinations Including MMR: A Systematic Review." *Vaccine* 28(26): 4235–4248.

Buttram, Harold. 2012. "The Ultimate Gamble: Do Childhood Vaccines Result in Genetic Hybridization from Alien Human and Animal DNA Contents?" *Vactruth. com*. March 13. http://vactruth.com/2012/03/13/vaccines-human-animal-dna/.

Centers for Disease Control and Prevention. 2005. *A Comprehensive Immunization Strategy to Eliminate Transmission of Hepatitis B Virus Infection in the United States*. Vol. 55 / No. RR-16. *Morbidity and Mortality Weekly Report*. December 23. www.cdc.gov/mmwr/preview/mmwrhtml/rr5416a1.htm.

Centers for Disease Control and Prevention. 2014a. "CDC – Chickenpox Web Site Home Page – Varicella." *Centers for Disease Control and Prevention*. February 26. www.cdc.gov/chickenpox/.

Centers for Disease Control and Prevention. 2014b. "Food Safety and Raw Milk | Food Safety | CDC." *Centers for Disease Control and Prevention*. May 16. www. cdc.gov/foodsafety/rawmilk/raw-milk-index.html.

Chapman, Hanah A., and Adam K. Anderson. 2013. "Things Rank and Gross in Nature: A Review and Synthesis of Moral Disgust." *Psychological Bulletin* 139(2): 300–327.

Charo, R. Alta. 2007. "Politics, Parents, and Prophylaxis – Mandating HPV Vaccination in the United States." *New England Journal of Medicine* 356(19): 1905–1908. doi:10.1056/NEJMp078054.

Colbin, Annemarie. 2011. "A Holistic Health Perspective." In *Vaccine Epidemic*, edited by Louise Kuo Habakus and Mary Holland, 192–210. Skyhorse Publishing.

Conis, Elena. 2015. *Vaccine Nation*. University of Chicago Press.

Converse, Judy. 2011. "Pediatrics: Sick Is the New Healthy." In *Vaccine Epidemic*, edited by Louise Kuo Habakus and Mary Holland, 105–110. Skyhorse Publishing.

Corvino, John, and Maggie Gallagher. 2012. *Debating Same-Sex Marriage (Point/ Counterpoint)*. Oxford University Press.

Curtis, Valerie, and Adam Biran. 2001. "Dirt, Disgust, and Disease: Is Hygiene in Our Genes?" *Perspectives in Biology and Medicine* 44(1): 17–31.

Darwin, Charles. 2004. *The Descent of Man*. Penguin Classics.

Deigh, John. 2008. *Emotions, Values, and the Law*. Oxford University Press.

Deisher, Theresa A. 2009. *Is Aborted Fetal DNA in Vaccines Linked to Autism?* Accessed June 17, 2015. www.all.org/article/index/id/NDAzOQ.

De Melo-Martín, Inmaculada, and Arleen Salles. 2011. "On Disgust and Human Dignity." *The Journal of Value Inquiry* 45(2): 159–168.

Douglas, Heather E. 2009. *Science, Policy, and the Value-Free Ideal*. University of Pittsburgh Press.

Douglas, Mary. 2002. *Purity and Danger: An Analysis of the Concepts of Pollution and Taboo*. Routledge.

Downs, Julie S., Wändi Bruine de Bruin, and Baruch Fischhoff. 2008. "Parents' Vaccination Comprehension and Decisions." *Vaccine* 26(12): 1595–1607.

Dreyfus, Hubert L. 1996. "Being and Power: Heidegger and Foucault." *International Journal of Philosophical Studies* 4(1): 1–16.

Dubé, Eve, Caroline Laberge, Maryse Guay, Paul Bramadat, Réal Roy, and Julie A. Bettinger. 2013. "Vaccine Hesitancy: An Overview." *Human Vaccines & Immunotherapeutics* 9(8): 1763–1773.

Durbach, Nadja. 2005. *Bodily Matters: The Anti-Vaccination Movement in England, 1853–1907.* Duke University Press.

Dworkin, Ronald. 1994. *Life's Dominion: An Argument about Abortion, Euthanasia, and Individual Freedom.* Vintage.

Fichman, Martin, and Jennifer E. Keelan. 2007. "Resister's Logic: The Anti-Vaccination Arguments of Alfred Russel Wallace and Their Role in the Debates over Compulsory Vaccination in England, 1870–1907." *Studies in History and Philosophy of Science Part C: Studies in History and Philosophy of Biological and Biomedical Sciences* 38(3): 585–607.

Flanagan, Caitlin. 2007. *To Hell with All That: Loving and Loathing Our Inner Housewife.* Back Bay Books.

Foucault, Michel. 2003. *The Birth of the Clinic.* Psychology Press.

Francl, Michelle M. 2013. "Don't Take Medical Advice from the *New York Times Magazine*." *Slate*, February 7. www.slate.com/articles/health_and_science/medical_examiner/2013/02/curing_chemophobia_don_t_buy_the_alternative_medicine_in_the_boy_with_a.html.

Gallup. 2012. "Honesty/Ethics in Professions." Poll. *Gallup.* November 26. www.gallup.com/poll/1654/honesty-ethics-professions.aspx#1.

Gillray, James. 1802. *The Cow-Pock – or – the Wonderful Effects of the New Inoculation! – Vide. the Publications of Ye Anti-Vaccine Society Print (color Engraving).* Color engraving. http://en.wikipedia.org/wiki/File:The_cow_pock.jpg.

Glanz, Jason M., Nicole M. Wagner, Komal J. Narwaney, Jo Ann Shoup, David L. McClure, Emily V. McCormick, and Matthew F. Daley. 2013. "A Mixed Methods Study of Parental Vaccine Decision Making and Parent–Provider Trust." *Academic Pediatrics* 13(5): 481–488.

Grabenstein, John D. 2013. "What the World's Religions Teach, Applied to Vaccines and Immune Globulins." *Vaccine* 31(16): 2011–2023.

Greene, Joshua. 2008. "The Secret Joke of Kant's Soul." In *Moral Psychology*, Vol. 3, edited by Walter Sinnott-Armstrong, 35–117. MIT Press.

Gust, D. A., N. Darling, A. Kennedy, and B. Schwartz. 2008. "Parents with Doubts about Vaccines: Which Vaccines and Reasons Why." *Pediatrics* 122(4): 718.

Haelle, Tara. 2014. "No More Formaldehyde Baby Shampoo." *Slate*, March 3. www.slate.com/articles/health_and_science/medical_examiner/2014/03/is_formaldehyde_dangerous_no_but_johnson_johnson_removed_it_from_baby_shampoo.html.

Haidt, Jonathan. 2012. *The Righteous Mind: Why Good People Are Divided by Politics and Religion.* Penguin.

Hayes, Christine E. 2002. *Gentile Impurities and Jewish Identities: Intermarriage and Conversion from the Bible to the Talmud.* Oxford University Press.

Healy, C. Mary, and Larry K. Pickering. 2011. "How to Communicate with Vaccine-Hesitant Parents." *Pediatrics* 127 (Supplement 1): S127–133.

Honest. 2013. "What Does 'Non-Toxic' Really Mean?" *Honestly... The Honest Company Blog.* March 28. http://blog.honest.com/what-does-non-toxic-really-mean/.

Hooper, Edward. 1999. *The River: A Journey to the Source of HIV and AIDS.* Little Brown & Co.

Inbar, Yoel, David A. Pizarro, and Paul Bloom. 2009. "Conservatives Are More Easily Disgusted than Liberals." *Cognition and Emotion* 23(4): 714–725.

Inbar, Yoel, David A. Pizarro, Joshua Knobe, and Paul Bloom. 2009. "Disgust Sensitivity Predicts Intuitive Disapproval of Gays." *Emotion* 9(3): 435.

International Forum for Steiner/Waldorf-Education. 2014. "Waldorf World List." November. www.freunde-waldorf.de/fileadmin/user_upload/images/Wa ldorf_World_List/Waldorf_World_List.pdf.

Isaacs, David, Henry A. Kilham, Shirley Alexander, Nick Wood, Adam Buck-master, and Jenny Royle. 2011. "Ethical Issues in Preventing Mother-to-Child Transmission of Hepatitis B by Immunisation." *Vaccine* 29(37): 6159–6162.

Jadrnak, Jackie. 2013. "Waldorf Has Most Vaccine Exempted." *Albuquerque Journal*. November 29. www.abqjournal.com/310942/news/waldorf-has-most-va ccine-exempted.html.

James, Walene. 1988. *Immunization: The Reality behind the Myth*. Greenwood Publishing Group.

Jenner, Edward. 1798. *An Inquiry into the Causes and Effects of the Variolæ Vaccinæ*. Sampson Low.

Kahan, Dan M. 1998. "The Anatomy of Disgust in Criminal Law." *Michigan Law Review* 96(6): 1621–1657.

Kahan, Dan M. 1999. "The Progressive Appropriation of Disgust." In *The Passions of Law*, edited by Susan A. Bandes, 63–79. Critical America. New York University Press.

Kahan, Dan M. 2014. *Vaccine Risk Perceptions and Ad Hoc Risk Communication: An Empirical Assessment*. SSRN Scholarly Paper ID 2386034. Accessed June 17, 2015. Social Science Research Network.http://papers.ssrn.com/abstract=2386034.

Kapferer, Jean-Noël. 1990. *Rumors: Uses, Interpretations and Images*. Transaction Publishers.

Kass, Leon R. 1997. "The Wisdom of Repugnance: Why We Should Ban the Cloning of Humans." *New Republic* 216(22): 17–26.

Kass, Leon R., and James Q. Wilson. 1998. *The Ethics of Human Cloning*. American Enterprise Institute.

Kelly, Daniel. 2011. *Yuck! The Nature and Moral Significance of Disgust*. MIT Press.

Kelly, Daniel, and Nicolae Morar. 2014. "Against the Yuck Factor: On the Ideal Role of Disgust in Society." *Utilitas* (26)2: 153–177.

Kirby, David. 2006. *Evidence of Harm: Mercury in Vaccines and the Autism Epidemic: A Medical Controversy*. St. Martin's Griffin.

Kitcher, Philip. 2011. *Science in a Democratic Society*. Prometheus Books.

Kitta, Andrea. 2012. *Vaccinations and Public Concern in History*. Routledge.

Kluger, Jeffrey. 2009. "Jenny McCarthy on Autism and Vaccines." *TIME*, April 1. www.time.com/time/health/article/0,8599,1888718,00.html.

Krieger, Lisa M. 2015. "Measles Outbreak Raises Fury over California's Vaccine Exemptions." *San Jose Mercury News*. January 31. www.mercurynews.com/health/ ci_27433439/measles-outbreak-raises-fury-over-californias-vaccine-exemptions.

Largent, M. A. 2012. *Vaccine: The Debate in Modern America*. Johns Hopkins University Press.

Leask, Julie, Paul Kinnersley, Cath Jackson, Francine Cheater, Helen Bedford, and Greg Rowles. 2012. "Communicating with Parents about Vaccination: A Framework for Health Professionals." *BMC Pediatrics* 12(1): 154.

Lewin, Tamar. 1991. "Measles and Faith Combine In 5 Deaths in Philadelphia." *The New York Times*, February 16, sec. Education. www.nytimes.com/1991/02/16/us/measles-and-faith-combine-in-5-deaths-in-philadelphia.html?src=pm.

Luño, Angel Rodríguez. 2006. "Ethical Reflections on Vaccines Using Cells from Aborted Fetuses." *The National Catholic Bioethics Quarterly* 6(3): 453–460.

Malthus, Thomas Robert. 1806. *An Essay on the Principle of Population: Or, A View of Its Past and Present Effects on Human Happiness; with an Inquiry into Our Prospects Respecting the Future Removal or Mitigation of the Evils Which It Occasions.* J. Johnson.

Matchar, Emily. 2013. "Is Michael Pollan a Sexist Pig?" *Salon.com*. April 27. www.salon.com/2013/04/28/is_michael_pollan_a_sexist_pig/.

May, Joshua. 2014. "Does Disgust Influence Moral Judgment?" *Australasian Journal of Philosophy* 92(1): 125–141.

Meigs, Anna S. 1984. *Food, Sex, and Pollution: A New Guinea Religion*. Rutgers University Press.

Mendelsohn, Robert S. 2003. "Foreword to Hans Ruesch's Slaughter of the Innocent." In *Slaughter of the Innocent: The Use of Animals in Medical Research*, edited by Hans Ruesch. Sling-Shot Press.

Messenger, Stephanie. 2012. *Melanie's Marvelous Measles*. Trafford.

Miller, Neil Z. 1996. *Vaccines: Are They Really Safe and Effective?* Landau & Associates.

Miller, William Ian. 1997. *The Anatomy of Disgust*. Harvard University Press.

Minardi, Margot. 2004. "The Boston Inoculation Controversy of 1721–1722." *The William and Mary Quarterly* 61(1): 47–76.

Mintz, Zoe. 2013. "Dutch 'Bible Belt' Measles Outbreak Reaches 161 Cases in Unvaccinated Children." *International Business Times*. July 2. www.ibtimes.com/dutch-bible-belt-measles-outbreak-reaches-161-cases-unvaccinated-children-1331617.

Mludzinski, Tom. 2011. *Doctors Are Most Trusted Profession – Politicians Least Trusted*. Research. www.ipsos-mori.com/researchpublications/researcharchive/2818/Doctors-are-most-trusted-profession-politicians-least-trusted.aspx.

Mnookin, Seth. 2011a. *The Panic Virus: A True Story of Medicine, Science, and Fear*. Simon & Schuster.

Mnookin, Seth. 2011b. "Anecdotal Amish-Don't-Vaccinate Claims Disproved by Fact-Based Study." *The Panic Virus*. June 28. http://blogs.plos.org/thepanicvirus/2011/06/28/anecdotal-amish-dont-vaccinate-claims-disproved-by-fact-based-study/.

Mooney, Chris. 2011. "More Polling Data on the Politics of Vaccine Resistance." *The Intersection*. April 27. http://blogs.discovermagazine.com/intersection/2011/04/27/more-polling-data-on-the-politics-of-vaccine-resistance/#.UYqjJbWPNd1.

Moseley, Benjamin. 1806. *Commentaries on the Lues Bovilla; or Cow Pox*. Longman, Hurst, Rees, and Orme; Asperne; Cuthell and Martin; Highley; Ridgeway; and Callow.

Nietzsche, Friedrich. 1996. *Nietzsche: Human, All Too Human: A Book for Free Spirits*. Translated by R. J. Hollingdale. Cambridge University Press.

Nussbaum, Martha C. 1998. *Sex and Social Justice*. Oxford University Press.

Nussbaum, Martha C. 2004. *Hiding from Humanity: Disgust, Shame and the Law*. Princeton University Press.

Nussbaum, Martha C. 2010. *From Disgust to Humanity: Sexual Orientation and Constitutional Law*. Oxford University Press.

Offit, Paul A. 2010. *Deadly Choices: How the Anti-Vaccine Movement Threatens Us All*. Basic Books.

Oliver, Stephen P., Kathryn J. Boor, Steven C. Murphy, and Shelton E. Murinda. 2009. "Food Safety Hazards Associated with Consumption of Raw Milk." *Foodborne Pathogens and Disease* 6(7): 793–806.

Olmsted, Dan. 2005. "The Age of Autism: The Amish Anomaly." *United Press International*, April 18. www.upi.com/Science_News/2005/04/19/The-Age-of-Aut ism-The-Amish-anomaly/UPI-95661113911795/.

Omer, S. B., D. A. Salmon, W. A. Orenstein, M. P. deHart, and N. Halsey. 2009. "Vaccine Refusal, Mandatory Immunization, and the Risks of Vaccine-Preventable Diseases." *New England Journal of Medicine* 360(19): 1981–1988.

Oshinsky, David M. 2006. *Polio: An American Story*. Oxford University Press.

Palfreman, John. 2010. "The Vaccine War." *Frontline*. PBS. Accessed June 17, 2015. www.pbs.org/wgbh/pages/frontline/vaccines/view/.

Parrella, Adriana, Michael Gold, Helen Marshall, Annette Braunack-Mayer, and Peter Baghurst. 2013. "Parental Perspectives of Vaccine Safety and Experience of Adverse Events Following Immunisation." *Vaccine* 31(16): 2067–2074.

Plakias, Alexandra. 2013. "The Good and the Gross." *Ethical Theory and Moral Practice* 16(2): 261–278.

Plotkin, Stanley A. 2011. "History of Rubella Vaccines and the Recent History of Cell Culture." In *History of Vaccine Development*, edited by Stanley A. Plotkin, 219–231. Springer.

Poinar, H., M. Kuch, and S. Paabo. 2001. "Molecular Analyses of Oral Polio Vaccine Samples." *Science* 292(5517): 743–744.

Pollan, Michael. 2009. "Out of the Kitchen, Onto the Couch." *The New York Times*, August 2, sec. Magazine. www.nytimes.com/2009/08/02/magazine/02cooking-t.html.

Prince, Rose. 2010. "Has Feminism Killed the Art of Home Cooking?" *Mail Online*, September 21. www.dailymail.co.uk/femail/article-1313528/Feminism-kill ed-art-home-cooking.html.

Prinz, Jesse. 2006. "The Emotional Basis of Moral Judgments." *Philosophical Explorations* 9(1): 29–43.

Prinz, Jesse. 2007. *The Emotional Construction of Morals*. Oxford University Press.

Reiss, Dorit Rubinstein. 2014. "Thou Shalt Not Take the Name of the Lord Thy God in Vain: Use and Abuse of Religious Exemptions from School Immunization Requirements." *Hastings Law Journal* 65: 1551–1602.

Robinson, J. L., L. Nations, N. Suslowitz, M. L. Cuccaro, J. Haines, and M. Pericak-Vance. 2010. *Prevalence Rates of Autism Spectrum Disorders among the Old Order Amish*. International Society for Autism Research. https://imfar. confex.com/imfar/2010/webprogram/Paper7336.html.

Rozin, Paul, and April E. Fallan. 1987. "A Perspective on Disgust." *Psychological Review* 94(1): 23–41.

Rozin, Paul, Jonathan Haidt, and Clark R. McCauley. 2000. "Disgust: The Body and Soul Emotion." In *Handbook of Cognition and Emotion*, edited by Tim Dalgleish and Mick J.Power,429–446. John Wiley and Sons.

Russell, Pascale Sophie, and Roger Giner-Sorolla. 2011. "Moral Anger, but Not Moral Disgust, Responds to Intentionality." *Emotion* 11(2): 233.

Russell, Pascale Sophie, and Roger Giner-Sorolla. 2013. "Bodily Moral Disgust: What It Is, How It Is Different from Anger, and Why It Is an Unreasoned Emotion." *Psychological Bulletin* 139(2): 328–351.

Sadaf, Alina, Jennifer L. Richards, Jason Glanz, Daniel A. Salmon, and Saad B. Omer. 2013. "A Systematic Review of Interventions for Reducing Parental Vaccine Refusal and Vaccine Hesitancy." *Vaccine* 31(40): 4293–4304.

Sahni, Vanita, Florence Y. Lai, and Shannon E. MacDonald. 2014. "Neonatal Vitamin K Refusal and Nonimmunization." *Pediatrics* 134(3): 497–503.

Salmon, Daniel A., Stephen P. Teret, C. Raina MacIntyre, David Salisbury, Margaret A. Burgess, and Neal A. Halsey. 2006. "Compulsory Vaccination and Conscientious or Philosophical Exemptions: Past, Present, and Future." *The Lancet* 367(9508): 436–442.

Sandel, Michael J. 2012. *What Money Can't Buy: The Moral Limits of Markets.* Farrar, Straus and Giroux.

Schaller, Mark, and Justin H. Park. 2011. "The Behavioral Immune System (and Why It Matters)." *Current Directions in Psychological Science* 20(2): 99–103.

Sheperd, Tori. 2013. "Controversial Anti-Vaccination Book Removed from Sale." *News.com.au*, January 11, online edition, sec. Health & Fitness. www.news.com.au/lifestyle/health-fitness/controversial-anti-vaccination-book-removed-from-sale/story-fneuzlbd-1226551911539.

Shweder, Richard A. 1990. "In Defense of Moral Realism: Reply to Gabennesch." *Child Development* 61(6): 2060–2067.

Shweder, Richard A., Nancy C. Much, Manamohan Mahapatra, and Lawrence Park. 1997. "The 'Big Three' of Morality (Autonomy, Community, Divinity) and the 'Big Three' Explanations of Suffering." In *Morality and Health*, edited by Allan M. Brandt and Paul Rozin, 119–171. Routledge.

Skepticat. 2013. "A Review of 'Melanie's Marvelous Measles'." *Skepticat UK*. January 6. www.skepticat.org/2013/01/a-review-of-melanies-marvelous-measles/.

Smith, Morgan, Annie Daniel, and Ryan Murphy. 2015. "See Vaccine Exemptions in Texas by School District." *The Texas Tribune*. February 5. www.texastribune.org/2015/02/05/school-vaccine-exemptions-high-pockets-texas/.

Specter, Michael. 2009. *Denialism: How Irrational Thinking Hinders Scientific Progress, Harms the Planet, and Threatens Our Lives.* Penguin Press.

Szabo, Liz. 2013. "Amid Measles Outbreak, Megachurch Scrutinized for Vaccine Teachings." *Gleanings | ChristianityToday.com*. September 16. www.christianitytoday.com/gleanings/2013/august/measles-outbreak-megachurch-kenneth-copelannd-vaccines.html.

Tafuri, S., M. S. Gallone, M. G. Cappelli, D. Martinelli, R. Prato, and C. Germinario. 2014. "Addressing the Anti-Vaccination Movement and the Role of HCWs." *Vaccine* 32(38): 4860–4865.

Ubelacker, Sheryl. 2009. "Doctors Nix Idea of 'Flu Parties' to Get Immunity in Case Virus Becomes Deadlier." *Winnipeg Free Press*, July 2, online edition, sec. Flu Fight. www.winnipegfreepress.com/special/flu/Doctors-nix-idea-of-_flu-parties_-to-get-immunity-in-case-virus-becomes-deadlier.html.

Udesky, Laurie. 2007. "Push to Mandate HPV Vaccine Triggers Backlash in USA." *The Lancet* 369(9566): 979–980.

Waldman, Paul, Elbert Ventura, Robert Savillo, Susan Lin, and Greg Lewis. 2008. *Fear and Loathing in Prime Time Immigration Myths and Cable News.* Media Matters. Accessed June 17, 2015. http://mediamattersaction.org/reports/fearandloathing/online_version.

Wallace, Alfred R. 1910. *Vaccination a Delusion, Its Penal Enforcement a Crime: Proved by the Official Evidence in the Reports of the Royal Commission.* National Anti-Vaccination League.

Wei, F., J. Mullooly, M. Goodman, M. McCarty, A. Hanson, B. Crane, and J. Nordin. 2009. "Identification and Characteristics of Vaccine Refusers." *BMC Pediatrics* 9(1): 18.

Wolfe, R. M., and L. K. Sharp. 2002. "Anti-Vaccinationists Past and Present." *British Medical Journal* 325(7361): 430–432.

Wong, Alvin. 2010. "Dignitas Personae and Cell Line Independence." *The National Catholic Bioethics Quarterly* 10(2): 273–280.

Yoder, Jonathan S., and Mark S. Dworkin. 2006. "Vaccination Usage among Old-Order Amish Community in Illinois." *The Pediatric Infectious Disease Journal* 25(12): 1182–1193.

Young, Leslie. 2010. *The Everything Parent's Guide to Vaccines: Balanced, Professional Advice to Help You Make the Best Decision for Your Child.* Adams Media.

Young, Liane, and Rebecca Saxe. 2011. "When Ignorance Is No Excuse: Different Roles for Intent across Moral Domains." *Cognition* 120(2): 202–214.

4 Parental prerogatives and the morality of vaccination

"[W]e have ceded the ethical high ground to the [vaccine] critics."

(Caplan 2011, 1207)

Are parents morally permitted to refuse vaccines if they reasonably think that would be good for their children? In the previous chapters of this book, I argued that parents may reasonably doubt whether vaccines are good for their children. In chapter one, I argued that parents sometimes become vaccine denialists because of their understandable refusal to defer to the expertise of pediatricians, and because of their sensible decision to join resistant epistemic communities. In chapter two, I argued that common cognitive biases may lead parents towards false beliefs about vaccines, if parents attempt to reason about vaccines on their own. But parents don't need to be vaccine denialists to think vaccines are bad for their children. At the end of chapter two, and continuing through chapter three, I argued that some parents may disagree with vaccine advocates about the non-epistemic values that ought to inform decisions about children's health care. For example, vaccine refusers may value avoiding 'toxins' and living 'naturally', and they may believe that government and pharmaceutical companies play too big a role in health care. The values that motivate vaccine refusers are not nonsense, but are considered accounts of what makes the lives of individuals and societies go well. Of course, we can criticize vaccine refusers and their values. In particular, my goal in this chapter is to criticize the popular presumption that vaccine refusers have a moral right to refuse vaccines – a presumption that vaccine advocates have done little to resist.

Consider what Dr. Bob Sears[1] says in *The Vaccine Book*:

> Some parents, however, aren't willing to risk the very rare side effects of vaccines, so they choose to skip the shots. Their children benefit from herd immunity (the protection of all the vaccinated kids around them) without risking the vaccines themselves. Is this selfish? Perhaps. But as parents you have to decide. Are you supposed to make decisions that are good for the country as a whole? Or do you base your

decisions on what's best for your own child as an individual? Can we fault parents for putting their own child's health ahead of other kids around him? ... [W]e can't really fault parents who think that vaccines are too risky and decide to put their own kids first. We all put our own children first in most situations.

(Sears 2007, 220)[2]

Dr. Bob's focus in this passage is on moral judgment, rather than on the safety and efficacy of vaccines. If Dr. Bob is a vaccine denialist, he is a moderate one, since he admits that vaccines have only "very rare side effects."[3] In this passage, Sears is not so much fomenting vaccine denialism as making a moral argument: We should not "fault parents" who refuse vaccines out of a reasonable concern for their children's well-being. On Dr. Bob's view, morality permits parents to prioritize the interests of their children over the "good of the country as a whole."[4]

If the popularity of *The Vaccine Book* is any indication, many people agree with Dr. Bob about the morality of vaccine refusal.[5] Like Dr. Bob, they do not think parents are morally required to vaccinate in order to promote community health. To be clear: Dr. Bob is not the first person to point to a possible tension between the well-being of vaccinated people and the health of the community. Indeed, writers for popular audiences have often argued that vaccine refusal may be justified by a parental prerogative to prioritize their children's interests over the greater good (Coulter 1991; Habakus and Holland 2011; Kirby 2006; Murphy 1993; Wakefield 2011).[6] And writers for academic audiences have often characterized the morality of vaccination in terms of an analogous tension between personal (or parental) autonomy and considerations of public health (Fine and Clarkson 1986; Last 1987; Spier 1998; Vermeersch 1999). For example, Mark Largent has written that vaccination decisions are occasions for conflicts between "individual rights and the public good" (Largent 2012, 152).

I use Dr. Bob's comments as a framing device for this chapter, since they express the common conviction that parents are morally permitted to refuse vaccines. I begin by arguing that Dr. Bob's remarks can best be understood (and defended) as a rejection of merely instrumental conceptions of permissible parental partiality. I think Dr. Bob is right to say that parents are permitted to prioritize their children's interests even when doing so does not promote the greater good. (Children are not merely tools for increasing overall well-being.) However, the fact that vaccination promotes overall well-being is not the only (or the weightiest) moral reason to vaccinate. A duty of *fairness* and a duty to show *concern for vulnerable and disadvantaged people* provide additional moral reasons to vaccinate. Neither of these two duties is reducible to a duty to promote the greater good, and neither can be defeated by the parental prerogative Sears and others defend.

Utilitarian morality and a parental prerogative

Mass vaccination generates individual and herd immunity, and both of these kinds of immunity generate and protect important goods, which I will discuss in the next section. For now, I take for granted that the value of the goods associated with individual and herd immunity exceeds the costs of vaccination programs. To be clear, this is a society-wide calculus. Some *individuals* will not realize a net benefit from vaccination, since some people will experience serious vaccine complications that will not be outweighed by the personal benefits of individual and herd immunity. These few people would likely have been better off without vaccines. But I take for granted that *society* will experience better net consequences with mass vaccination than without it.

I also take for granted that we have a moral reason to act to bring about good (or better) states of the world. If one of our potential actions will cause or contribute to a greater good, this is a moral reason for us to undertake that action, especially if we can do so at minimal expected cost to our own well-being. This is the morality of beneficence.

It follows that individuals have a moral duty to vaccinate. This is not an exciting conclusion, since it follows from premises I assumed. Instead, what interests me – and what will get us back to Dr. Bob Sears – are questions about the *strength* (or the *stringency* or *weightiness*) of a moral duty to promote the greater good. Dr. Bob can agree that parents have a moral duty to vaccinate their children, but he certainly doesn't think they have a moral obligation to vaccinate. Why? Because he thinks parents may choose to do what they think is best for their children, rather than what would be best for society. To use Dr. Bob's words, we should not "fault parents for putting their own child's health ahead of other kids around him."

I think we can best understand Dr. Bob's position as a criticism of a Utilitarian way of thinking about parenting (and vaccination choices). For that reason, I hope the reader will forgive a short detour into (some oversimplified) moral theory. At its core, classical Utilitarianism (which I associate with philosophers such as Jeremy Bentham and Henry Sidgwick) claims that an act is right as it tends to promote the happiness of all who are affected by the act. Of course, almost everyone thinks that we ought sometimes to act to bring about good (or better) all-things-considered consequences. But Utilitarianism goes further than this, since it asserts that our *supreme moral obligation* is always to act to bring about good (or better) consequences. On such a view, the fact that vaccination promotes the good of public health is not just one moral reason (perhaps among many) for us to vaccinate. Rather, it is the only moral reason that matters. It follows that vaccine refusal is always immoral, under conditions when vaccination would contribute to greater overall well-being. In this way, Utilitarianism offers a strong, and perhaps the strongest, defense of a moral (and a legal) obligation to vaccinate (see e.g. Field and Caplan 2008).[7]

Utilitarianism is the dominant – though often unstated – moral backbone of much public policy, including public health policy. Consider the following comments from Tim Dare, which reflect upon the background Utilitarian moral commitments Dare finds in John Last's textbook on public health policy:

> The more traditional utilitarian justification of immunisation programmes will be obvious: if we accept as practically certain the standard claims for the benefits and risks of immunisation, then immunisation promises great benefits to large numbers of people, albeit at the cost of perhaps very serious harms to a small number of people. Hence John Last writes that "[t]he ethical issues that arise when we seek to protect the population by immunising have long been clearly defined. The risks of adverse effects to individuals have to be balanced against the benefits to the community."
>
> (Dare 1998, 134)[8]

But as Dare observes, the ethical issues surrounding vaccination choices have only been 'clearly defined' in the way Last suggests if you take Utilitarianism for granted. At the very least, then, we should be explicit about what Utilitarianism requires of us, and we should consider the familiar objections that have been leveled against Utilitarian approaches to ethics and social policy (Dare 1998, 135).

One of the most attractive aspects of Utilitarianism is that it encourages us to take up an impartial perspective towards the happiness of all people. Utilitarianism says that moral judgments should not be biased by our personal feelings or interests, since morality is about the all-things-considered consequences of our actions. For this reason, some have argued that Utilitarianism is a uniquely reasonable (or rational) moral theory (see e.g. Sidgwick 1981, III.13).[9] One way to make the point that Utilitarianism is a rational moral theory is to show that there is a deep analogy between the Utilitarian moral calculus and an individual's rational pursuit of her own happiness. John Rawls sets up the analogy this way:

> Just as an individual balances present and future gains against present and future losses, so a society may balance satisfactions and dissatisfactions between different individuals ... The principle of choice for an association of men is interpreted as an extension of the principle of choice for one man ... [I]t does not matter, except indirectly, how this sum of satisfactions is distributed among individuals any more than it matters, except indirectly, how one man distributes his satisfactions over time.
>
> (Rawls 1999, 21, 23)

It is rational for me to redistribute my pleasures and pains across my lifetime to promote my overall well-being. I save money so I will be comfortable in my retirement. It would be irrational for me to spend all of my money now, if that left me impoverished in old age. In much the same way, Utilitarian morality may seem to be a rational strategy for weighing the gains and losses of all people against each other, so as to realize the greatest aggregate good. The moral perspective is supposed to be an unbiased view from everywhere (or from nowhere), and it demands that we treat everyone's happiness with impartial concern. (Here, consider John Stuart Mill's claim that we ought to judge our actions from the point of view of a 'disinterested spectator'.)[10]

It seems straightforward that public health policy would be informed by Utilitarian moral theory and that public health officials would take up Utilitarianism's disinterested perspective. Public health programs ought to aim at achieving the best consequences for the community, without sexist, racist, or other discriminatory intent. Public health officials certainly regret that some people suffer vaccine complications, but they may try to justify these harms by claiming they are more than offset by the great benefits that individual and herd immunity provide. From a public health perspective, it would be irrational to be so concerned about avoiding vaccine complications for a few individuals that we sacrificed the community's protection against communicable diseases. I suspect that one reason vaccine refusal can seem irrational to public officials is because vaccine refusers may reject the impartial point of view that Utilitarianism requires, and on which public health policy may rely. Some vaccine refusers have chosen to focus on their children's well-being, rather than on public health. But this supposed parental 'bias' or 'irrationality' results from a disagreement about morality, rather than a rejection of mainstream scientific views.

Like most parents, I devote far more resources to my children than I do to other people's children. This is because my children's happiness matters more to me than their children's happiness. A classical Utilitarian can approve of this common form of parental partiality, but only if it is the best means for promoting overall happiness. On such a view, normal parental love is morally acceptable only because it brings more happiness into the world than alternative parenting practices do. But this is an odd way to think about parental love, and I agree with Bernard Williams that a Utilitarian justification for the partiality we show to our loved ones introduces "one thought too many" into our discourse (Williams 1981, 17–18). For Williams, and for me, parents ought to be entitled to show (some) partiality towards their children *just because they are their children*. And a person who points to the instrumental benefits of parental partiality seems to have too much to say on the topic. He seems not to understand what matters in the parent-child relationship.[11]

Let's return now to Dr. Bob's question: "Can we fault parents for putting their own child's health ahead of other kids around him?" A Utilitarian will say 'yes', we can fault such a parent, if acting on the basis of parental partiality will lead to suboptimal outcomes, all things considered. The fact that Dr. Bob answers 'no' to this question may show that he rejects a Utilitarian justification of parental partiality. If that's the case, I think he's right. But does rejecting a Utilitarian justification of parental partiality lead to the conclusion that vaccine refusal is morally permitted? It would, if the only weighty moral reason in favor of vaccination were a duty to promote overall well-being. But there are other weighty moral reasons to vaccinate, and the parental prerogative Sears defends is unlikely to defeat those other moral reasons.

Fairness and free-riding on herd immunity

We have a duty of fairness to contribute towards valuable public goods, such as herd immunity, when we are able to do so at a reasonable cost to ourselves. Becoming vaccinated is a way to contribute to herd immunity at a reasonable cost to ourselves. Therefore, we have a moral duty of fairness to vaccinate. If we don't vaccinate, then we will unfairly 'free-ride' on the socially productive labor of others.[12] A duty of fairness is distinct from a duty to promote overall happiness.[13] It is one thing for me to give greater weight to the interests of my children than I give to the interests of other children. But it is something else entirely to advance my children's interests by making unfair use of other people's efforts to promote public goods such as herd immunity (Dawson 2007; Hoven 2012).

A number of things may be unclear: Why do we have a moral reason to contribute to public goods? Why does the fact that herd immunity exists mean that I have to contribute to it? Consider the commonsense conviction that we ought to pay for goods we request, but that we don't need to pay for unsolicited goods. For example, I ought to pay for books I order online, but I do not have to pay for books someone else orders and has shipped to my house (Nozick 1974). Even when unsolicited goods emerge within the context of existing relationships, I remain morally free not to contribute towards the cost of those goods. For example, if my neighbor decides to mow my lawn unprompted by me, his gift does not make me morally liable to contribute to the maintenance of his lawnmower. The fact that we are neighbors gives rise to associative duties, including a duty of mutual aid, but these duties are not grounded in the mere fact that my neighbor has done something kind for me.

Why isn't herd immunity like a gifted book or a mowed lawn? If I am not obligated to contribute to schemes for the public distribution of books or the neighborly distribution of lawn-mowing services, why should I be required to contribute to schemes for generating and maintaining herd immunity? I did not ask to receive the benefits of herd immunity; I did not sign a contract for an exchange of goods and services. So, if members of societies that possess herd immunity have not asked to receive the benefits of herd immunity, and if they have not agreed to contribute to its production and maintenance, why should we think they have a duty to support herd immunity?

The short answer is that we sometimes have a stringent moral duty to contribute to the maintenance of public goods, and herd immunity is both a public good in itself and an essential means for promoting many other public goods. I will not attempt to resolve ongoing debates about the conceptual content of public goods, nor will I attempt to identify necessary and sufficient conditions for the public goods that are valuable enough to give people moral reasons to contribute to their maintenance. There is, of course, an extensive literature on public goods (in economics, philosophy, and in other disciplines), but I will keep my discussion at a fairly general level, so as to sidestep debates in the literature (Arneson 1982; Boran 2006; Cullity 1995; Cullity 2008; Klosko 1987).[14] My goal is to show that parents have a moral duty of fairness to contribute to herd immunity, since some of the goods that herd immunity provides meet many of the criteria of valuable public goods.

A good is public when it cannot be private. First, it is (nearly) impossible to prevent people (or for people to prevent themselves) from making use of a public good. For example, there is no feasible scheme by which citizens of the United States could be prevented, or could prevent themselves, from enjoying the benefits of national security or clean air. In contrast, there are possible (and existing) schemes for controlling access to hamburgers and houses. Air and security are, therefore, public in a way that hamburgers and houses are not. Herd immunity produces goods that are more like air and security in this way than they are like hamburgers and houses. You cannot prevent people (and people cannot prevent themselves) from making use of the community's protection against disease transmission.

Second, a public good has no marginal costs. The costs of one person enjoying a public good are the same as the costs of all people enjoying it. For example, the price for one member of society to enjoy the benefits of national security is the same as the price for all members of society to enjoy national security. Once you have national security for one, you have it for all. In contrast, it costs more money for more people to eat hamburgers. Here, again, herd immunity provides goods that are more like national security than like hamburgers. The cost for *one* person to enjoy the increased social trust that exists in communities that do not fear massive disease outbreaks is the same as the cost for *all* members of society to enjoy this good. Once enough people are vaccinated to provide this good for one person, there is no added cost to provide this good to every member of society.

Third, and relatedly, a public good has no marginal benefits. The benefits to the first person who enjoys the good are the same as the benefits to the last person who enjoys the good. Again, this is a feature that herd immunity and its associated goods share with clean air and national security, and this is a feature of herd immunity and its associated public goods that hamburgers and houses do not possess.

The special nature of public goods means that ideas about the fair production and consumption of private goods do not (indeed, cannot) apply to them. A fair distribution of the costs of a public good cannot depend on voluntary contracts, since one cannot voluntarily accept or refuse a public good. The fair cost of these goods cannot be determined by reference to the marginal costs of production or the marginal benefits of consumption, because there are no marginal costs, and because the benefits are the same to all. Instead, a public good is a product of social cooperation, and the responsibility for creating and maintaining it falls to the members of the community. The members of a community have a duty to establish fair schemes by which people may contribute to the public goods that social cooperation generates.[15] And, when a fair scheme exists for people to contribute to public goods, then members of the community have a moral duty to contribute.

I will not offer a general account of fair contribution schemes for public goods. However, it may be worthwhile to make two general points about fair contribution schemes in relation to questions about vaccination and herd immunity. First, a fair contribution scheme imposes a reasonable cost on the individual. Since the risks of vaccine complications are very low for most people, vaccination likely imposes reasonable costs on most people. Second, a fair contribution scheme imposes equitable costs among participants in the scheme. The costs of vaccination, e.g. a low risk of complications, are the same for almost all people. Of course, a generally fair contribution scheme for herd immunity may not be fair for people who are at elevated risk of vaccine complications. Accordingly, these people may not have a duty of fairness to become vaccinated.

Here it may be helpful to say something about the various public goods that herd immunity creates and protects by preventing (or lessening the severity of) outbreaks. These goods include reduced burdens on the public health system; protection against economic losses (including decreased tax revenues); increased social trust; and contributions to public safety, political stability, and national security. Herd immunity also produces more amorphous public goods, such as the sense that we live in a society in which people look out for one another. I suppose some of this latter idea falls under the category of 'public trust', but I also mean something less explicit and less conscious than that, e.g. a sense that we live in a community where we identify with other citizens as fellow participants in public projects.

All of these results of mass vaccination programs are entirely *public*, in the ways I described above. Once they exist, people cannot be excluded from making use of them; these goods also lack either marginal benefits or marginal costs. More importantly, these are all very valuable goods. This is a significant point because we may not have a duty of fairness to contribute to less valuable public goods. For example, imagine a community effort to put on fireworks displays every night of the week. These performances would be public goods, since there would be no way to prevent someone in the community from seeing the displays, and there would be no marginal costs or benefits. But I don't think these spectacular displays and fantastic explosions would be valuable enough to generate a moral reason for members of the community to pay for community fireworks every night of the week. In contrast, the public goods that mass vaccination generates are especially valuable. If the political community is going to promote any public goods at all, surely public safety, political stability, and national security should be among them. Therefore, members of a community that possesses herd immunity have a moral reason of fairness to contribute to their community's herd immunity.[16]

Someone who does not contribute to a fair cooperative scheme for the production of a valuable public good takes unfair advantage of the work that others have done to create that good. She is a 'free-rider' (Arneson 1982, 622; Boran 2006, 99; Cullity 1995, 5–7). A free-rider not only prioritizes her own interests, but she uses her fellow human beings as means to promote her own good.[17]

Some vaccine refusers (and their allies) admit that vaccine refusal is a form of free-riding. For example, Dr. Bob Sears says that he tells his non-vaccinating patients "not to share their fears with their neighbors, because if too many people avoid the MMR [the measles, mumps, and rubella vaccine], we'll likely see the disease increase significantly" (Sears 2007, 96–97). This is clearly immoral free-riding. It demonstrates a willingness to make unfair use of the contributions others have made to socially valuable goods. It's telling that Sears invites parents to be secretive or deceptive about their decision to refuse vaccines. He knows vaccine refusers need other people to continue to vaccinate in order for it to be safe for some people not to get vaccinated. I am reminded of one of the most famous ideas from Immanuel Kant's *Groundwork for the Metaphysics of Morals*: At the core of immorality is an expectation of special treatment – that I should be able to act in a way that it is only possible for me to act because most other people will not act in that way – where this moral violation is (supposed to be) equivalent to treating people in ways they could not agree to be treated (Kant 1998). I do not want to commit myself to any particular claim about (the equivalence of) Kant's formulations of the core principles of morality. But his work provides helpful context for the argument I have been making: Free-riding cannot survive publicity, but it requires secrecy or deception, and it is intrinsically immoral.

Free-riding is unfair, and acting unfairly is wrong not (only) because it may reduce overall happiness. Indeed, low levels of free-riding may result in higher levels of overall welfare than universal compliance would achieve. If few enough people free-ride, then the public good may be maintained, but the free-riders will also benefit by not having to bear the costs of vaccination (including the risks of vaccine complications). For this reason, some people have argued that there is no moral duty to become vaccinated when herd immunity exists, as long as vaccine refusal would not compromise herd immunity (e.g. Dawson 2007). How can it be immoral to free-ride if our contributions to public goods will be superfluous?

I have four responses to this objection. First, this objection begs the question against people who are committed to non-Utilitarian moral duties of fair play. The fact that there are some forms of cheating that optimize overall consequences does not make cheating morally permissible. Of course, Utilitarians may accuse me of begging the question by responding this way, and I don't have the space to adequately defend non-Utilitarian moral duties of fair play. So, the next three responses point to other reasons to resist the claim that free-riding on herd immunity can sometimes be morally permissible.

My second response is that the circumstances that this objection describes may never arise, and if they do, we may never know it when they do. This is because herd immunity requires very high levels of vaccination (sometimes up to 95%). When we consider that some people have medical conditions that make vaccination unsafe and others are restrained by inadequate resources (time, transportation) from vaccinating, there may be little (if any) room for people to free-ride without compromising herd immunity.[18] Also, we may have imperfect information about when there *is* room for harmless free-riding. Furthermore, herd immunity is not static; we do not create it once and possess it forever. Today's superfluous vaccinations may be required for herd immunity tomorrow. Furthermore, vaccination and vaccine refusal are not randomly distributed. Since vaccine refusers are often geographically clustered, even very low overall rates of vaccine refusal may compromise herd immunity. What may seem to be a superfluous vaccination in the aggregate may be necessary for herd immunity in local communities.

Third, fairness-based moral obligations help to solve a classic problem about the instability of cooperation, even when they generate excessive costs (or are otherwise inefficient). We may endorse a fairness-based moral obligation to vaccinate because its existence (and wide endorsement) communicates to people who have vaccinated that others are doing their part (and are not free-riding). Consider that social cooperation may become unstable if it becomes widely known that some members of the community are failing to make equitable contributions or to bear equitable costs. Indeed, one of the most effective ways to discourage vaccination is to tell people that other people are free-riding (Hershey et al. 1994). Many people would rather act against their own interests than have the costs and benefits of cooperation distributed unfairly. Since herd immunity is immensely valuable, and since it tolerates only the smallest levels of vaccine refusal, we ought to embrace a fairness-based moral obligation, even at some cost to utility.[19]

Fourth, and finally, there is a fairness-based moral obligation to vaccinate (even when herd immunity exists) because vaccine refusal often contributes to existing unjust forms of inequality. In particular, vaccine refusers are often socially privileged people, and they make unfair use of the contributions to herd immunity that are made by members of disadvantaged social groups. (These concerns about the fair distribution of the benefits and burdens of vaccination between social groups also cannot be straightforwardly reduced to concerns about aggregate goods.)

I want to say some more about this fourth response to the claim that non-harmful free-riding is morally permitted. The practice of free-riding is often more available to members of privileged social groups, and less available to members of disadvantaged groups.[20] Members of disadvantaged groups may lack the knowledge, money, time, or confidence necessary to refuse routine childhood vaccines or to negotiate alternate vaccination schedules with their physicians. (Recall that vaccine refusers often refuse only some vaccines, and they often insist on customized slowed-down schedules for the vaccines they accept.) Members of disadvantaged groups may find it especially difficult to resist authoritarian physician-patient relationships or to insist on modifications to standard vaccination protocols (Cooper-Patrick 1999; Roter et al. 1997). For example, Annette Lareau has shown that there are pervasive class-based differences in the ways parents interact with authority figures, such as physicians, on behalf of their children (Lareau 2003). Furthermore, members of disadvantaged groups may depend on the public health system and, consequently, they may lack access to the sorts of pediatricians who are willing (or able) to customize vaccine schedules. Because of the ways in which members of disadvantaged groups engage with the health care system, they are very unlikely to become free-riders on the goods that herd immunity provides. When they have access to vaccines, they are unlikely to refuse them. And when they lack access to vaccines, their failure to become vaccinated cannot be characterized as free-riding, since under such conditions they lack a means by which to make a fair contribution to herd immunity.

Free-riding is more available to members of privileged social groups because it is less available to members of disadvantaged groups. Recall that, to preserve herd immunity, we can tolerate only very small numbers of free-riders. Therefore, free-riding is not only an unearned advantage primarily enjoyed by otherwise privileged people; it is also an unearned advantage that makes unfair use of the socially cooperative labor of members of otherwise socially disadvantaged groups (among others). In this way, free-riding compounds existing injustices rooted in social inequalities.

The practice of privileged people free-riding on the mass vaccination of disadvantaged people is as old as the history of vaccination. Mass disease outbreaks have often been accompanied by a disproportionate focus on vaccinating immigrants, the poor, and racial minorities.[21] For example, Eula Biss reflects on the burdens borne by disadvantaged groups during mass vaccination efforts against smallpox in the United States:

> When the last nationwide smallpox epidemic began in 1898, some people believed that whites were not susceptible to the disease. It was called "nigger itch" or, where it was associated with immigrants, "Italian itch" or "Mexican bump." When smallpox broke out in New York City, police officers were sent to help enforce the vaccination of Italian and Irish immigrants in the tenements. And when smallpox arrived in Middlesboro, Kentucky, everyone in the black section of town who resisted immunization was vaccinated at gunpoint. These campaigns did limit the spread of the disease, but most of the risk of vaccination, which at that time could lead to infection with other diseases, was absorbed by the most vulnerable. The poor were forced into the service of the privileged.
>
> (Biss 2013)

Well-off white people have often taken advantage of the mass vaccination of *others*. Dr. Bob's advocacy of this 'privilege of vaccine refusal' is only the latest episode in a sordid history.

Some facts about Dr. Bob Sears and his practice may be relevant to this discussion of vaccine-refusal privilege. Dr. Bob is the son of Dr. Bill Sears (who is author of multiple best-selling books) and he is the brother of Dr. Jim Sears (host of the CBS television show *The Doctors*). He practices pediatrics at his family's private clinic in Capistrano Beach, an especially wealthy community of Orange County, California. His notable achievement is an alternative 'slowed-down' vaccine schedule. This schedule is a template for parents to use when selecting which vaccines their children will refuse and how to delay the vaccines their children will receive. Sears admits that his schedule will likely be useful only to the privileged *and* that the limited availability of his schedule is a good thing, since its widespread implementation would likely undermine herd immunity:

> This schedule would probably drive public health officials crazy. In large cities, where some families don't have good access to health care (whether from lack of insurance, language barriers, or financial reasons), it's already a challenge to get kids fully vaccinated. If we double the number of visits needed, we can forget the goal of achieving high vaccination levels in some areas. Yet, ultimately, the choice is yours if you think the precautions are worth it.
>
> (Sears 2007, 241)

Importantly, the 'choice' to forgo or customize vaccination is 'yours' only if you are privileged. If the poor asked for this special treatment from the public health system, they would likely be denied, since public health officials lack the resources to create and manage customized vaccination schedules. However, on Sears's view, that's a good thing, since restricting vaccine refusal and customization to a privileged few makes it possible for society to achieve high rates of vaccination and herd immunity. Sears's comments illustrate both of the ways in which free-riding intersects with existing forms of social inequality. First, on his view, the ability to refuse routine childhood vaccines (or to otherwise deviate from mainstream treatments) is likely available only to members of society who already enjoy economic, social, and intellectual advantages. Second, the privilege of (relatively) risk-free vaccine customization (and refusal) is available to these few members of society only because members of disadvantaged groups have received routine vaccines. Those who customize or refuse aspects of childhood vaccination not only make unfair use of a social good others have created. They also make unfair use of the social cooperation of *otherwise disadvantaged members of society.*

Does the fact that many people vaccinate for selfish reasons undermine the claim that people have a duty of fairness to vaccinate?[22] Consider that public health efforts to promote vaccination usually emphasize the benefits of *individual* immunity. One list of ten reasons to vaccinate identifies nine ways in which the vaccinated individual will benefit (and just one way in which becoming vaccinated helps others) (National Foundation for Infectious Diseases 2012). Additionally, physicians in the United States are required by the National Childhood Vaccine Injury Act of 1986 to provide a Vaccine Information Statement (VIS) whenever a vaccine is administered. These statements usually highlight the *personal* benefits and risks of vaccines (Centers for Disease Control and Prevention 2012; English et al. 2008). So, public health officials seem to think that people who vaccinate are often motivated by selfish interests. If they are right, then vaccinated people have already gotten what they wanted from vaccines – individual immunity – and vaccine refusers don't take anything from them. How can this be unfair?

In response, I agree that it makes a moral difference whether a public good is merely an unintended byproduct of an individual's (or many individuals') selfish pursuit of private ends, rather than an intentional result of other-regarding acts. For example, consider a billionaire who builds a lighthouse for his private purposes. Suppose he enjoys sitting on the deck of his shorefront mansion at night, while watching his artificial light shine across the water. I think it would be unjust of the billionaire to demand that local ship captains pay him for the cost of building and maintaining the lighthouse, even though the lighthouse generates a public good from which the ship captains benefit, i.e. safer maritime navigation. In this case, the people who have benefited from a public good do not seem to have a duty of fairness to contribute to the costs of that public good.[23]

I accept the general principle that one does not have a duty of fairness to support public goods that are the unintentional result of self-interested acts, as in the case of our billionaire lighthouse builder. But the fact that many people vaccinate for selfish reasons does not mean that herd immunity is merely an unintended side effect of selfish acts (Cullity 1995; Hoven 2012). Throughout its history, vaccination has almost always been part of public and political efforts to promote the health of the community, and the architects of mass vaccination programs have consistently aimed at the generation of herd immunity. So, even if many individuals have agreed to become vaccinated for private and selfish reasons, they did so against the backdrop of a set of institutions and incentives that aimed at the generation of a public good. I do not deny that there may be little moral worth in the self-regarding choices many individuals make to become vaccinated (or to vaccinate their children). But the duty of fairness to vaccinate does not depend on the moral worth of the actions of individuals. Instead, it exists because the community has acted (often without the knowledge or intention of many of its members) to create herd immunity through vaccination programs. And it is these public efforts that generate a duty of fairness to vaccinate. For a similar example, consider that many people pay taxes only because they have to, but this does not absolve citizens from a moral duty to pay taxes (at least when taxes finance valuable public goods). Of course, public efforts to promote public goods raise important questions about the legitimate use of state coercion to ensure compliance with cooperative schemes. I take up questions about state coercion in the next chapter.

Another way to resist the claim that vaccine refusers are immorally free-riding is to point to the fact that most vaccine refusers are unaware that they are free-riding. While some vaccine refusers act with an intention to free-ride on herd immunity, many others may be indifferent to herd immunity, but may be motivated primarily by worries about the potential harms of vaccination. The fact that these vaccine refusers do not consciously intend to free-ride on herd immunity may seem to mitigate (or eliminate) the moral wrongness of what they are doing.[24]

I agree that vaccine refusers who are unaware that they are making unfair use of herd immunity may be less morally blameworthy than they might otherwise be. (I assume, for the purpose of making this point, that these unaware vaccine refusers are not culpably ignorant.) However, even though ignorance may sometimes be a reason to forgo blaming a person for what she has done, it is less commonly a reason to think that otherwise wrong acts are right. In particular, one can act unfairly even if one is not acting from an intention to treat other people as mere instruments, and even if one attempts to show appropriate respect for others. Consider that I might accidentally 'cut' into a line because I do not know where the back of the line is located. Or, when playing cards, I may unknowingly play out of turn. In these cases, I do not deserve (much) blame. I would hope that people would not react with (much) anger or resentment to my accidental line-cutting or turn-taking. After all, moral anger is usually sensitive to our judgments about the intentions of those who we believe have acted wrongly. But these claims about blame and the moral emotions do not change the fact that I have acted unfairly, or that I ought to correct myself when other people call me out for what I have done. Similarly, vaccine refusers who do not intend to free-ride perhaps are not very blameworthy, but they still make unfair use of the public goods that herd immunity creates, and they have a stringent moral duty not to free-ride.[25]

Concern for the vulnerable

Another moral reason to vaccinate is grounded in the fact that some members of society are especially vulnerable to infection and to the secondary negative consequences of mass disease outbreaks. Here, I am not talking about a moral reason of fairness, but a reason to show special concern for people who are at heightened risk of harm.[26] There may be many different reasons to show special concern for the vulnerable, and I won't pretend to work out the foundational issues in this chapter. Instead, I claim only that our duties to the vulnerable are not exhausted by a general duty to promote aggregate well-being. The vulnerable are people whose interests ought to be given special consideration.

In this section, I focus on two kinds of vulnerability. First, some people are especially vulnerable to infection, because they are unable to develop individual immunity through vaccination. These vulnerable members of society include people for whom vaccines fail to generate or maintain individual immunity (Grubeck-Loebenstein et al. 2009), and people who are too young or too sick to be safely vaccinated (American Academy of Pediatrics 2012; Centers for Disease Control and Prevention 2011). Second, some people – particularly, women and the poor – are especially vulnerable to negative consequences of mass disease outbreaks. I argued in the last section that herd immunity generates many public goods. But many of the *bads* that result from failures of herd immunity are relatively *private*, since mass disease outbreaks will cause different harms to different people, depending on their social and economic positions.

On the first kind of vulnerability, consider people who are unable to acquire individual immunity, or who are unable to do so at a reasonable cost. By definition, these people cannot usually contribute to herd immunity, even though they benefit from it.[27] The fact that some people are especially vulnerable to infection gives rise to a distinct moral reason to vaccinate. By becoming vaccinated, people can demonstrate concern for the vulnerable, since being vaccinated contributes to herd immunity, and since the vulnerable rely on herd immunity to avoid infection. The fact that the vulnerable depend on us to help keep them safe speaks to the existence of a relationship of social dependency between vulnerable people and those who can contribute to herd immunity. To use Eula Biss's phrase, "we owe each other our bodies," since other people depend upon our bodies, and since our bodies depend upon other people's bodies, too (Biss 2014). A parental prerogative to sometimes prioritize the interests of our children is not enough to defeat a duty to show concern for the vulnerable.

Some people live in countries that have very low vaccination rates. These people are especially vulnerable to disease outbreaks. One way to show concern for them is to support global immunization efforts. But at the very least, we ought not to undermine mass vaccination efforts in their societies. However, domestic vaccine refusal movements may undermine vaccination efforts abroad (Kata 2012; Leach and Fairhead 2007). This is a further reason why concern for the vulnerable should incline us to vaccinate.

So far, I have argued that people have a moral duty to contribute to the herd immunity that vulnerable people rely on. But we need not appeal to herd immunity to show that vaccination helps protect vulnerable people. Vaccination is a way to prevent yourself (or your child) from directly infecting a vulnerable person. And we have a duty to take reasonable steps – such as becoming vaccinated – to avoid infecting other people.[28] For example, the San Diego measles outbreak of 2008 began when a non-vaccinated child became infected during a visit to Switzerland. This child infected students at his school and he infected other children (including an infant) who were in the waiting room when he went to get treated (Sugerman et al. 2010). (Notably, his pediatrician was Dr. Bob Sears.)

We also have a moral duty to protect people who are especially vulnerable to the secondary harms of disease outbreaks. The primary harm of a disease outbreak is infection – and the suffering, disability, and death it may cause. The secondary harms of disease outbreaks include the various social, economic, and political disruptions that outbreaks can cause. These harms are more diffuse and they can afflict both vaccinated and unvaccinated persons. For example, the fact that a poor single mother vaccinated her child will not protect her from losing her minimum wage job if she has to stay home with her child when quarantines shut down schools and daycare centers.

It's worth focusing on the harms that quarantine may cause, especially for women and people who have non-professional jobs. When outbreaks occur, daycare centers and schools will be shuttered within affected communities, and parents will have to take leave from work – or quit their jobs entirely – to stay at home with their children (Ferguson et al. 2006; Longini et al. 2005; Stern and Markel 2008). Parents, including parents of vaccinated children, will have to find other ways to provide childcare. Often, the only feasible childcare solution during disease outbreaks will be for parents (usually mothers) to stay home with their children. In this way, a decision not to vaccinate one's child is also a decision to contribute towards the creation of a world in which it will be more difficult for women (specifically, mothers) to participate in formal labor markets. But women's equal access to formal labor markets has long been part of the goal of achieving greater flourishing and equality for women. Therefore, vaccine refusers show insufficient concern for the ways in which their actions may undermine the goals of gender justice.

Someone could reply that we should blame existing gender injustices – not vaccine refusers – for the negative effects women may experience from widespread outbreaks and quarantines.[29] After all, if we lived under conditions of egalitarian gender relations, then women would not bear a disproportionate share of the costs of quarantines, etc. This may be true, but I do not think that it gets vaccine refusers off the hook. All of our decisions take place against the background of existing injustices, and it counts against the moral permissibility of an act if it would exacerbate existing injustices. For example, a decision by government officials to cut per-pupil public school funding will disproportionately harm students who live in poor communities (since wealthier school districts have additional resources to make up lost revenues). These cuts would not disproportionately harm students from poorer communities if their communities were not so poor. But that does not change the fact that cutting school funding will exacerbate the poverty of already unjustly impoverished people.

Recent outbreaks of previously (nearly) eradicated childhood diseases make it clear that worries about future quarantines (and the requirements of additional parental labor) are not merely dystopian speculations. For example, the 2008 San Diego measles outbreak inconvenienced thousands of parents. In the words of one mother:

> [Y]ou're getting ready to drop your child off at their child care place, and you're greeted by a public health nurse who says your child has been exposed to measles, and we'd like you to *go home and be there for the next three weeks* while we monitor you for symptoms.
>
> (Knox 2010, emphasis added)

Few parents are able to take off three weeks of work on short notice. Instead, the choice to stay home and care for one's child during extended quarantines may also be a choice to lose one's job. Since the increased domestic labor associated with quarantines will fall primarily on mothers, we have reason to think that quarantines will place pressure on women to exit the formal workforce. If levels of routine childhood vaccination continue to decline, mothers may face increasingly burdensome barriers to their full participation in formal labor markets. To be clear: Quarantines and school closures during disease outbreaks often apply to *all children*, including those who are vaccinated. So, parents may not be able to protect themselves from the disruptive impact of quarantines and the closures of schools/daycares by vaccinating their own children.

The burdens of quarantine will fall even harder on parents (and especially mothers) who are economically disadvantaged. The well-off can afford to quit their jobs or hire people to look after their children, and many professionals will be able to restructure their work around their childcare responsibilities. But people who are working minimum wage jobs usually cannot afford to quit their jobs (or to hire full-time caregivers for school-age children). And you cannot 'work from home' if you work at McDonalds. Quarantines are likely to be burdensome and these burdens will be disproportionately borne by women and, in particular, economically disadvantaged women.

I argued in the first three chapters of this book that *scientific ignorance* does not fully explain vaccine refusal. Vaccine refusers tend to know more about vaccines than parents who vaccinate do, even if vaccine refusers often have some false beliefs about vaccines, too. I suspect that *social ignorance* (or social indifference) is often an important contributor to vaccine refusal. Parents may be unaware of the consequences of mass disease outbreaks or of the immense public goods that mass vaccination defends. Or, parents might think that individuals don't have to consider the social consequences of their actions.

Some parents claim a moral right to disregard the ways vaccine refusal can affect other people. Jennifer Margulis says:

> It's my responsibility as a parent to keep my child safe, I think, and I don't think it's your responsibility to take a vaccine because I might be at the same party with you and you might cough on her. Honestly, I think your job is to protect your own health. And I mean, maybe I sound—I really don't mean to be sounding selfish in that way.
>
> (Palfreman 2010)[30]

Margulis expresses an intuitive idea: Parents have a right to care only about their kids. When they decide whether to vaccinate, parents are permitted to consider only whether vaccination is likely to benefit their children. Other people should look after themselves. Margulis might not mean it, but what she says sounds selfish to me. What is selfishness other than an exclusive focus on your own interests? (Here, I assume that your 'own interests' may include the interest of your child.)

Maybe Margulis's view is redeemed by the fact that she thinks every parent has an equal moral right to focus only on the interests of their own children. They are just as entitled to disregard the interests of her children as she is entitled to disregard the interests of their children. (Consider: "I don't think it's your responsibility to take a vaccine because … you might cough on [my child].") This seems less immoral than free-riding, since Margulis does not expect other people to treat her interests with greater concern than she treats theirs. She embraces reciprocal indifference. But the fact that Margulis accepts other people's selfishness does not justify selfishness. It is immoral to place others at risk of serious harm when you can easily avoid doing so. It is morally negligent not to take reasonable means to prevent yourself (and your children) from hurting other people. But even if I'm wrong, and even if there is no such thing as moral negligence, it would still be immoral to harm people, especially if you could have taken easy steps to avoid harming them. Even if it is not immoral to shoot my gun into the air, it is certainly wrong for the bullets from my gun to hit someone.

Barbara Loe Fisher responds to the claim that vaccine refusers are morally responsible when they harm other people (even if their choice to refuse vaccines is not itself morally negligent). She says "if vaccines are as effective as they are touted to be, then those who are vaccinated will not face any risk from those who are not" (Offit 2010, 76). Fisher accuses vaccine advocates of hypocrisy. If vaccines are as effective as public health officials claim they are, then vaccinated people have nothing to worry about from unvaccinated persons. But if vaccinated people are at risk of harm from unvaccinated people, then public health officials have overstated the effectiveness of vaccines. For Fisher, the fact that public health officials think that vaccines are effective *and* that vaccine refusers can harm people shows that public health officials are either ignorant or lying. This is a very popular argument. I have seen a version of it on almost every website that encourages parents to refuse vaccines, and in the comments section of almost every online article about vaccine refusal.

I am not convinced by Fisher's defense of the moral permissibility of vaccine refusal. First, the fact that a person *could* protect herself, but does not do so, is not always a sufficient reason to let someone else off the hook for harming her.[31] I admit that the common law principle of *volenti non fit injuria* ("to a willing person, injury is not done") may seem to support Fisher. But this is a principle of the law of torts, not of moral philosophy. Even if a deliberately unvaccinated person would not be allowed to *sue* a vaccine refuser who infected her, this fact does not make vaccine refusal morally permissible. For example, if a drunk driver causes an automobile accident with another drunk driver, the fact that the second drunk driver could have avoided the accident had she been sober does not extinguish the first drunk driver's moral responsibility for the accident. Even if one is insufficiently protective of one's own interests, it may still be morally wrong for another person to act in a way that places one's interests at further risk.

A second and more powerful objection to Fisher's argument is that it relies on a set of (perhaps willful) false beliefs about vaccination. Some people remain unvaccinated because they lack the resources to become vaccinated, e.g. transportation, time, accessible medical care, money. These people may not have a reasonable means to avoid becoming infected by vaccine refusers. Other people cannot safely become vaccinated. These include the very young, the very sick, and the otherwise immunocompromised.

Further, some vaccinated people will not acquire individual immunity from vaccines. They have taken reasonable means to avoid becoming infected – by getting vaccinated – but they will not achieve their goal. However, these people will not normally know that they have failed to develop individual immunity, since post-immunization titer testing is not standard practice. All of these kinds of people can be harmed by vaccine refusers, even if they do everything reasonable to protect themselves. Finally, even people who develop individual immunity from vaccination can be harmed by vaccine refusers. Mass quarantines can be very burdensome, even for people who do not become sick, as I discussed earlier in this chapter. Infection is only one of the many harms that vaccine refusers may bring to their communities.[32] Therefore, we should not be convinced by Fisher's defense of permissible indifference to the consequences of vaccine refusal. Merely appealing to the value of personal responsibility will be insufficient to block moral objections to vaccine refusal.

Conclusion

Some people think that vaccine refusal is morally permissible, regardless of what they think about vaccine science. Since moral disagreements need not rest on factual disagreements, it follows that efforts to better educate the public about vaccines may not be as effective at increasing vaccination rates as we might hope they would be. And even committed vaccine denialists may retreat to moral arguments when their factual claims fall apart. Consider the following exchange:

> Vaccine refuser: Vaccines cause high rates of serious complications.
>
> Public health advocate: Here is some evidence that shows you are wrong.
>
> Vaccine refuser: Well, it's my right as a parent to do what I think is best for my kid.

This kind of exchange is all too familiar in science denialism contexts (Michaels 2008; Oreskes and Conway 2011).[33] For example, people who resisted public health efforts to restrict smoking started to lean more heavily on arguments based on consumer freedom after evidence about the harms of smoking became overwhelming. Today's climate change skeptics seem to be in the middle of a similar retreat: As the scientific consensus about anthropogenic climate change becomes impossible to resist, they are retreating to the claim that individuals and businesses have a right to emit carbon. When their factual arguments start to fail, people who reject science-based views often retreat to claims about their moral or political freedom. But this means that public health advocates ought to be prepared to make moral arguments on behalf of vaccination, even if their immediate target includes forms of vaccine refusal that arise from false beliefs about science, and even if they are more comfortable invoking scientific evidence than moral values.

Parents have wide moral discretion when it comes to their children. But I have argued that a moderate parental prerogative to sometimes prioritize the interests of one's children is insufficient to morally justify vaccine refusal. Instead, it is often morally wrong for parents to refuse childhood vaccines. But even if I have succeeded, these arguments may not do much to persuade vaccine refusers. They could bite the bullet and insist that they are willing to act immorally on behalf of their children. However, many vaccine refusers are unlikely to be persuaded that they are acting immorally. Like everyone else, they are experts at rationalizing their choices. In either case, public health advocates may have to do more than invoke moral values. They may also need assistance from the state. In the next chapter, I argue that parents do not have an absolute political right to refuse routine childhood vaccines.

Notes

1 I use the terms 'Dr. Bob' and 'Dr. Bob Sears' to distinguish the author of *The Vaccine Book* from his father (Dr. Bill Sears) and from his brother (Dr. Jim Sears), both of whom are media personalities in their own right. Also, Dr. Robert Sears uses the term 'Dr. Bob' to identify himself, e.g. "Dr. Bob's Alternative Vaccine Schedule," (Sears 2007, 236).

2 See Cave and Mitchell (2010, xiv, 17) and Tenpenny (2008, 2) for similar quotations in support of parental permission to choose their children over the aggregate well-being of society. There is some reason to think that Sears has distanced himself from his earlier views on vaccination. See Mnookin (2011).

3 Dr. Sears's support for a slowed-down and selective vaccine schedule qualifies him as a vaccine denialist, as I discuss in the Introduction. But much of the appeal of Dr. Bob's alternative vaccination schedule seems grounded in the fact that it occupies a "refreshing middle ground" in debates about vaccination, since many people prefer a comfortable centrism between 'extremes' (Woo 2012).

4 I reject (what I take to be) Dr. Bob's claim that the scope of the morality of vaccination extends only to the borders of one's own country. The relevant moral community is humanity as a whole. Of course, my advocacy of an expanded scope for the morality of vaccination is not, by itself, a challenge to Sears's characterization of the (supposed) tension between a prerogative of parental partiality and a duty to promote the public good.

5 Many physicians report that parents often bring Sears's book (or his ideas) with them to office visits (Offit and Moser 2009). Sears's book has been a best seller since its release (Parikh 2010).

6 One might also consider a recent anti-vaccine movie, entitled *The Greater Good* (Nelson and Pilaro 2011).

7 In a different article, Field and Caplan argue that ethical decision making about vaccines must engage a variety of moral values, and not merely the cost-benefit analyses that are at the center of Utilitarian forms of evidence-based medical decision making (Field and Caplan 2012).

8 Dare is quoting from Last (1987, 353–354).

9 For a contemporary example, Joshua Greene draws upon work in cognitive science and neuroscience to conclude that Utilitarianism (which he calls 'deep pragmatism') offers more reliable moral guidance than do more deontological forms of moral reasoning (Greene 2013).

10 John Stuart Mill writes that "the happiness which forms the utilitarian standard of what is right in conduct, is not the agent's own happiness, but that of all concerned. As between his own happiness and that of others, utilitarianism requires him to be as strictly impartial as a disinterested and benevolent spectator" (Mill 2002, II.8.1–4). Mill may have been drawing on the views of Adam Smith, who wrote that "[w]e endeavour to examine our own conduct as we imagine any other fair and impartial spectator would examine it. If, upon placing ourselves in his situation, we thoroughly enter into all the passions and motives which influenced it, we approve of it, by sympathy with the approbation of this supposed equitable judge. If otherwise, we enter into his disapprobation, and condemn it" (Smith 2002, III.1.2). (Amartya Sen notes that the Rawlsian interpretation of Smith as a proto-Utilitarian is "extremely odd," but of course nothing in my book depends upon a particular interpretation of Smith (Sen 2009, 137).)

11 To be clear, the worry I have raised is not primarily about moral *motivation*, but about moral *justification*. The worry is not that Utilitarianism demands that people be motivated by unreasonably impartial goals, i.e. aggregate well-being, but that Utilitarianism's rule for assessing moral rightness or wrongness ignores relevant facts about an agent's relationship to those who are affected by his acts. Indeed, Utilitarians have a good response to the worry about motivation, though (as I suggest later) their response to worries about justification may not be so convincing. Utilitarians have long argued that people are morally permitted to be motivated by self-love, love for their family and friends, or other considerations that are not directly about aggregate well-being, whenever doing so promotes the overall good. For example, John Stuart Mill wrote that critics of Utilitarianism who object to its supposed demand for impartial motivation "confound the rule of action with the very motive of it. It is the business of ethics to tell us what are our duties, or by what test we may know them; but no system of ethics requires that the sole motive of all we do shall be a feeling of duty; on the contrary, ninety-nine hundredths of all our actions are done from other motives, and rightly so done, if the rule of duty does not condemn them" (Mill 2002, II.19.7–12). For Mill, permissible motivations can be of any sort, as long as they lead to good consequences. Henry Sidgwick went even further in embracing the moral permissibility of non-Utilitarian motivation. He argued that under certain conditions people should not be motivated by a commitment to Utilitarianism (and that this moral theory should be a merely 'esoteric morality', i.e. a morality known only to society's elite). He supposed that acting on the basis of other motivations – including a commitment to non-Utilitarian moral principles – would best promote the aggregate good (Sidgwick 1981, IV.5).

12 The fact that one has failed to vaccinate is evidence that one is making an unfair use of herd immunity only if vaccination would have been a fair method by which one could have contributed to herd immunity, and only if one did not undertake an alternative means for making a fair contribution to herd immunity. I leave aside questions about whether alternative methods of making fair contributions to herd immunity exist (or what would be required for them to exist).

13 One does not have a reason of fairness to vaccinate against diseases for which herd immunity is not possible, e.g. tetanus. (This disease is not contagious and

the bacterium that causes it is ubiquitous in the environment.) The only goods that tetanus generates are *private*, i.e. individual immunity for the vaccinated person. Tetanus vaccination does not create *public* goods; therefore, one cannot free-ride on tetanus vaccination.

14 The appendix in Cullity (1995) contains an extensive list of publications on 'public goods', with discussion of the different attributes that have been ascribed to this phenomenon.

15 A further question is whether a particular public good is sufficiently valuable to be worth the support of the community. I assume that herd immunity meets this condition.

16 Importantly, not all of the goods created by mass vaccination are public goods. In particular, individual immunity is a private good. It is something that one possesses (or does not) depending on one's choice to become vaccinated, or on one's successful recovery from a disease. The direct benefits of individual immunity accrue only to the individual.

17 For the purposes of this chapter, I remain agnostic about how best to characterize the 'unfairness' of free-riding. Whether it ought best to be characterized in terms of treating someone as a 'mere means', treating someone disrespectfully, treating someone in a way he could reasonably reject being treated, etc., is beyond the scope of this chapter.

18 Dawson acknowledges this as a source of skepticism about the claim that some levels of vaccine refusal will not compromise herd immunity (Dawson 2007, 173).

19 A moral obligation may be insufficient to solve problems about the instability of cooperation. Political coercion may also be required. I take up this possibility in chapter five.

20 There is empirical evidence that families of vaccine denialists are, on average, wealthier and better educated than families of vaccinated children, as I discuss in the Introduction.

21 See the disproportionate burdens borne by the poor and working class from the mandatory vaccination laws (the Vaccination Acts) in the late 19th and early 20th centuries (Albert, Ostheimer, and Breman 2001; Colgrove 2004).

22 Here (and elsewhere) I characterize a parent who considers only the interests of her child when deciding whether to vaccinate as a 'self-interested' agent. Admittedly, this is an idiosyncratic use of the term 'self-interest', since one's child is not part of oneself. However, I use the language of self-interest because this is the language Sears uses, and because using this language allows me to treat parent-and-child as a single moral agent for the purposes of my chapter. By obscuring the division between parent and child – and the prudential and moral duties parents have to their children – I can focus more clearly on the (supposed) tension between permissible 'self-interest' and the duties one owes to others.

23 Thanks to Karl Martin Adam for this example.

24 Dare observes that "it seems unlikely that those who fail to immunize on grounds of ignorance, apathy, inconvenience, or the like will properly be counted as deliberately taking advantage of immunization schemes, though the conduct may be morally blameworthy on other grounds" (Dare 1998, 146).

25 We may make a similar response in the case of parents who would refuse vaccination even in the absence of herd immunity. These parents are not motivated by a desire to make unfair use of the contributions of others, since they are not counterfactually responsive to such contributions. These parents may be less morally blameworthy for free-riding than they would be if they

were inclined to vaccinate under conditions in which there were no herd immunity. However, the fact that these parents are indifferent to the existence of the public good of herd immunity does not change the fact that they are, in fact, making use of this public good without making a fair contribution towards it.

26 Consider Angus Dawson, who says that "the mere fact that there is a fore-seeable increase in the probability of causing harm is enough to impose an obligation to act" (Dawson 2011, 1030).

27 Of course, they are not immorally free-riding. It is not unfair for them to benefit from herd immunity without contributing to it, since there is no rea-sonable method by which such people could contribute to herd immunity. Vaccinated vulnerable people may be treated *unfairly* by vaccine refusers, since people who vaccinate but do not develop individual immunity have done what they can to contribute to herd immunity. Indeed, free-riding on herd immunity may be *more unfair* to vaccinated people who fail to develop individual immunity, since these people paid all of the private costs of vacci-nation (e.g. risks of complications) without enjoying any of the private benefits (e.g. individual immunity).

28 The duty to avoid infecting other people has limits. As Verweij observes, we do not have to lock ourselves in our homes to avoid infecting people (Verweij 2005). Instead, the duty to avoid infecting others requires only that we take reasonable steps to avoid getting people ill. I take for granted that vaccination is such a reasonable step.

29 Thanks to Karl Martin Adam for pushing me on this point.

30 Margulis claims that views were misrepresented on the *Frontline* episode, since she does vaccinate her children against a handful of diseases (Margulis 2010). But the fact that she vaccinates her children against some diseases does not protect her from being criticized for her indifference to the harms vaccine refusal may cause. For a similar quote, see Habakus and Holland (2011, 1).

31 See Dare: "Perhaps it will seem, however, that even if the unimmunised do threaten harm to others, it will only be to those who have 'consented' to that risk by themselves choosing not to immunise" (Dare 1998, 140).

32 And it is just false to claim, as Fisher does, that vaccine proponents have "touted" vaccines to be (1) safe for all to receive, (2) effective at producing individual immunity for all who receive them, or (3) sufficient protection against the systemic harms that could result from the mass vaccine refusal of others.

33 For a psychological account of this phenomenon, see Friesen et al. (2014).

Bibliography

Albert, Michael R., Kristen G. Ostheimer, and Joel G. Breman. 2001. "The Last Smallpox Epidemic in Boston and the Vaccination Controversy, 1901–1903." *New England Journal of Medicine* 344(5): 375–379.

American Academy of Pediatrics. 2012. "Recommended Childhood and Adoles-cent Immunization Schedules – United States, 2012." *Pediatrics* 129(2): 385–386.

Arneson, R. J. 1982. "The Principle of Fairness and Free-Rider Problems." *Ethics* 92(4): 616–633.

Biss, Eula. 2013. "Sentimental Medicine." *Harper's Magazine*, January, 33–40.

Biss, Eula. 2014. *On Immunity: An Inoculation.* Graywolf Press.

Boran, I. 2006. "Benefits, Intentions, and the Principle of Fairness." *Canadian Journal of Philosophy* 36(1): 95–115.

Caplan, Arthur. 2011. "Vaccination: Facts Alone Do Not Policy Make." *Health Affairs* 30(6): 1205–1208. doi:10.1377/hlthaff.2011.0472.

Cave, Stephanie, and Deborah R. Mitchell. 2010. *What Your Doctor May Not Tell You About Children's Vaccinations.* Wellness Central.

Centers for Disease Control and Prevention. 2011. *General Recommendations on Immunization.* Centers for Disease Control and Prevention. Accessed June 17, 2015. www.cdc.gov/mmwr/preview/mmwrhtml/rr6002a1.htm.

Centers for Disease Control and Prevention. 2012. "Vaccines: Pubs/VIS/Fact Sheet." January 20. www.cdc.gov/vaccines/pubs/vis/vis-facts.htm.

Colgrove, James Keith. 2004. "Between Persuasion and Compulsion: Smallpox Control in Brooklyn and New York, 1894–1902." *Bulletin of the History of Medicine* 78(2): 349–378.

Cooper-Patrick, L. 1999. "Race, Gender, and Partnership in the Patient-Physician Relationship." *JAMA: The Journal of the American Medical Association* 282(6): 583–589. doi:10.1001/jama.282.6.583.

Coulter, H. 1991. *A Shot in the Dark.* Avery Trade.

Cullity, G. 1995. "Moral Free Riding." *Philosophy & Public Affairs* 24(1): 3–34.

Cullity, G. 2008. "Public Goods and Fairness." *Australasian Journal of Philosophy* 86(1): 1–21.

Dare, Tim. 1998. "Mass Immunisation Programmes: Some Philosophical Issues." *Bioethics* 12(2): 125–149.

Dawson, Angus. 2007. "Herd Protection as a Public Good: Vaccination and Our Obligations to Others." In *Ethics, Prevention, and Public Health*, edited by Angus Dawson and Marcel Verweij, 160–178. Clarendon Press.

Dawson, Angus. 2011. "The Moral Case for the Routine Vaccination of Children in Developed and Developing Countries." *Health Affairs* 30(6): 1029–1033.

English, A., F. E. Shaw, M. M. McCauley, D. B. Fishbein, and others. 2008. "Legal Basis of Consent for Health Care and Vaccination for Adolescents." *Pediatrics* 121 (Supplement 1): S85–87.

Ferguson, N. M., D. A. T. Cummings, C. Fraser, J. C. Cajka, P. C. Cooley, and D. S. Burke. 2006. "Strategies for Mitigating an Influenza Pandemic." *Nature* 442(7101): 448–452.

Field, Robert I., and Arthur L. Caplan. 2008. "A Proposed Ethical Framework for Vaccine Mandates: Competing Values and the Case of HPV." *Kennedy Institute of Ethics Journal* 18(2): 111–124.

Field, Robert I., and Arthur L. Caplan. 2012. "Evidence-Based Decision Making for Vaccines: The Need for an Ethical Foundation." *Vaccine* 30(6): 1009–1013. doi:10.1016/j.vaccine.2011.12.053.

Fine, P. E. M., and J. A. Clarkson. 1986. "Individual versus Public Priorities in the Determination of Optimal Vaccination Policies." *American Journal of Epidemiology* 124(6): 1012–1020.

Friesen, J. P., T. H. Campbell, and A. C. Kay. 2014. "The Psychological Advantage of Unfalsifiability: The Appeal of Untestable Religious and Political Ideologies." *Journal of Personality and Social Psychology* 108(3): 515–529.

Greene, Joshua. 2013. *Moral Tribes: Emotion, Reason and the Gap between Us and Them.* Atlantic Books.

Grubeck-Loebenstein, B., S. Della Bella, A. M. Iorio, J. P. Michel, G. Pawelec, R. Solana, and others. 2009. "Immunosenescence and Vaccine Failure in the Elderly." *Aging Clinical and Experimental Research* 21(3): 201–209.

Habakus, Louise Kuo, and Mary Holland. 2011. *Vaccine Epidemic: How Corporate Greed, Biased Science, and Coercive Government Threaten Our Human Rights, Our Health, and Our Children*. Skyhorse Publishing.

Hershey, John C., David A. Asch, Thi Thumasathit, Jacqueline Meszaros, and Victor V. Waters. 1994. "The Roles of Altruism, Free Riding, and Bandwagoning in Vaccination Decisions." *Organizational Behavior and Human Decision Processes* 59(2): 177–187. doi:10.1006/obhd.1994.1055.

Hoven, Mariëtte van den. 2012. "Why One Should Do One's Bit: Thinking about Free Riding in the Context of Public Health Ethics." *Public Health Ethics* 5(2): 154–160. doi:10.1093/phe/phs023.

Kant, Immanuel. 1998. *Groundwork of the Metaphysics of Morals*. Edited by Mary Gregor. Cambridge University Press.

Kata, Anna. 2012. "Anti-Vaccine Activists, Web 2.0, and the Postmodern Paradigm – An Overview of Tactics and Tropes Used Online by the Anti-Vaccination Movement." *Vaccine* 30(25): 3778–3789.

Kirby, David. 2006. *Evidence of Harm: Mercury in Vaccines and the Autism Epidemic: A Medical Controversy*. St. Martin's Griffin.

Klosko, George. 1987. "Presumptive Benefit, Fairness, and Political Obligation." *Philosophy & Public Affairs* 16(3): 241–259.

Knox, Richard. 2010. "Measles Resurgence Tied to Parents' Vaccine Fears." NPR. Accessed June 17, 2015. www.npr.org/templates/story/story.php?storyId=125570056.

Lareau, Annette. 2003. *Unequal Childhoods: Class, Race, and Family Life*. University of California Press.

Largent, M. A. 2012. *Vaccine: The Debate in Modern America*. Johns Hopkins University Press.

Last, John M. 1987. *Public Health and Human Ecology*. Appleton and Lange.

Leach, Melissa, and James Fairhead. 2007. *Vaccine Anxieties: Global Science, Child Health and Society*. Routledge.

Longini, I. M., A. Nizam, S. Xu, K. Ungchusak, W. Hanshaoworakul, D. A. T. Cummings, and M. E. Halloran. 2005. "Containing Pandemic Influenza at the Source." *Science* 309(5737): 1083.

Margulis, Jennifer. 2010. "Letter from Jennifer Margulis." *Frontline*. May 17. www.pbs.org/wgbh/pages/frontline/vaccines/etc/margulis.html.

Michaels, David. 2008. *Doubt Is Their Product: How Industry's Assault on Science Threatens Your Health*. Oxford University Press.

Mill, John Stuart. 2002. *Utilitarianism*. Edited by George Sher. 2nd ed. Hackett Publishing Company.

Mnookin, Seth. 2011. "Is 'Dr. Bob' Sears Moving Away from His Profitable Anti-Vaccine Pandering?" *The Panic Virus*. June 3. http://blogs.plos.org/thepanicvirus/2011/06/03/is-dr-bob-sears-moving-away-from-his-profitable-anti-vaccine-pandering/.

Murphy, Jamie. 1993. *What Every Parent Should Know About Childhood Immunization*. Edited by Carol White. Earth Healing Products.

National Foundation for Infectious Diseases. 2012. "10 Reasons to Be Vaccinated." Accessed August 7. www.adultvaccination.org/10-reasons-to-be-vaccinated.

Nelson, Kendall, and Chris Pilaro. 2011. *The Greater Good*. BNP Pictures.

Nozick, R. 1974. *Anarchy, State, and Utopia*. Basic Books.

Offit, Paul A. 2010. *Deadly Choices: How the Anti-Vaccine Movement Threatens Us All*. Basic Books.

Offit, Paul A., and Charlotte A. Moser. 2009. "The Problem with Dr Bob's Alternative Vaccine Schedule." *Pediatrics* 123(1): e164–169. doi:10.1542/peds.2008-2189.

Oreskes, Naomi, and Erik M. Conway. 2011. *Merchants of Doubt: How a Handful of Scientists Obscured the Truth on Issues from Tobacco Smoke to Global Warming.* Bloomsbury Press.

Palfreman, John. 2010. "The Vaccine War." *Frontline.* PBS. www.pbs.org/wgbh/pages/frontline/vaccines/view/.

Parikh, Rahul K. 2010. "Face-off with the Bestselling Vaccine Guru." *Salon.com.* October 13. www.salon.com/2010/10/13/vaccine_book_sears/.

Rawls, John. 1999. *A Theory of Justice.* Rev. ed. Belknap Press of Harvard University Press.

Roter, D. L., M. Stewart, S. M. Putnam, M. Lipkin, W. Stiles, and T. S. Inui. 1997. "Communication Patterns of Primary Care Physicians." *JAMA: The Journal of the American Medical Association* 277(4): 350–356. doi:10.1001/jama.1997.03540280088045.

Sears, R. 2007. *The Vaccine Book: Making the Right Decision for Your Child.* Little, Brown and Company.

Sen, A. K. 2009. *The Idea of Justice.* Harvard University Press.

Sidgwick, Henry. 1981. *The Methods of Ethics.* 7th Edition. Hackett Publishing Company.

Smith, Adam. 2002. *Adam Smith: The Theory of Moral Sentiments.* Edited by Knud Haakonssen. Cambridge University Press.

Spier, R. E. 1998. "Ethical Aspects of Vaccines and Vaccination." *Vaccine* 16(19): 1788–1794.

Stern, A. M., and H. Markel. 2008. "Influenza Pandemic." In *From Birth to Death and Bench to Clinic: The Hastings Center Bioethics Briefing Book for Journalists, Policymakers, and Campaigns,* 89–92. The Hastings Center.

Sugerman, David E., Albert E. Barskey, Maryann G. Delea, Ismael R. Ortega-Sanchez, Daoling Bi, Kimberly J. Ralston, Paul A. Rota, Karen Waters-Montijo, and Charles W. LeBaron. 2010. "Measles Outbreak in a Highly Vaccinated Population, San Diego, 2008: Role of the Intentionally Undervaccinated." *Pediatrics* 125(4): 747–55.

Tenpenny, Sherri J. 2008. *Saying No to Vaccines: A Resource Guide for All Ages.* Edited by NMA Media Press. NMA Media Press.

Vermeersch, E. 1999. "Individual Rights versus Societal Duties." *Vaccine* (Supplement 17(3)): S14–17.

Verweij, Marcel. 2005. "Obligatory Precautions against Infection." *Bioethics* 19(4): 323–335.

Wakefield, Andrew J. 2011. *Callous Disregard: Autisms and Vaccines: The Truth Behind a Tragedy.* Skyhorse Publishing.

Williams, Bernard. 1981. *Moral Luck.* Cambridge University Press.

Woo, Michelle. 2012. "Dr. Robert Sears Takes on Both Sides of the Great Vaccination Divide." *OC Weekly,* August 9. www.ocweekly.com/2012-08-09/news/doctor-robert-sears-vaccine-debate/.

5 Coercive vaccination

"In America, vaccination is the first act the state requires of a person; without it, or a legal exemption, a kid can't even get into nursery school."

(Allen 2007, 15)

If most people acted on the basis of the moral duties I discussed in the previous chapter, we might not have to consider using state coercion to ensure mass vaccination. Like Angus Dawson, I think "something has gone wrong" when we have to talk about whether the government should use force to promote public health (Dawson 2011, 151).[1] But something has gone wrong, as much of my discussion in earlier chapters indicates. So we should reflect on whether the state may use coercion to ensure mass vaccination, since coercion may be the only way to achieve that goal. Of course, we should not take coercion lightly. There are weighty *pro tanto* reasons against it: Coercion constrains liberty, undermines autonomy, and often causes psychological harms. We do not have to be students of history to know that state power can be oppressive. Even so, state coercion may be permitted when it is necessary to achieve especially valuable political goals. But we should permit only as much coercion as is necessary, and we should prefer less coercive measures whenever they are effective.

The political arguments I make in this chapter sometimes overlap with the moral arguments I made in the last chapter. But it does not follow from the fact that vaccination is required by morality that the state may coerce people to be vaccinated. One reason to resist reducing political justice to morality is because the state is in principle unable to ensure that people act morally. The state acts by externally coercing the members of society – by compelling them to act in particular ways or by seizing some of their property for public purposes. But external coercion is insufficient to guarantee morality, since the state is unable to directly compel me to cultivate virtuous character traits or to act for moral intentions. Another reason to treat questions about permissible state coercion as a separate subject from interpersonal morality is because political justice has a different purpose. Political justice focuses on the use of state power to promote safety and security, and to establish stable conditions for cooperative behavior. These are not the primary tasks of interpersonal morality, and so they require their own set of justificatory principles.

How should we identify principles for the permissible use of state coercion to promote vaccination? One way to proceed is to try to identify a *true* theory of justice. We might consider which political principles would best protect individual liberties, or promote well-being, or do whatever else we think justice requires. And we could go on to identify the liberties the state ought to protect, or the conception of well-being the state ought to promote, or whatever other goods our theory of justice requires the state to be concerned about. Then, we could show that state coercion to ensure mass vaccination is (or is not) consistent with these true principles of justice. For example, if we were committed to a Utilitarianism theory of justice, then we could defend a legal obligation to vaccinate by showing that coercive vaccination programs sometimes promote better outcomes than voluntary vaccination programs.

I do not think we should try to justify coercive vaccination by appealing to one true theory of justice. This is because rules that govern political life ought to be, in some sense, acceptable or justifiable to the people who are coerced by those rules, and because no one theory of justice is likely to be acceptable to all members of a pluralistic society.[2] Here, I endorse *public reason liberalism*, a tradition that has its origins in the work of Hobbes, Rousseau, and Kant; but that has found more recent defenders in John Rawls and Gerald Gaus, among many others. As is the case for any interesting view, there are many versions of public reason liberalism. I will try to keep my discussion as general as possible, and I hope that what I sacrifice in specificity is made up for with greater clarity.

One reason public reason liberals believe that political rules should be acceptable or justifiable to the people who are coerced by those rules is because they think people are free when they are governed only by laws they give to themselves. But more generally, public reason liberals think that we cannot respect people as moral persons if we use only threats of force to get them to conform to laws. We must also be able to give people reasons they could (or should) accept for why state coercion may be used against them. But – and here is a key point – it is unreasonable to expect everyone to endorse one true theory of justice. Reasonable people disagree about fundamental moral, political, and religious values; and this disagreement seems intractable under anything like current conditions. (This is what Rawls calls the 'fact of reasonable pluralism' (Rawls 2005, 36–37).) Of course, we might be able to structure society so that everyone would be led to support one true theory of justice, but this would likely require significant restrictions of fundamental liberties, e.g. freedoms of speech and religion, and liberal justice would prohibit exactly those sorts of restrictions. Therefore, we cannot justify coercion by invoking a common theory of justice, but instead we must support laws that people with diverse values and beliefs will have reasons to accept.

To be clear: Public reason justifications do not require universal consent. If they did, then we would be unable to justify coercive vaccination, since some people object to it. Most other forms of state coercion would be unjustified, too. Instead, we show that laws are justified by demonstrating that sufficiently *idealized* members of the community would accept them. And we idealize the members of the community by assuming that they have (reasonably) good information, that they have engaged in adequate reasoning about their views, and that they are sufficiently immune to selfishness or other forms of undue bias when they consider potential laws.[3] So, when we ask whether people have a reason to accept a law, we are inquiring whether they would accept that law if they had sufficiently good information, reasoning practices, and character traits.

My primary goal in this chapter is to show that coercive vaccination laws can be justified by general political principles that diverse members of society have reasons to accept. In particular, I argue that people with diverse moral, political, and religious views should agree that the state may (1) intervene in family life to protect children's fundamental interests, (2) prevent people from causing significant harms to others, and (3) ensure the fair distribution of the costs of valuable social programs. It is possible that some people may have a reason to reject one of these general principles, though this would depend on how much we idealized people for the purposes of public justification – and this is something that public reason liberals disagree about. For example, someone committed to an expansive conception of parental rights may have a reason to reject (1), and a libertarian may have a reason to reject (a version of) (3). But I argue that both of these people have reasons to endorse other principles that can justify coercive vaccination. The defender of expansive parents' rights has a reason to accept (2) and (3), while the libertarian has a reason to accept (2), and maybe (1). But these are outliers. Most members of society have a reason to accept all three principles.

The majority of this chapter focuses on the sorts of reasons people have for accepting the three general principles for state coercion that I argue can justify coercive vaccination. But there is a gap in my argument and I will try to fill some of it here. (Some of the gap will remain unfilled, which will lead to the next chapter's discussion of *exemptions* to coercive vaccination laws.) Consider that some people have factual beliefs that prevent them from agreeing that coercive vaccination laws protect children's interests, or prevent people from harming each other, or ensure the fair distribution of the costs of social cooperation. Other people may have normative commitments that lead them to reject vaccination, and they think these normative commitments trump the three general principles I will defend. People with these factual beliefs or normative commitments have a reason to accept my three general principles of permissible state coercion, but they do not think these principles justify coercive vaccination laws. This is because they think vaccines are ineffective at generating individual immunity, or cause very high rates of complications, or are otherwise unsafe, unnecessary, or immoral. Do these people have a reason to support coercive vaccination laws?

When we idealize members of the community – when we ask whether they would accept laws under better epistemic and moral conditions – we may assume that they have true beliefs about widely known consensus scientific views and that they have reasoned about scientific views in relatively epistemically virtuous ways. This means that someone who is a vaccine denialist because he is committed to pseudo-skeptical conspiracy thinking does not thereby have a reason to reject coercive vaccination laws.[4] But what about the mothers I discussed in chapter one? I argued that they sometimes have good reasons to be skeptical of their pediatricians' testimony, and that they sometimes have good reasons for participating in resistant epistemic communities that encourage vaccine denialism and refusal. These mothers may seem to be a harder case. However, I argued that these vaccine denialist mothers are often committed to poor reasoning practices. For example, they fail to recognize differences in expertise and competence, and they try to avoid circumstances in which their views may be challenged. I think that once we idealize away these serious epistemic vices, many vaccine denialist mothers would agree that coercive vaccination laws are justified by the general principles I defend in this chapter.

I am not as confident about how to handle the case of parents who reject the *values* that vaccination policy is based on. For example, in chapter three I argued that some parents may reject vaccines because they think it is important for their children to avoid unnatural interventions, and because they think it is natural (and, therefore, not too problematic) for their children to be infected with vaccine-preventable diseases. These people may agree that the state is permitted to use coercion to protect children, to prevent harms, and to ensure fairness. But they don't think children need to be protected against infectious diseases, or that infectious diseases are very harmful to anyone else. They may also claim that herd immunity is not a valuable public good and, therefore, that there is no need to fairly distribute the costs of maintaining it. Another kind of parent may think that vaccine-preventable diseases are very bad, but she may think that God commands her not to vaccinate, and she may think that it is far worse to violate God's commands than for her child to be at a higher risk of infection from vaccine-preventable diseases. In all of these cases – of value-based vaccine refusal – it is not obvious that moderate idealization would suffice to get parents to agree that they have reasons to vaccinate. Religious and secular values may sometimes be reasonable bases for rejecting public laws.

We might respond that the fact that coercive vaccination laws coerce *children* complicates matters. Even though an adult's values may give him reasons to reject laws that would coerce him, it's not as clear that a parent's values always give him reasons to reject laws that would coerce his child. Indeed, my discussion in the next section addresses the justification of expansive parental rights.

Before moving on, it may help to say something quickly about what I mean by 'coercion'. Forcible constraint is clearly coercive, but other uses of state power to influence behavior can be coercive, too. In particular, I think it is coercive for the state to bar children from school or daycare if their parents do not vaccinate their children. (Here, then, I treat some forms of state 'manipulation' as forms of coercion.) In contrast, I think it may be non-coercive for the state to use deliberation and emotional appeals to try to get someone to act in a particular way. Of course, there are likely to be intermediate cases about which we may not have clear intuitions, e.g. conditional offers that it may be difficult to refuse. But for my purposes it does not much matter where the line between coercion and non-coercion is drawn, since I will argue that some clear cases of coercive vaccination are justified, but that less coercive (and, indeed, non-coercive) measures are preferable when they are effective.[5] (In the concluding section of this chapter, I survey a spectrum of more and less coercive vaccination policies.)

Against coercion: informed consent and parents' rights

Two important values may seem to ground a definitive rejection of coercive vaccination policies: *informed consent* and *parents' rights*.

First, using state power to ensure mass vaccination may seem to violate the fundamental bioethical ideal of informed consent. Coercing a person into medical treatment is widely considered to be a violation of human dignity (and human rights), since patients have a right to make informed decisions about their medical care, and since they have a human right to be free from non-consensual medical treatment. For example, the UN Committee on Economic, Social and Cultural Rights has found that the right to health identified in the International Convention on Economic, Social and Cultural Rights includes "the right to control one's health and body ... such as the right to be free from torture, non-consensual medical treatment and experimentation" (UN Committee on Economic, Social and Cultural Rights 2001, 130). Since vaccination is a form of medical treatment, coercive vaccination may seem to violate human dignity and human rights.

Vaccine refusers often invoke the ideal of informed consent to defend their right to refuse vaccines (Fisher 1997). And they sometimes compare coercive vaccination programs to prominent historical examples of coercive medical treatment and experimentation. For example, Vera Sharav argues that coercive mass vaccination and Nazi medical experiments show a similar disregard for human rights (Sharav 2011). In her view, both of these practices are (or were) efforts to promote a 'greater good' through massive violations of informed consent. Another vaccine refuser invokes a contemporary example: Richard Rovet compares coercive mass vaccination programs to the American torture of prisoners at the Abu Ghraib prison in Iraq (Rovet 2011).

I think this sort of objection goes astray because vaccination is not merely a personal medical treatment. Vaccination prevents individuals from becoming ill, but it is also a means by which people may make a fair contribution to public goods and by which they may prevent themselves from harming others. As Jessica Flanigan argues (following Onora O'Neill), "the principle of informed consent does not go so far as to justify harming others with one's medical choices" (Flanigan 2014, 17; O'Neill 2004). Furthermore, as Margaret Battin et al. observe, patients are not only victims of disease; they are also disease vectors (Battin et al. 2009).[6] This means that we cannot simply apply the bioethical principles that are appropriate to medical treatment to the case of vaccination. To be clear: The mere fact that people with contagious diseases are both victims and vectors does not justify coercive vaccination. But it means that we cannot invoke 'informed consent' and quickly conclude that coercive vaccination is unjustified.

The value of informed consent may seem out of place in discussions about *childhood* vaccines. Infants and very young children are not capable of informed consent. Instead, we generally allow parents to make health care decisions for their children. So, if informed consent matters in the case of childhood vaccines, it is because parents have a right to informed consent regarding their children's medical treatments. But this raises a question about the role parents ought to play in decisions about their children's health care, and it points us to another claim that is popular among vaccine refusers: Parents have the right to decide whether their children get vaccinated.

Some vaccine refusers invoke an expansive conception of parental rights and make common cause with participants in broader movements aimed at protecting the internal norms and practices of the family from government interference.[7] One group with which vaccine refusers have sometimes worked is *Parentalrights.org*. This is a high-powered non-governmental organization. Its leadership includes Grover Norquist, the president of the influential Americans for Tax Reform.[8] *Parentalrights.org* and other organizations have used their political sway to prevent the United States from ratifying the United Nations Convention on the Rights of the Child (UNCRC). This convention identifies a minimal set of children's rights (including a right to health care) as worthy of protection by the state. It has been ratified, accepted, or acceded to by every member state of the United Nations, *except for Somalia, South Sudan, and the United States* (United Nations 2015).[9] According to the extreme version of parents' rights that has led the United States to reject the UNCRC, it may seem like state coercion of childhood vaccination should be ruled out without further consideration.

In response, I think it's unlikely that any more than a few of the most radical parents' rights advocates entirely reject legal interventions in family life. In the case of the movement to reject the UNCRC, most of the concern seems limited to protecting parents' rights to raise their children in the family's religion, where this includes sending them to private schools or using homeschooling methods (Farris 2009). Even the critics of the UNCRC likely believe that the law may sometimes intervene in family life. Consider the views of Murray Rothbard, a prominent 20th-century libertarian scholar and activist, who had a famously expansive conception of parents' rights. Rothbard thought that "the parent should have the legal right not to feed the child, i.e., to allow it to die" (Rothbard 2002, 100). But even Rothbard thought that the law could sometimes get involved in family life. For example, he said that "the parent ... may not murder or mutilate his child, and the law properly outlaws a parent from doing so" (Rothbard 2002, 100). I assume that most parents' rights advocates embrace an even larger scope for legitimate state involvement in family life than does Rothbard. But this means that even people who are sympathetic to claims about parents' rights should not quickly conclude that coercive vaccination is unjustified, without first considering whether vaccination choices fall in the scope of the state's legitimate exercise of coercion in the family.

Paternalism

Many laws have paternalistic aims. It is illegal to purchase and use some dangerous drugs; other drugs are legal but restricted or heavily taxed. In 2012, New York City tried to ban the sale of sweetened drinks in containers larger than sixteen ounces. And many communities require motorcyclists to wear helmets. (These are often controversial laws – and for good reason – as I discuss below.) The state intervenes more frequently, and more significantly, to protect the interests of children. States may require school attendance, impose curfews, and mandate child car seats.[10]

Paternalism exists when one agent restrains the liberty of another agent, without the second agent's consent, for the purpose of promoting the welfare of the second agent (Dworkin 2014). Paternalism is at best a weak reason to coerce *adults*. This is because adults should usually have a legal right to act in ways that cause themselves harm, as long as they do not harm others or otherwise violate the demands of social justice. John Stuart Mill famously wrote that

> [A person's] own good, either physical or moral, is not a sufficient warrant [for state coercion]. He cannot rightfully be compelled to do or forbear because it will be better for him to do so, because it will make him happier, because, in the opinion of others, to do so would be wise, or even right.
>
> (Mill 1998a, I.9)

Mill embraced anti-paternalism as a consequence of his Utilitarian liberalism. Mill believed individuals care more about making their lives go well than the government does. He also supposed that individuals generally know more about what will make them happy.[11] Furthermore, Mill believed that a self-directed life (one that manifests what he called 'individuality') is, in itself, a happier life than one that is directed by outside forces (Mill 1998a, III).

Anti-paternalism is not limited to Utilitarian liberalism. For example, Immanuel Kant wrote that

> *paternalistic government* (*imperium paternale*), in which the subjects, like minor children who cannot distinguish between what is truly useful or harmful to them, are constrained to behave only passively, so as to wait upon the judgment of the head of state as to how they *should be* happy ... is the greatest *despotism* thinkable.
> (Kant 1996, 8: 290–291, emphasis in original)

Kant grounded his rejection of paternalism in a fundamental commitment to the value of autonomy – a way of life that is governed by rules that one gives to oneself. This way of life is impossible when the state uses coercion to try to make the lives of its citizens go well. There are many other flavors of liberalism, but a resistance to (at least some kinds of) paternalism is a central feature of them all.

Some people think we should allow paternalistic state constraint of adult behavior when people are not acting fully voluntarily. This is what Joel Feinberg has called 'soft paternalism' (Feinberg 1986). Soft paternalism constrains people only to ensure that their potentially self-harmful choices are voluntary and sufficiently well-informed. The classic case is John Stuart Mill's example of a person who is about to cross an unsafe bridge. Mill says that we may "seize him and turn him back, without any real infringement of his liberty; for liberty consists in doing what one desires, and he does not desire to fall into the river" (Mill 1998a, V.5).[12] Soft paternalism may count in favor of requiring vaccine refusers to attend education sessions about vaccines, such as the ones that Michigan has recently required for parents who want their children to be exempted from mandatory school immunization requirements. But soft paternalism is unlikely to count in favor of mandatory school immunization requirements, since these do more than try to ensure that people are well-informed about the choices they make. Paternalistic justifications of mandatory school vaccinations will have to appeal to the value of *strong* paternalism, i.e. paternalism that uses state power to interfere with the ends that people have chosen.

Strong paternalism is not a weighty reason to constrain the activities of adults, but it is a weighty reason to constrain the activities of *children*, and to constrain what parents and others may do to children.[13] A child has less claim than an adult to make self-destructive choices.[14] Children often lack the ability to use liberty in ways that contribute to their well-being, e.g. through deliberation and long-term planning. Children may also lack the rational capacities that are necessary for autonomous action. Instead, they are likely to use liberty to satisfy pre-reflective desires or instinctual drives. I acknowledge that some people who are technically children may have a moral right to liberty, even to pursue potentially imprudent choices. For example, if two sixteen-year-olds aim to engage in consensual sexual activity with each other, I do not think it is obvious that either the state or their parents have a right to forcibly prevent them from doing so. This is the case even though it may be imprudent for these sixteen-year-olds to have sex, and even though their parents (and others) may have a moral right to try to talk them out of it.

It is fortunate that we do not need to resolve questions about the demarcation between childhood and adulthood to consider whether paternalism counts in favor of the coercive vaccination of children. This is because the overwhelming majority of vaccines are routinely administered in the first four years of life, to people who are clearly children. Therefore, the relevant question is not *whether* one may treat vaccination-aged children paternalistically, but *who* is best suited to exercise paternalistic power over children in the context of vaccine decisions. Should it be parents or the state?

There are good reasons to defer to parents when it comes to the care of children. Parents are almost always in the best position to know what to do to help their children's lives go well. And they are usually more motivated to care for their children than other people are. Also, when we protect a large parental prerogative, we promote values – including intimacy, security, and spontaneity – that autonomous parent-child relationships often cultivate (Brighouse and Swift 2009).

The fact that there are good reasons for the state to defer to parents when it comes to the care of children does not mean that the family is a private association, or that it ought to be free from public accountability. Parents have a public responsibility to raise children to become free and equal citizens, and to protect their children's ongoing interests as moral persons, e.g. their interest in avoiding suffering (Brennan and Noggle 1997; Mill 1998b; Morse 1999; Okin 1989). When parents fail to achieve these central goals of parenthood, society has a right and a responsibility to intervene. Since children are future citizens, society has an obligation to ensure the conditions for children to develop political autonomy. If parents are not adequately preparing children to participate in social cooperation in a pluralistic liberal democratic society, then the state may need to interfere. For example, the state has an obligation to ensure that children receive a basic education that preserves their right to an 'open future' (Feinberg 1980). For example, even if the state permits homeschooling, it has a responsibility to ensure that homeschooling parents provide an education that is adequate to prepare children to become free and equal members of society. Second, children are moral persons (even if they are not yet citizens), and society has a responsibility to protect the welfare of moral persons (Brighouse 2002).[15] Ordinarily, parents are the best custodians of their children's welfare, but when they're not, society may intervene. For example, children have a moral right not to be physically or sexually abused. In serious cases, society has a responsibility to remove abused children from the custody of their parents.

How far must parents fall short before state intervention is justified? I do not know, but I will provide a partial response, on the hope that it may inform our thinking about paternalism-based reasons for the coercive vaccination of children. First, what is in children's interests cannot be determined by the beliefs of parents (Dawson 2005; Moran, Gainotti, and Petrini 2008). The fact that a parent believes that vaccine refusal is the best choice for her child does not mean that it is. Parents are not entitled to impose their own values (or their own 'facts') on their children, when doing so fails to adequately protect children's future and current interests. And children's interests are objective, even if they are sometimes context dependent. For example, it will count in favor of the claim that routine vaccination is in a child's interests if diseases are more prevalent or if "public health policy … is based upon assumptions that the welfare baseline of their citizens includes immunization" (Dare 1998, 140). I argued in chapters two and three that there may be reasonable disagreements about what is in children's interests. But it does not follow that the state must grant equal weight to all parental claims about children's interests. For example, parents who think that it is essential for children to eat a vegetarian or paleo diet have more reasonable conceptions of their children's well-being than parents who think it is good for children to get measles.

We are looking for a minimum standard, below which the care for children should not be allowed to fall, rather than a standard of optimal (or even good) parenting. The mere fact that one is not the best parent (or even a very good parent) is not enough reason for the state to intervene, nor is the fact that a parent's conception of a good childhood deviates somewhat from mainstream views. I do not know what should be the precise standard for paternalistic state intervention in family life, and I acknowledge that reasonable people may disagree. But, by way of a general principle, I offer the following, which I believe has some intuitive force:

> The state has a responsibility to prevent parents from placing their children at a significant risk of serious harm, if those risks can be avoided at a reasonable cost.[16]

For example, it seems obvious to me that the state should prevent parents from letting their children die of treatable disorders. It is unfortunate that courts and legislatures in the United States have often disagreed with me. Parents are regularly allowed to escape punishment for resisting medical care for their children, especially if they claim to do so for a religious reason (Antommaria et al. 2013; Asser and Swan 1998; Offit 2015). Milder cases of parental negligence warrant state intervention, too. For example, I think that a police officer (acting on behalf of the state) has an obligation to remove a child from the busy street where she finds the child playing, even if the child was allowed to play in the street by his parents. The police officer may place the child in her cruiser, bring the child back home to his parents, and insist that the child's parents not allow the child to play in the street in the future. These actions are not without risk. The police officer could have a serious automobile accident while driving the child home, causing the child to be injured or to die. But this is a reasonable risk, and I think that it is a risk that the state is allowed to impose on the child, in order to rescue him from the much more risky circumstances in which the policer officer found him.

Vaccine refusal may place a child at a significant risk of serious harm. Routine vaccination avoids that risk at a reasonable cost. On my view, parental refusal of routine vaccines is like letting a child play in a busy street, and coercive vaccination is like a police officer driving a child home.[17] Like parents who allow their children to play in busy streets, parents who do not vaccinate their children may fail to protect their children's future political autonomy and their current welfare. Accordingly, the state may use coercion to ensure vaccination, since doing so protects a child's interests, by protecting the child from serious diseases with only minimal risk of vaccine complications.

Many of the vaccines that children routinely receive offer protection against diseases that cause suffering, disability, and death. Children who are not vaccinated against these diseases are much more likely to suffer and die than are vaccinated children. For examples, non-vaccinated children are six times more likely to become infected with pertussis (whooping cough) and thirty-five times more likely to become infected with measles (Feikin et al. 2000; Salmon et al. 1999).

For some vaccines, paternalism may be the only moral reason that could justify coercive vaccination. Consider tetanus. This disease causes painful muscle spasms and, in some cases, death. Paternalism is a good reason to use coercion to ensure that children are vaccinated against tetanus. However, this disease is not contagious, so vaccination will not prevent people from infecting each other, since under ordinary conditions it is not possible to infect another person with tetanus. For this reason, herd immunity against tetanus is not nearly as valuable as herd immunity against contagious diseases would be. Finally, the tetanus bacterium, *Clostridium tetani*, is ubiquitous in the environment, and there is no hope of eradicating it. It follows that neither a commitment to prevent harm to others nor a commitment to fairly distribute the costs of herd immunity (or disease eradication efforts) will count in favor of using coercion to vaccinate against tetanus. If states are going to use coercion to ensure high vaccination rates for tetanus, they will have to justify their efforts in terms of paternalism.

But not all vaccines protect against diseases that are very harmful to healthy children. Children are routinely vaccinated against varicella (chicken pox), even though chicken pox almost always causes only mild symptoms to healthy children. However, chicken pox can be fatal for people with compromised immune systems. Rubella vaccination presents a similar case. Rubella usually causes only minor symptoms in children, but can cause significant harm to fetuses if pregnant women are exposed to rubella. Congenital Rubella Syndrome often causes deafness, vision problems, and heart disease. Accordingly, paternalism is a less weighty reason to coerce vaccination against chicken pox and rubella than it is for vaccinating against tetanus. Furthermore, if paternalism were the only reason to coerce vaccination against chicken pox and rubella, then coercive vaccination against these diseases would not generally be justified. However, there are other reasons to coerce vaccination against chicken pox and rubella, as I will discuss in later sections of this chapter.[18]

Even well-meaning parents sometimes fail to protect their children's best interests. Consider that the most common reason parents give for refusing the HPV vaccine is that their eleven-year-old children are 'too young' to get a vaccine against a sexually transmitted disease (Charo 2007). I suspect that some of these parents view their children only *as children*, and that they give insufficient consideration to the fact that a choice not to vaccinate may cause their children harm later in life. I understand. It is not easy for me to think that my children – ages four, six, and eight as I write this – are almost certain to have multiple sexual partners and that they may use intravenous drugs. Even when I can imagine these possibilities, I locate them in the far distant future. I suspect that any choices I would be forced to make based on these future possibilities would be hindered by my reluctance to dwell for long on the idea of my children engaging in sexual and drug-related activities. (Even writing these words causes me a negative visceral reaction.) I suspect my vulnerability to this sort of epistemic deficit is common among parents. If this tendency is widespread, then there is even more reason to place some choices about the care of children in the hands of the state. It may 'take a village' to know what is best for a child, even if parents are usually experts about their children, since parents may sometimes have a hard time making good choices for their children.

Preventing harm

The state often uses its power to restrain and punish people who harm each other. Assault is a crime, as is theft. And the state may force someone who defames you to pay damages. But the state does not only intervene after harms have occurred. It also uses coercion to prevent harms before they take place. For example, the state makes it illegal to drive at very high speeds, to own automatic weapons, or to sell rat poison as a food product.

Preventing harm is usually thought to be a paradigm case of permissible state coercion. John Stuart Mill famously said that preventing harm was "[t]he only purpose for which power can be rightfully exercised over any member of a civilized community, against his will" (Mill 1998a, IV.3). We do not have a moral right to harm others, regardless of whatever else our liberties entitle us to do. Furthermore, since harming people restricts their liberty, the state promotes liberty when it uses coercion to prevent harms. It restricts the liberty of a person who would harm another in order to protect the liberty of a person who would otherwise be harmed.

Many instances of state coercion could reduce my chances of harming other people, but not all of them are justified. For example, the state could prevent me from causing automobile accidents if it placed me under house arrest for the remainder of my life. But we would be right to object to this abuse of state power. I do not have a complete account of when states may use coercion to prevent harm, but the following has some intuitive appeal:

> The state may use coercion to prevent harms only when the harms prevented are serious, coercion significantly reduces the risk of harm, and coercion does not cause very bad side effects.[19]

First, the state should only use coercion to constrain acts that increase the risk of *serious* harms. For example, wearing sunglasses while walking in the city at night increases my risk of bumping into other pedestrians, but the state should not constrain my choices about nocturnal eyewear if bumping into other people is unlikely to cause them much harm. Second, a commitment to prevent harm could justify constraints only when those constraints *significantly* reduced the risk that others would be harmed. For example, suppose that the state could reduce automobile accident fatalities by 0.1% if it made it mandatory for all drivers to get eight hours of sleep each night. Such a small decrease in the risk of harm would not warrant dramatic interference in people's sleep schedules or driving practices.

Third, the state may constrain behavior in the name of preventing harm only when doing so is unlikely to generate large amounts of harmful side effects. For example, I take for granted that girls and boys are often harmed by being raised in families with especially patriarchal values (Mill 1998b; Okin 1989). These sorts of families often stunt the intellectual development of their girl children, and they distort the moral personalities of children of both sexes. For example, girls and boys from these families are likely to believe that the social subordination of women is natural or divinely ordained, and they are likely to have diminished capacities to participate as free and equal members of liberal democratic societies. But I don't think the state should outlaw patriarchal parenting or remove children from the care of parents who are committed to the social subordination of women, since these radical interventions in family life would likely cause serious political blowback and, ultimately, do more harm than good.

Many people have argued that the state may use coercion to promote vaccination, on the grounds that vaccine refusal may harm others. For example, Jessica Flanigan has recently defended the use of coercion to promote vaccination, since she thinks that vaccine refusal is like shooting bullets into the air, which is a harmful practice that the state may legitimately restrict (Flanigan 2014). Others also use the metaphor of gun violence to describe vaccine refusal, and they invoke the permissibility of constraints on firearms as a reason to use coercion to promote vaccination (see e.g. Francis et al. 2005).[20] Even though WHO endorses a presumption in favor of voluntary vaccination, it endorses coercive vaccination when doing so will "prevent a concrete and serious harm" (Moodley et al. 2013; quoting Verweij and Dawson 2004).

Vaccination often meets the three conditions I identified above for using state coercion to prevent harms. First, unvaccinated people may cause *serious harms* to others. These harms include death, permanent disability, pain, and the many other costs and inconveniences associated with illness. Unvaccinated people also contribute to broader outbreaks, which cause diminished public trust, economic losses, and many other social and political harms. Second, vaccination significantly *reduces the odds* that one will harm others. Vaccinated people are far less likely to infect other people because they, themselves, are far less likely to become infected.

Third, vaccine complications are infrequent and usually mild, and the most serious vaccine complications are extremely rare. But vaccine complications are not the only potential negative side effects of coercive vaccination programs. Some parents may be so resistant to vaccination that they are willing to pull their children out of school rather than have them vaccinated. Other parents may be initially indifferent to childhood vaccination, but they may be so opposed to *coercive* medical interventions that they become vaccine refusers. In the next chapter I discuss these (and other) reasons to permit some parents to be *exempted* from vaccine mandates. For now, the important point is that worries about parental blowback do not count against coercive vaccination programs, per se, since these bad side effects are limited to relatively few families, and since selective exemption programs may allow us to avoid bad side effects even in these cases.

Arguments in favor of coercive vaccination for the purpose of preventing harm need to be disease specific. For example, as I discussed earlier, tetanus is not contagious. Therefore, a commitment to prevent people from harming each other does *not* count in favor of using coercion to vaccinate against tetanus. In contrast, measles is extremely contagious and harmful. A commitment to prevent people from harming each other does count in favor of using coercion to vaccinate against measles.

Criminal or civil liability

Some people have argued that it should be a crime or a tort when vaccine refusers (or, rather, their unvaccinated children) infect people (Caplan 2013; Caplan et al. 2012; Lipinski 2013; Reiss 2013; Stewart 2009). For example, Art Caplan says:

> I can choose to drink but if I run you over it is my responsibility. I can choose not to shovel the snow from my walk but if you fall I pay. Why should failing to vaccinate your children or yourself be any different?
>
> (Caplan 2013)

Caplan argues that the law ought to hold vaccine refusers accountable for negligently infecting people, just as the law holds people accountable for other harms they avoidably cause. This is a bold claim, since we ordinarily think that getting someone sick is a non-culpable accident, rather than an occasion of a tort or a crime. It may seem unreasonable for the government to prosecute you (or for your fellow citizens to sue you) just because you gave someone an illness. We have social norms about covering up coughs and sneezes, but we do not usually think that a failure to abide by social norms is sufficient to make you liable to punishment or reparations.

Vaccine refusal complicates matters. Vaccines are a low-risk means by which people may significantly reduce their odds of causing serious harms to others. In a similar way, driving sober is a low-risk means of significantly reducing the odds of causing dangerous automobile accidents. In the case of drunk driving, we allow the criminal and civil law to hold people accountable for the harms that result from their negligence. I think Caplan and others are right to argue that similar reasoning may apply in the case of vaccine refusers.

Making vaccine refusers criminally or civilly liable for infecting people with vaccine-preventable diseases may incentivize vaccination. If people know that they will be held accountable for the harmful consequences of their negligent vaccine refusal, then they may be more likely to vaccinate. We might wonder whether this incentive would be sufficient to make coercive vaccination unnecessary. Perhaps we could ensure high rates of vaccination, even in the absence of coercive vaccination programs, by expanding criminal and civil liability for vaccine refusers. Consider that the state does not require drivers to pass a breathalyzer test each time they get behind the wheel, nor does the state send the police to your house to ensure you shovel on snowy days. In a similar way, perhaps we could make vaccination voluntary, but hold vaccine refusers responsible for the harms they cause?

I agree that increased criminal and civil liability for vaccine refusers is a good idea, but I think it is unlikely to be able to replace other instances of state coercion, e.g. school immunization mandates.[21] First, it is doubtful whether epidemiologists will be able to identify who has infected whom during disease outbreaks, or that they will be able to do so with the sort of precision and reliability that would be necessary for that information to serve as evidence in criminal or civil proceedings (Ciolli 2008; Rubin and Kasimow 2009). However, even if epidemiology could adequately establish responsibility for infections, it would likely be able to do so only in cases with few possible disease vectors (Caplan et al. 2012). For example, it is much easier to identify the cause of a child's measles infection when she has been exposed only to one or two people who have had measles. If she were exposed to dozens of people it would be (nearly) impossible to determine who had infected her. Therefore, societies are less likely to be able to use the law to hold people responsible for infecting other people in the context of large disease outbreaks.[22] But during outbreaks the state needs as many tools as possible to constrain vaccine refusal. Furthermore, only the wealthiest litigants in civil trials would likely be able to afford to bring the relevant epidemiological evidence to bear on their behalf, since in civil trials litigants finance their lawsuits, and they are not usually able to use the resources of the state to gather evidence. The general epistemic problem therefore entails a moral problem: Only a privileged few would be able to receive redress for the harms that vaccine refusers caused them. (Of course, if it were a crime to infect someone, the state would bear the burden of collecting the relevant evidence.)

I also have a general worry about prioritizing compensation over coercive prevention. If the fact that the law can punish or otherwise hold accountable someone who negligently harms another is a reason for the state not to use coercion to prevent harms, then we may have reason to discard many legal forms of *ex ante* coercion which seem to be justified by a commitment to preventing harms. These include coercive safety standards for workplaces, commercial food preparation, and manufactured goods. They also include laws preventing unlicensed persons from driving cars or practicing medicine, and legal prohibitions on the ownership of machine guns and armored assault vehicles. But the fact that I can sue a quack for injuring my body or the owner of a filthy restaurant for making me sick does not count against the coercive imposition of safety standards for medical or food service businesses. Likewise, the fact that I may be able to sue someone who infects my infant with measles does not count against coercive vaccination aimed at preventing that person from infecting my infant in the first place.

Fairness

The state often uses its power to ensure that members of society make fair contributions to public efforts. Taxes finance the activities of the state; they are not voluntary. Conscription supports public safety; it is coercive. The state promotes clean air and unpolluted space by making it illegal for individuals to smoke or for businesses to release industrial byproducts into the air and water. The idea of fair play – of society as a fair system of cooperation among free and equal members – points us towards an equitable distribution of the burdens of community life. Importantly, fairness is distinct from harm prevention, since it is sometimes possible to make unfair use of shared goods without harming others. For example, if I do not pay my tax bill, my choice will have almost no effect on my government's ability to operate. My US federal income tax payments amount to only about one one-billionth of the US federal government's revenue. No one is going to be harmed if I don't pay my taxes (if I can get away with it). But it would be unfair for me to enjoy the benefits of being a member of US society – benefits that others have paid for – without doing my part. One reason to make taxation coercive is to ensure that the costs of valuable public programs are fairly distributed, even when doing so does little to prevent harm.

John Stuart Mill agreed that the state is permitted to coerce people to contribute to public projects:

> [E]very one who receives the protection of society owes a return for the benefit, and the fact of living in society renders it indispensable that each should be bound to observe a certain line of conduct towards the rest. This conduct consists, *first*, in not injuring the interests of one another; or rather certain interests, which, either by express legal provision or by tacit understanding, ought to be considered as rights; and *secondly*, in each person's bearing his share (to be fixed on some equitable principle) of the labors and sacrifices incurred for defending the society or its members from injury and molestation.
>
> (Mill 1998a, IV.3, emphasis added)

Mill identifies two distinct political duties: non-malfeasance and contributions to efforts aimed at protecting people from various harms or bad circumstances. To be clear, Mill is not talking merely about moral duties, but personal principles of justice which the state may enforce. Mill says that "[t]hese conditions society is justified in enforcing, at all costs to those who endeavor to withhold fulfilment" (Mill 1998a, IV.3). On such a view, making a fair contribution to public projects is not only morally right but legally obligatory.

Even though the duties of fairness and non-malfeasance are distinct, we may sometimes harm people through a failure to make a fair contribution.

If one's non-contribution compromises community projects that protect people from being harmed, then a decision to unfairly refuse to contribute may harm others. Jeroen Luyten et al. seem to have something like this in mind when they write that "not-contributing [to herd immunity] undercuts this joint effort and is in itself a harmful act" (Luyten et al. 2011, 283). I agree with Luyten et al. that vaccine refusal may be harmful when it "undercuts" herd immunity and places people at greater risk of infection. But I am not sure that non-contribution is always "in itself a harmful act," since vaccine refusal does not always undercut herd immunity. Instead, refusing to contribute to herd immunity is in itself *unfair*, where the fact that it is unfair is a distinct reason (i.e. distinct from *preventing harm*) for the state to use coercion to promote vaccination. I understand the tendency to try to reduce fairness to harm prevention. Talking about harms allows us to focus on the rights and interests of individuals. Almost everyone cares about these core ideals of classical liberal political thought. Even libertarians think that legal authorities may use force to prevent harms. 'Fair play' has the disadvantage of being both less clear and less popular, which may explain Viens, Bensimon, and Upshur's observation that discussions about coercion on behalf of public health often "do not pay adequate attention to ... reciprocity," or to the ideal of "fair play" (Viens, Bensimon, and Upshur 2009, 208, 211; see also Viens, Coggon, and Kessel 2013).[23]

State coercion may be necessary to promote fair play because a moral duty of fairness (which I discussed in chapter four) may be insufficient to ensure widespread cooperation in fair cooperative schemes. In particular, people may abstain from cooperative acts because they are selfish or because they doubt that other people will act cooperatively. These are the problems of *egoism* and *assurance*. In his *Leviathan*, Thomas Hobbes famously argued that state coercion can solve both of these problems. First, coercion protects against egoistic free-riding. In the absence of external coercion, a selfish person may benefit from a less selfish person's contributions to cooperative efforts without making a contribution of her own. Hobbes says that "[f]or he that performeth first has no assurance the other will perform after, because the bonds of words are too weak to bridle men's ambition, avarice, anger, and other passions, without the fear of some coercive power" (Hobbes 1996, XIV). The fact that it is in someone's interest not to cooperate may undermine the possibility of cooperation. But if non-cooperation can be punished by the state, then it may be in everyone's interest to contribute to cooperative efforts.

I am not so worried about the *egoist* challenge, and scholars in recent generations (e.g. Gert 1967; Kavka 1986) have argued that Hobbes was not as worried about it as his earlier readers sometimes thought he was.[24] Most people have a sense of justice. They are willing to pay for valuable public goods, even at some cost to themselves. The main problem is not selfishness, but the fact that people only have a reason to pay their fair share when they have *assurance* that others are also paying their fair share. Of course, I *could* still contribute even if other people did not contribute, but then my contribution would be altruistic (or foolish), rather than fair. (A duty of fair play does not demand that people selflessly contribute when others abstain.) Furthermore, contributing to public goods when other people do not would be foolish if non-contribution were widespread enough to undermine the public good that contributions were supposed to support.[25] Here, the Hobbesian insight is not that people are generally *selfish*, but that their moral duties depend on their *epistemic* circumstances. If they cannot be assured that most other people are complying with fair terms for cooperation, then they do not have a moral duty of fairness to cooperate.

Individuals are unlikely to be able to solve the epistemic problem of assurance through interpersonal and associational relationships. As John Rawls says, members of a large society are unlikely to experience a "degree of mutual confidence in one another's integrity that renders enforcement superfluous" (Rawls 1999, 237). Instead, state coercion is likely to be necessary to solve the assurance problem. Rawls says:

> Even if all citizens were willing to pay their share, they would pre-sumably do so only when they are assured that others will pay theirs as well ... But in normal circumstances a reasonable assurance in this regard can only be given if there is a binding rule effectively enforced. Assuming that the public good is to everyone's advantage, and one that all would agree to arrange for, the use of coercion is perfectly rational from each man's point of view.
>
> (Rawls 1999, 236)

Here, state coercion solves the problem of assurance that may otherwise prevent people from making a fair contribution to public efforts.

State coercion may help to solve an assurance problem in the case of mass vaccination programs. I have a duty of fairness to contribute to herd immunity only if most other members of my community act on the basis of this duty. If they do not, then herd immunity will not exist and, therefore, I will not have a duty of fairness to contribute to it. My knowledge that the state is willing to use coercion to ensure high vacci-nation rates secures my moral duty to vaccinate, since it assures me that compliance will be sufficiently widespread to generate herd immunity.

I have assumed something that I argued for in chapter four: Herd immunity provides and protects essential public goods. In particular, herd immunity results in massively reduced risks of disease outbreaks, and this saves money for the public health system, avoids economic losses (including decreased tax revenues), and helps keep kids in school. Preventing outbreaks also protects social trust and promotes public safety, political stability, and national security. The history of disease – and, in particular, the history of massive outbreaks – should make it clear how valuable it can be for a community to possess herd immunity.

I hope that states will not have to use much (or any) coercion to promote mass vaccination. The fact that vaccination also provides a private good – individual immunity – means that most people have self-interested reasons to contribute to herd immunity. And this fact may be enough to guarantee that enough people vaccinate to protect herd immunity (see e.g. Dare 1998, sec. VI). I have argued only that the value of fairness is a reason for the state to *ensure* that most people are vaccinated. Coercive vaccination may be permitted if it is the only means available to ensure that people make fair contributions to herd immunity.

No coercion for public goods?

One way to object to the argument I have been making in this section is to claim that the state is authorized to use coercion only to protect the private rights of individuals, but not to promote the so-called public rights of the community. For example, someone might think that the state should enforce laws against murder and theft – and use coercion to collect taxes to fund the enforcement of these laws – but should not use coercion to ensure that everyone has enough to eat. Someone who makes the objection I have in mind may deny that citizens have rights to general or public goods, such as education or health care or herd immunity. This is because guaranteeing people's putative rights to these goods would require violating the private rights of individuals.

Robert Nozick makes something like this objection, when he argues that people cannot have rights to public or general goods, if these rights would require violations of the rights that individuals have to particular objects. And since "particular rights over things fill the space of rights," guaranteeing putative general or public rights (e.g. to welfare, education, herd immunity) would necessarily violate the rights of individuals (Nozick 1974, 238). Nozick continues:

> Other people's rights and entitlements to particular things (that pencil, their body, and so on) and how they choose to exercise these rights and entitlements fix the external environment of any given individual and the means that will be available to him … No rights exist in conflict with this substructure of particular rights. Since no neatly contoured right to achieve a goal will avoid incompatibility with this substructure, no such rights exist.
>
> (Nozick 1974, 238)

On this view, the state may violate an individual's right to the freedom of her person if it used coercion to ensure that everyone made a fair contribution to the costs associated with herd immunity. Coercive vaccination involves the use of state power to control what is done to people's bodies, and the freedom to control what is done to one's body is a funda-mental liberty (see e.g. Nozick 1974, 206). And, the objection continues, the state may not violate a person's individual liberty merely to provide the community-at-large with a valuable good. So, it looks like the state may not use coercion to ensure a fair distribution of the costs of herd immunity.

To be clear: The libertarian position I'm exploring is consistent with the *voluntary* creation of public goods. It finds no fault when herd immunity results from the uncoerced choices of free persons. Even more, advocates of this libertarian position may endorse *coercive* vaccination policy, when it aims at preventing people from harming each other. As I discussed in an earlier section, coercion in the name of preventing harm is often liberty preserving, since it aims to protect the liberty of (potential) victims of harm.

But now it may be unclear why this sort of libertarian must reject the use of state coercion to ensure that people make a fair contribution towards herd immunity. If herd immunity is the means by which the state can most effectively prevent people from infecting each other, then a libertarian may endorse the state's use of coercion to ensure herd immunity. And since the state is permitted to use coercion to ensure that people make a *fair contribution* to the activities that the state is permitted to pursue, it follows that the state may use coercion to ensure that people make a fair contribution to herd immunity. Consider the analogous case of taxation-funded military and police forces: The libertarians I have in mind believe that the state should protect national security and public safety, since this is a way to prevent members of the community from being harmed. But this entails that the state may use coercive taxation schemes to ensure that everyone pays her fair share towards military and police forces. So, the difference between the arguments I have made and the arguments that could be made by the libertarians I have in mind is that I have argued that the state may promote herd immunity because herd immunity promotes a variety of public goods, e.g. public trust, economic stability, education. In contrast, the libertarians I have in mind will argue that the only reason for the state to promote herd immunity (and to ensure that people make fair contributions to it) is that herd immunity prevents people from being harmed.

This sort of response is unlikely to convince anarchists and others who reject even a minimal state, since these people object to all forms of public coercion. For example, Murray Rothbard rejects the public provision of security and safety, and instead supports a free market of private security companies (Rothbard 1978). Advocates of this position may consistently reject the use of state coercion to ensure fair contributions to herd immunity. Of course, they could claim that ill individuals may be coercively restrained from infecting others, e.g. through quarantine or enforced social distancing. They could even endorse *ex ante* restraint, where this may include coercive vaccination programs run by individuals and associations. But the people I have in mind would reject the state (or anyone else) using coercion to ensure that people make a fair contribution to herd immunity since, among other reasons, they object to the existence of a state.

Coercion and bodily integrity

I assume there are many ways the state may permissibly use its power to protect the interests of children, to prevent people from harming each other, and to fairly distribute the costs of supporting public goods. Throughout this chapter, I have compared coercive vaccination to examples of state coercion that should be unobjectionable to most people – keeping children from playing in traffic, preventing people from shooting bullets into the air, raising money to pay for the military and police. Even in the contemporary US, where distrust of government is at historical highs, most people support many kinds of state coercion, including taxation, regulations on business activity and property rights, and licensing both for professions and for common activities such as driving and fishing. People often complain about the particular forms that these kinds of state coercion take. They think their taxes are too high or their driver's license costs too much, but they nonetheless believe that coercive taxation and licensing are legitimate state activities.

But perhaps vaccination involves a fundamentally more objectionable kind of state coercion. Vaccine refusers may insist that coercive vaccination violates bodily integrity, which is something that the state may not do. I suspect that this sort of conviction motivates some people who oppose coercive vaccination, so I want to consider how strong an objection it is.

First, you might think that coercive interventions on a person's body do much more to constrain liberty than do seizures of a person's property or restrictions on a person's business activities. But this seems unlikely. A 95% flat income tax rate would do much more to constrain my choices than a momentary vaccination would do. Or consider laws that require dental hygienists to practice under the supervision of a dentist, and which cost dental hygienists tens of thousands of dollars over the course of their careers (Kleiner and Park 2010). In contrast, coercive vaccination requires only a momentary inconvenience. Therefore, if coercive bodily intervention is less justified than other forms of state coercion, it is not because coercive bodily intervention always does much more to restrict a person's liberty.

Second, you might think that the body is, in principle, not an appropriate object for state coercion. I think this is an unpersuasive objection, too. Clearly, conscription involves the coercive treatment of a person's body, i.e. through training, deployment, and combat. But we need not invoke such a dramatic example. Mandatory jury duty coerces bodily activity, too, and I don't think that anyone who cares about the right to a jury trial should object to that. So, the 'bodily integrity' objection to coercive vaccination is unlikely to succeed if it is focused on the claim that there is something especially objectionable about coercing someone to do something with their body.

Third, the 'bodily integrity' objection may focus on the state using its power to *put things in a person's body*. According to this version of the objection, the worry is not that coercive acts upon a body do much more to constrain someone's liberty than other forms of coercion, or that it is always unjust to compel someone to do something with their body. Instead, the worry is about using state coercion to violate the protective barriers that separate a person's pure self from a dirty world.[26] I think this objection has more intuitive force than the other versions of the 'bodily integrity' objection, but I do not find it convincing. Bodily purity is an unreasonable and unrealizable ideal. We fail to achieve it (or even promote it) in everyday activities and in non-controversial interactions with government. For example, things were forcibly put into and against my body whenever I have gone to the Department of Motor Vehicles (DMV) to get a driver's license. I have had to smell the perfume and the body odor of people around me. I have had to touch the dirty fabric on the chair on which I was forced to sit. When someone sneezed, she projected diseased water droplets from her mouth into my eyes. Therefore, when the government forces me to go to the DMV to get a driver's license, it forces me to undergo violations of my bodily integrity.[27] Clearly, I am being overdramatic in describing the contamination I experienced at the DMV. But that's the point. Someone who objects to coercive vaccination because it involves the state 'putting things into her body' is also overreacting, on the basis of an unreasonable ideal of bodily purity.

The contingent weights of reasons for coercive vaccination

Coercive vaccination is a means to protect the interests of children, to prevent foreseeable significant harms to others, and to fairly distribute the costs of social cooperation. Whether and how each of these three reasons counts in favor of coercive vaccination depends on the particular circumstances in which vaccine policy operates.

First, I agree with Luyten et al. that "[j]ustifications based upon the harm principle are often unstable" (Luyten et al. 2011, 288). If herd immunity is vulnerable or nonexistent, then my decision to refuse a vaccine significantly increases my odds of infecting someone. In these circumstances, a commitment to prevent harm weighs more heavily in favor of coercing vaccination. However, if herd immunity exists and is robust (and will survive my decision to refuse vaccines), then it may be "hard to see how harm to others considerations can be used to justify an obligation to vaccinate" (Dawson 2007, 171). The problem Dawson identifies is that it is unclear whether people harm others (or contribute towards harms) if their acts do not cause harms or directly contribute to harmful conditions, but only make it (slightly) more likely that harmful conditions will exist in the future.

I agree with Dawson that it may be hard to see how vaccine refusal could be harmful when herd immunity is robust. Of course, if enough people refused vaccines, then herd immunity would fail. And when herd immunity fails, people are much more likely to be harmed by vaccine refusal. But who is responsible for the harms that result after herd immunity fails? Is it only the people whose acts of vaccine refusal caused vaccination rates to drop below the threshold for herd immunity? If herd immunity for a particular disease requires a 92% vaccination rate, then the people who cause the rate to drop from 92% to 91% seem to have contributed to harmful conditions. But what about people whose decisions not to vaccinate caused vaccination rates to drop from 95% to 94%? Their acts did not cause herd immunity to fail, but they did make it possible for later acts of vaccine refusal to undermine herd immunity. Did these previous vaccine refusers also contribute to harmful conditions?

Consider a fanciful example. Three people are holding a tiger on a leash and two of them must hold the leash to keep the tiger under control. If one person lets go, then I think he shares some responsibility for the harms the tiger will cause when a second person later lets go, and leaves the third person to be devoured. To make use of a popular saying: It seems unfair to lay all of the blame for 'breaking the camel's back' (or setting the tiger free) on the person who burdened the animal with its 'last straw' (or was last to let go of the leash). Surely those who placed previous straws (like the first person who dropped the leash) share responsibility, though I admit it is unclear how to think about their relative responsibility for the harmful circumstances they indirectly contribute to. For the same reason, I think that vaccine refusers can be responsible for causing harmful conditions even if herd immunity survives their decisions to refuse vaccines, though it is not clear to me how responsible they are.

Second, the weights of the different reasons for coercive vaccination vary depending on the net balance of benefits and harms that particular vaccines provide. If a disease is very nasty – if it spreads easily, has high morbidity, causes severe symptoms, etc. – then this makes paternalism, preventing harm, and fairness weightier reasons to coerce vaccination against that disease than if the disease were less nasty. For example, these three moral reasons provide a stronger justification for coercive vaccination against polio, measles, and pertussis than they do against varicella (chicken pox). The vaccines against the first three diseases provide a much higher net benefit (both to vaccinated individuals and society) than does the vaccine against the last disease. The reasons in favor of coercive vaccination against chicken pox may still be sufficiently weighty to justify coercion, but they are likely to be less weighty than the reasons to coerce vaccination against the other diseases I just mentioned. It is unfortunate that vaccination advocates sometimes talk as if every vaccine is equally important or that the case for coercive vaccination is equally strong for every vaccine.[28]

Conclusion: from compulsory to voluntary vaccination

There are weighty reasons to think the state may sometimes use coercion to promote mass vaccination. But, of course, there are also weighty reasons to think the state should use coercion to promote vaccination only when doing so is necessary, i.e. necessary to protect children's best interests, to prevent people from harming each other, and to ensure a fair distribution of the costs of creating herd immunity. And even when coercion is necessary for these purposes, the state should use the least amount of coercion that is sufficient to achieve these goals.

My focus has been on questions about political morality and justice, but pragmatic considerations also loom large. In particular, it is vital to keep major social and political groups on the side of mass vaccination. It would be a grave problem if opinions about coercive vaccination became politically polarized. Depending on the disease, herd immunity requires between 80% and 95% vaccination rates, so herd immunity will not survive if vaccination programs become politically controversial. For this reason, we ought to be willing to use *less coercion* than may be necessary to generate the most robust herd immunity, if using less coercion would prevent forms of political and social backlash that could weaken herd immunity even more. Clearly, these are complicated political issues and they require much wisdom to resolve. My central point is that coercive vaccination programs should tolerate suboptimal results if doing so will have the best consequences for public health in a particular political context.

I close this chapter with a quick taxonomy of the ways in which public vaccination programs may be more or less coercive. On one extreme, vaccination is *compulsory* when members of society have a legal obligation to become vaccinated. Compulsory vaccination need not entail the forcible imposition of vaccination on those who do not 'voluntarily' accede to the state's lawful demand that they become vaccinated (though it may and it sometimes has). However, compulsory vaccination always entails that vaccine refusers are lawbreakers, and that the state may respond to their violations of the law with punitive action. Historically, very few communities have practiced compulsory vaccination, and almost none do today. (Wynia 2007).[29]

In contrast to compulsion, other forms of coercive vaccination are more 'indirect' and are now much more prevalent (Dawson 2011, 151). Paul Offit distinguishes between compulsory and mandatory vaccination:

Compulsory vaccination is you force someone to get a vaccine … We [the US] have mandatory vaccination, which is to say that if you choose not to get a vaccine, that you pay a societal cost, which can be, for example, not being allowed to go to school.

(Palfreman 2010)

Mandatory vaccination exists when vaccine refusal is legal, but when the state withholds from vaccine refusers social goods to which they would otherwise be entitled.[30] For example, unvaccinated children may be prevented from attending school or state-recognized daycare. Also, the state may sanction employment discrimination against vaccine refusers, i.e. by allowing some employers to make vaccination a condition of employment, such as in hospitals or the military. Vaccination is currently mandatory for public school attendance throughout the United States, Australia, and some parts of Canada.[31] In recent years, Italy has transitioned from mandatory school vaccination to a more voluntary vaccination program, and it has retained high vaccination rates (Molinelli et al. 2009; Moran, Gainotti, and Petrini 2008).[32] Australia has recently moved in the opposite direction. It now requires children to be 'fully vaccinated' for parents to receive their full tax refund for childcare expenses (Australian Government – Department of Human Services 2014; Ngo 2014).

Some states offer (or have offered) *incentives* to people who become vaccinated or to their health care providers. For example, aid programs in Nicaragua and India have given people small cash payments or gifts of food if they become vaccinated (Banerjee et al. 2010; Barham and Maluccio 2009). The United Kingdom's National Health Service has provided incentive payments to general practitioners who achieved high levels of vaccination in their communities (Smith and York 2004). The distinction between incentivized vaccination and mandatory vaccination is that the former allows vaccine refusers to continue to make use of all of the public goods that are ordinarily afforded to people in virtue of their membership in the community. For example, incentive programs do not make vaccine refusers ineligible to attend public school or daycare, nor do they permit vaccine refusers to be subject to employment discrimination because of their non-vaccinated status. Instead, vaccination programs that include incentives attempt to promote vaccination by providing vaccinated persons with goods that they would not otherwise be entitled to receive.[33] We might worry that incentive programs disproportionately influence the decisions of the poor, i.e. people who are less able to refuse 'supplemental' goods (Moran, Gainotti, and Petrini 2008). But this worry generalizes: The poor are also less able to pay the fines associated with *compulsory* vaccination, and they are less able to afford private or homeschooling, if they refuse public school vaccine *mandates*. The poor also report that they experience voluntary vaccination programs (including programs with incentives) as being less voluntary than socially advantaged people experience them being (Colgrove 2004).

States ought to try to protect herd immunity through vaccination programs that are as voluntary as possible.[34] They should prefer mandatory vaccination to compulsory vaccination, and incentivized vaccination to mandatory vaccination. In particular, states should cultivate conditions under which citizens will choose to vaccinate. One might object that it is coercive for the state to manipulate the 'choice architecture' for citizens' (supposedly) voluntary vaccination choices, e.g. in the ways that Richard Thaler and Cass Sunstein have suggested. I agree that 'libertarian paternalism' can be coercive. But, since I have argued that coercive vaccination policies are justified (when they are necessary), the fact that it may be coercive to manipulate people's choices is not an objection to using libertarian paternalism in vaccine policy. And since pragmatic considerations may tell in favor of vaccination policies that do as little as possible to trigger vaccine refusal among people who are already sensitive to state coercion, we should embrace libertarian paternalism, if it protects herd immunity while preserving free choice.

Notes

1 To be clear, Dawson's focus is on state *compulsion* of vaccination, rather than coercive state acts more generally.
2 My discussion in the following paragraphs has benefited from Quong (2013) and Vallier and D'Agostino (2014).
3 Here, I commit myself to a moderate form of idealization, like the one that Gaus defends (Gaus 2011, 232–260). But my argument in defense of the public justification of coercive vaccination policy is consistent with a more radical idealization, e.g. the one specified by Rawls's 'original position' (Rawls 2005, 23–28).
4 On the relationship between pseudo-skepticism and public justification, see Torcello (2011).
5 Consider what Vermeersch writes about coercion and vaccination: "[T]he exercise of coercion may in general be equaled to the infliction of injury or harm. This of course can only be justified if ample proof has been provided that the harm to others which is prevented by the coercion, is much greater than that which is inflicted" (Vermeersch 1999, S16).
6 *The Patient as Victim and Vector*, by Margaret Battin, Leslie Francis, Jay Jacobson, and Charles Smith, is the definitive treatment of the moral complexities raised by the dual role of the person who is infected with a contagious disease (Battin et al. 2009). In an earlier article, the authors of this book (joined by J. Botkin) observed that "[i]f we consider the patient's status as victim, or as vector, the emphasis might shift, from the health care that might be most desirable for the individual patient to broader social concerns and the worldwide distribution of care that might enable all to achieve opportunities over a reasonable life span" (Francis et al. 2005, 314). Also, "[a]s vector, the patient may ignore his/her effects on others, thus worsening the problem of achieving a decent minimum of care for them by his/her individual choices" (Francis et al. 2005, 315).
7 The idea that the family is not in the purview of the state – because it is essentially *private* or *natural* – has a long philosophical history. Consider, for

example, Rousseau's claim that the division of labor between men and women in the family emerged from pre-political ('natural') facts about gender, rather than from social or political forces (Rousseau 1987). Or, consider Christopher Lasch's insistence that the goods that the family makes available to its members (and to society, more generally) are at risk when the family becomes the object of state intervention (Lasch 1995).

8   On the political power of Grover Norquist, consider this reflection on the US budget crisis of 2012: "Virtually every Republican in Congress has taken the pledge, pushed by Grover Norquist's *Americans for Tax Reform*, never to vote for a tax increase – a pledge both parties see as a serious impediment to a tax compromise" (Weisman 2012).

9   Parents' rights activists are also pursuing an amendment to the US Constitution which would include the following text: "The liberty of parents to direct the upbringing and education of their children is a fundamental right ... Neither the United States nor any state shall infringe upon this right" (Parentalrights 2014).

10 There may also be non-paternalistic reasons for some of these policies. For example, requiring helmets for motorcyclists may decrease the costs to the public of caring for people who suffer brain injuries in motorcycle accidents. My point is only that there may (also) be paternalistic reasons to support these policies.

11 In *The Subjection of Women*, Mill writes that "things in which the individual is the person directly interested, never go right but as they are left to his own discretion ... freedom of individual choice is now known to be the only thing which procures the adoption of the best processes" (Mill 1998b, I.13).

12 The common cognitive deficits I discussed in chapter two may give us a reason to think that we could justify a great deal of coercion under the banner of soft paternalism. For example Richard Thaler and Cass Sunstein have defended a form of public policy that they call 'libertarian paternalism' (Thaler and Sunstein 2009). On their view, government ought to structure the conditions in which people make decisions so as to "influence choices in a way that will make choosers better off, *as judged by themselves*"; these are decisions that people would have made on their own, if they "paid full attention and possessed complete information, unlimited cognitive abilities, and complete self-control" (Thaler and Sunstein 2009, 5). For instance, Thaler and Sunstein recommend that retirement savings programs automatically deduct money from people's paychecks, and that people have to 'opt-out' to avoid making contributions. I am sympathetic with Thaler and Sunstein's project, though I worry that it understates the ways in which policymakers may also be influenced by their cognitive biases.

13 There is unfortunately not a uniform terminology for the sort of paternalism that one may use against children. Some use the term *weak paternalism* to describe making choices for children (see e.g. Dawson 2011, 144). Here, 'weak' seems to denote that paternalism over children does not have to override a presumption in favor of liberty, as a more robust (or *strong*) paternalism would. This is because children (supposedly) do not have liberty rights that would have to be overridden for paternalism to be permissible. However, others mean something else by the *weak/strong* divide, such that *strong* paternalism involves interference with the ends that agents choose (or do not choose), while weak paternalism involves only interference with the means that agents choose (see e.g. Dworkin 2014). In this case, paternalistic treatment of children may be *strong*, since it may interfere both with the means and the ends that children would otherwise choose.

14 For example, John Stuart Mill says: "It is, perhaps, hardly necessary to say that this doctrine is meant to apply only to human beings in the maturity of

their faculties. … Liberty, as a principle, has no application to any state of things anterior to the time when mankind have become capable of being improved by free and equal discussion" (Mill 1998a, I.10).

15   Importantly, we need not claim that children have *rights* in order to argue that the state ought to protect their interests (see e.g. Schoeman 1980).

16   Compare with Dawson, who says: "Where the parents make a decision about an infant's care which is likely to result in substantial risk of significant harm to that infant then third parties (such as the state) have an obligation to intervene to protect the infant from the consequences of that decision" (Dawson 2011, 146). Dawson is addressing the permissibility of state *compulsion* of vaccination, while I am interested more generally in questions about coercion.

17   I credit Galliott (2013) with the idea that vaccine refusal is like letting a child play in a busy street.

18   Wynia has argued that coercive public health interventions *must always* benefit the individuals who are coerced (Wynia 2007). It follows that the state might not be permitted to use coercion against healthy children to promote mass vaccination against rubella, if vaccination against rubella is not a net benefit for healthy children. I disagree. If the net harm to the vaccinated person is minimal, then they may be coerced into vaccinating, if vaccination is an essential means for preventing harm and promoting herd immunity.

19   Compare with Flanigan (2014).

20   "Like firearms, infectiousness poses a danger to others. As such, it may even legitimate legal or social interference with what we do" (Francis et al. 2005, 316).

21   Vaccine refusers are not usually clamoring for increased civil or criminal liability as an alternative to coercive vaccination. They tend to reject both (see e.g. Holland 2013).

22   For some skepticism about relying upon class action lawsuits to hold vaccine refusers responsible, see Ciolli (2008).

23   The sort of coercive acts Viens et al. have in mind are quarantine and forced isolation during disease outbreaks, but I think their arguments work for mandatory vaccination, too, given that mandatory vaccination is often much less coercive than quarantines and forced isolation.

24   Even Hobbes may agree with Rawls that the (Hobbesian idea) "[t]hat political rule is founded solely on men's propensity to self-interest and injustice is a superficial view" (Rawls 1999, 237).

25   I do not mean that individuals are absolved from their moral responsibilities in the absence of assurance of the contributions of others. Instead, they are absolved only from a duty to contribute to *cooperative* efforts. So, for example, imagine that some children are drowning in a nearby pond. Suppose that the best way to save the children is to participate in a collective activity (e.g. hiring a rescue boat). But if I lack assurance that others are going to contribute to the 'boat fund', I do not have a duty to contribute. (No one gets saved by a boat that we are unable to hire.) However, I still have a moral duty to try to save at least some children by myself, if I can do so at reasonable cost.

26   Here, it may help to recall my discussion in chapter three about contamination, disgust, and sanctity.

27   The bodily violation experienced through vaccination is different from the bodily violation experienced while at the DMV, since the violation is essential to the activity of the former but merely an accidental attribute of the latter. (It is possible to go to the DMV without smelling foul odors or receiving diseased water droplets into one's eyes, but it is not possible to be vaccinated without having material placed into one's body.) I do not think that this distinction makes a moral difference. In both cases, the violations are regular and predictable aspects of coercive state activity.

28 Mark Largent has a nice discussion of this phenomenon (Largent 2012, 166–168).
29 For one example of especially oppressive and degrading forms of compulsory vaccination, see Albert, Ostheimer, and Breman (2001).
30 Mandatory vaccination has proven to be effective at generating high rates of herd immunity. However, it is much less coercive than compulsory vaccination. So, it is helpful to keep these terms distinct.
31 This chart has comprehensive data on which vaccines are mandatory or voluntary in Europe: www.eurosurveillance.org/images/dynamic/EE/V17N22/DAncona_tab1.jpg
32 For some worries about Italy's program, see Attena, Abuadili, and Marino (2014).
33 We cannot assess whether a particular vaccination program is mandatory or voluntary with incentives merely by looking at the goods that it withholds from those who refuse vaccines. This is because the difference between these two kinds of programs hinges on whether the goods that are withheld from vaccine refusers are properly thought of as something extra, i.e. as something beyond what persons are entitled to as citizens. But making this assessment depends on facts about the social and political conditions in which people are making decisions about vaccines. Vaccination programs that may properly be considered voluntary in one context may be mandatory in other contexts. For example, Nicaragua's program of giving food products to people who receive vaccines is usually described as an incentives-based voluntary vaccination program. It is not obvious to me that this is correct. Nicaragua has a minimal social safety net and many of its citizens experience chronic food insecurity. Since people have a fundamental right to food security, vaccination programs that withhold food from food insecure persons may properly be described as *mandatory* vaccination programs, since they withhold goods to which people are otherwise entitled. The context dependency of the coerciveness of vaccination programs is worth keeping in view, especially when we reflect on international vaccination policies. Incentive-based vaccination programs in poorer societies deserve significant scrutiny, since many of these programs are financed and run by agents from outside of the local community, e.g. global institutions, transnational NGOs. Unfortunately, I lack the space in this book to address ethical issues raised by international immunization programs.
34 See Girard (2012) on whether mandatory or voluntary vaccination policies are more effective in developing societies.

Bibliography

Albert, Michael R., Kristen G. Ostheimer, and Joel G. Breman. 2001. "The Last Smallpox Epidemic in Boston and the Vaccination Controversy, 1901–1903." *New England Journal of Medicine* 344(5): 375–379.
Allen, Arthur. 2007. *Vaccine: The Controversial Story of Medicine's Greatest Lifesaver.* W. W. Norton & Company.
Antommaria, Armand H. Matheny, Kathryn L. Weise, Mary E. Fallat, Aviva L. Katz, Mark R. Mercurio, Margaret R. Moon, Alexander L. Okun, Sally A. Webb, and others. 2013. "Conflicts between Religious or Spiritual Beliefs and Pediatric Care: Informed Refusal, Exemptions, and Public Funding." *Pediatrics* 132(5): 962–965.
Asser, S. M., and R. Swan. 1998. "Child Fatalities from Religion-Motivated Medical Neglect." *Pediatrics* 101(4): 625–629.
Attena, Francesco, Amanda Valdes Abuadili, and Sara Marino. 2014. "The Informed Consent in Southern Italy Does Not Adequately Inform Parents about Infant Vaccination." *BMC Public Health* 14(1): 211.

Australian Government – Department of Human Services. 2014. "Immunising Your Children." *Australian Government – Department of Human Services.* Accessed June 21. www.humanservices.gov.au/customer/subjects/immunising-your-children.

Banerjee, Abhijit Vinayak, Esther Duflo, Rachel Glennerster, and Dhruva Kothari. 2010. "Improving Immunisation Coverage in Rural India: Clustered Randomised Controlled Evaluation of Immunisation Campaigns with and without Incentives." *British Medical Journal* 340 (May): c2220. http://dx.doi.org/10.1136/bmj.c2220.

Barham, Tania, and John A. Maluccio. 2009. "Eradicating Diseases: The Effect of Conditional Cash Transfers on Vaccination Coverage in Rural Nicaragua." *Journal of Health Economics* 28(3): 611–621.

Battin, M., L. P. Francis, J. A. Jacobson, and C. B. Smith. 2009. *The Patient as Victim and Vector: Ethics and Infectious Disease.* Oxford University Press.

Brennan, S., and R. Noggle. 1997. "The Moral Status of Children: Children's Rights, Parents' Rights, and Family Justice." *Social Theory and Practice* 23(1): 1–26.

Brighouse, Harry. 2002. "What Rights (If Any) Do Children Have?" In *The Moral and Political Status of Children*, edited by David Archard and Colin M. Macleod, 31–53. Oxford University Press.

Brighouse, Harry, and Adam Swift. 2009. "Legitimate Parental Partiality." *Philosophy and Public Affairs* 37(1): 43–80. Oxford University Press.

Caplan, Arthur L. 2013. "Liability for Failure to Vaccinate." *Bill of Health.* May 23. https://blogs.law.harvard.edu/billofhealth/2013/05/23/liability-for-failure-to-vaccinate/.

Caplan, Arthur L., David Hoke, Nicholas J. Diamond, and Viktoriya Karshenboyem. 2012. "Free to Choose but Liable for the Consequences: Should Non-Vaccinators Be Penalized for the Harm They Do?" *The Journal of Law, Medicine & Ethics* 40(3): 606–611.

Charo, R. Alta. 2007. "Politics, Parents, and Prophylaxis – Mandating HPV Vaccination in the United States." *New England Journal of Medicine* 356(19): 1905–1908. doi:10.1056/NEJMp078054.

Ciolli, Anthony. 2008. "Mandatory School Vaccinations: The Role of Tort Law." *Yale Journal of Biology and Medicine* 81(3): 129–137.

Colgrove, James Keith. 2004. "Between Persuasion and Compulsion: Smallpox Control in Brooklyn and New York, 1894–1902." *Bulletin of the History of Medicine* 78(2): 349–378.

Dare, Tim. 1998. "Mass Immunisation Programmes: Some Philosophical Issues." *Bioethics* 12(2): 125–149.

Dawson, Angus. 2005. "The Determination of the Best Interests in Relation to Childhood Immunisation." *Bioethics* 19(1): 72–89.

Dawson, Angus. 2007. "Herd Protection as a Public Good: Vaccination and Our Obligations to Others." In *Ethics, Prevention, and Public Health*, edited by Angus Dawson and Marcel Verweij, 160–178. Clarendon Press.

Dawson, Angus. 2011. "Vaccination Ethics." In *Public Health Ethics*, edited by Angus Dawson, 143–153. Cambridge University Press.

Dworkin, Gerald. 2014. "Paternalism." In *The Stanford Encyclopedia of Philosophy*, edited by Edward N. Zalta, Summer. http://plato.stanford.edu/archives/sum2014/entries/paternalism/.

Farris, Michael P. 2009. "Nannies in Blue Berets: Understanding the U.N. Convention on the Rights of the Child." *HSLDA.* January. www.hslda.org/docs/news/20091120.asp.

Feikin, D. R., D. C. Lezotte, R. F. Hamman, D. A. Salmon, R. T. Chen, and R. E. Hoffman. 2000. "Individual and Community Risks of Measles and Pertussis Associated with Personal Exemptions to Immunization." *JAMA: The Journal of the American Medical Association* 284(24): 3145–3150.

Feinberg, Joel. 1980. "The Child's Right to an Open Future." In *Whose Child? Children's Rights, Parental Authority and State Power*, edited by William Aiken and Hugh La Follette, 124–153. Rowman and Littlefield.

Feinberg, Joel. 1986. *Harm to Self: The Moral Limits of the Criminal Law*. Oxford University Press.

Fisher, Barbara Loe. 1997. "Informed Consent – National Vaccine Information Center." *National Vaccine Information Center (NVIC)*. May 2. www.nvic.org/informed-consent.aspx.

Flanigan, Jessica. 2014. "A Defense of Compulsory Vaccination." *HEC Forum* 26(1): 5–25.

Francis, L. P., M. P. Battin, J. A. Jacobson, C. B. Smith, and J. Botkin. 2005. "How Infectious Diseases Got Left Out – and What This Omission Might Have Meant for Bioethics." *Bioethics* 19(4): 307–322.

Galliott, Emma. 2013. "Vaccination Refusal: Like Putting a Child on a Freeway." *Tweed Daily News*. June 1. www.tweeddailynews.com.au/news/vaccination-re fusal-like-putting-a-child-on-a-free/1890374/.

Gaus, Gerald. 2011. *The Order of Public Reason: A Theory of Freedom and Morality in a Diverse and Bounded World*. Cambridge University Press.

Gert, Bernard. 1967. "Hobbes and Psychological Egoism." *Journal of the History of Ideas* 28(4): 503–520.

Girard, Dorota Zdanowska. 2012. "Recommended or Mandatory Pertussis Vaccination Policy in Developed Countries: Does the Choice Matter?" *Public Health* 126(2): 117–122.

Hobbes, Thomas. 1996. *Leviathan*. Edited by Richard Tuck. Rev. stu. ed. Cambridge University Press.

Holland, Mary. 2013. "Guest Post: Crack Down on Those Who Don't Vaccinate? A Response to Art Caplan." *Bill of Health*. June 21. http://blogs.law.harvard. edu/billofhealth/2013/06/21/guest-post-crack-down-on-those-who-dont-vaccina te-a-response-to-art-caplan/.

Kant, Immanuel. 1996. "On the Common Saying: That May Be Correct in Theory but It Is of No Use in Practice." In *Practical Philosophy*, edited and translated by Mary J. Gregor, 273–309. Cambridge University Press.

Kavka, Gregory S. 1986. *Hobbesian Moral and Political Theory*. Princeton University Press.

Kleiner, Morris M., and Kyoung Won Park. 2010. *Battles Among Licensed Occupations: Analyzing Government Regulations on Labor Market Outcomes for Dentists and Hygienists*. National Bureau of Economic Research. www.nber. org/papers/w16560.

Largent, M. A. 2012. *Vaccine: The Debate in Modern America*. Johns Hopkins University Press.

Lasch, Christopher. 1995. *Haven in a Heartless World*. W. W. Norton & Company.

Lipinski, Jed. 2013. "Endangering the Herd." *Slate*. August 13. www.slate.com/a rticles/news_and_politics/jurisprudence/2013/08/anti_vaxxers_why_parents_ who_don_t_vaccinate_their_kids_should_be_sued_or.html.

Luyten, Jeroen, Antoon Vandevelde, Pierre Van Damme, and Philippe Beutels. 2011. "Vaccination Policy and Ethical Challenges Posed by Herd Immunity, Suboptimal Uptake and Subgroup Targeting." *Public Health Ethics* 4(3): 280–291.

Mill, John Stuart. 1998a. "On Liberty." In *On Liberty and Other Essays*, edited by John Gray, 5–130. Oxford University Press.

Mill, John Stuart. 1998b. "The Subjection of Women." In *On Liberty and Other Essays*, edited by John Gray, 471–582. Oxford University Press.

Molinelli, A., A. Bonsignore, A. Querci, G. Icardi, M. Martini, and P. Durando. 2009. "Towards the Suspension of Compulsory Vaccination in Italy: Balancing Between Public Health Priorities and Medico-Legal and Juridical Aspects." *Journal of Preventative Medicine and Hygiene* 50(3): 135–140.

Moodley, Keymanthri, Kate Hardie, Michael J. Selgelid, Ronald J. Waldman, Peter Strebel, Helen Rees, and David N. Durrheim. 2013. "Ethical Considerations for Vaccination Programmes in Acute Humanitarian Emergencies." *Bulletin of the World Health Organization* 91(4): 290–297.

Moran, Nicola E., S. Gainotti, and C. Petrini. 2008. "From Compulsory to Voluntary Immunisation: Italy's National Vaccination Plan (2005–2007) and the Ethical and Organisational Challenges Facing Public Health Policy-Makers across Europe." *Journal of Medical Ethics* 34(9): 669–674.

Morse, J. R. 1999. "No Families, No Freedom: Human Flourishing in a Free Society." *Social Philosophy and Policy* 16(1): 290–314.

Ngo, Cindy. 2014. "Vaccine Objectors Rise as Parents Skirt 'No Jab, No Play' Law." *The Sydney Morning Herald*, January 11. www.smh.com.au/national/health/vaccine-objectors-rise-as-parents-skirt-no-jab-no-play-law-20140110-30mi1.html.

Nozick, R. 1974. *Anarchy, State, and Utopia*. Basic Books.

Offit, Paul. 2015. *Bad Faith: When Religious Belief Undermines Modern Medicine*. Basic Books.

Okin, Susan Moller. 1989. *Justice, Gender, and the Family*. Basic Books.

O'Neill, Onora. 2004. "Accountability, Trust and Informed Consent in Medical Practice and Research." *Clinical Medicine* 4(3): 269–276.

Palfreman, John. 2010. "The Vaccine War." *Frontline*. PBS. Accessed July 31, 2015. www.pbs.org/wgbh/pages/frontline/vaccines/view/.

Parentalrights. 2014. "Understanding the Parental Rights Amendment." *Parental-rights.org*. Accessed June 19. www.parentalrights.org/index.asp?SEC=%7BDE675888-E60A-4219-8A5E-000083244D13%7D&.

Quong, Jonathan. 2013. "Public Reason." In *The Stanford Encyclopedia of Philosophy*, edited by Edward N. Zalta, Summer 2013. http://plato.stanford.edu/archives/sum2013/entries/public-reason/.

Rawls, John. 1999. *A Theory of Justice*. Rev. ed. Belknap Press of Harvard University Press.

Rawls, John. 2005. *Political Liberalism*. 2nd ed. Columbia University Press.

Reiss, Dorit Rubinstein. 2013. "Compensating the Victims of Failure to Vaccinate: What Are the Options?" *Cornell Journal of Law and Public Policy* 23(3): 595.

Rothbard, Murray Newton. 1978. *For a New Liberty: The Libertarian Manifesto*. Ludwig von Mises Institute.

Rothbard, Murray Newton. 2002. *The Ethics of Liberty*. NYU Press.

Rousseau, Jean-Jacques. 1987. "Discourse on the Origin of Inequality." In *The Basic Political Writings*, translated by Donald A. Cress, 25–109. Hackett Publishing Company.

Rovet, Richard. 2011. "Who Will Defend the Defenders?" In *Vaccine Epidemic*, edited by Louise Kuo Habakus and Mary Holland, 121–126. Skyhorse Publishing.

Rubin, Daniel B., and Sophie Kasimow. 2009. "The Problem of Vaccination Noncompliance: Public Health Goals and the Limitations of Tort Law." *Michigan Law Review* 107(114): 114–119.

Salmon, D. A., M. Haber, E. J. Gangarosa, L. Phillips, N. J. Smith, and R. T. Chen. 1999. "Health Consequences of Religious and Philosophical Exemptions from Immunization Laws." *JAMA: The Journal of the American Medical Association* 282(1): 47–53.

Schoeman, F. 1980. "Rights of Children, Rights of Parents, and the Moral Basis of the Family." *Ethics* 91(1): 6–19.

Sharav, Vera H. 2011. "Medical Ethics and Contemporary Medicine." In *Vaccine Epidemic*, edited by Louise Kuo Habakus and Mary Holland, 71–80. Skyhorse Publishing.

Smith, Peter C., and Nick York. 2004. "Quality Incentives: The Case of UK General Practitioners." *Health Affairs* 23(3): 112–118.

Stewart, Alexandra M. 2009. "Challenging Personal Belief Immunization Exemptions: Considering Legal Responses." *Michigan Law Review* 107(105): 105–109.

Thaler, Richard H., and Cass R. Sunstein. 2009. *Nudge: Improving Decisions about Health, Wealth, and Happiness.* Penguin Books.

Torcello, Lawrence. 2011. "The Ethics of Inquiry, Scientific Belief, and Public Discourse." *Public Affairs Quarterly* 25(3): 197–215.

UN Committee on Economic, Social and Cultural Rights. 2001. *Report on the Twenty-Second, Twenty-Third and Twenty-Fourth Sessions.* United Nations. Accessed June 23, 2015. www.un.org/documents/ecosoc/docs/2001/e2001-22.pdf.

United Nations. 2015. "United Nations Treaty Collection." Accessed March 10. https://treaties.un.org/Pages/ViewDetails.aspx?src=TREATY&mtdsg_no=IV-11&chapter=4&lang=en.

Vallier, Kevin, and Fred D'Agostino. 2014. "Public Justification." In *The Stanford Encyclopedia of Philosophy*, edited by Edward N. Zalta, Spring 2014. http://plato.stanford.edu/archives/spr2014/entries/justification-public/.

Vermeersch, E. 1999. "Individual Rights versus Societal Duties." *Vaccine.* 17(Supplement): S14–17.

Verweij, Marcel, and Angus Dawson. 2004. "Ethical Principles for Collective Immunisation Programmes." *Vaccine* 22(23–24): 3122–3126. doi:10.1016/j.vaccine.2004.01.062.

Viens, A. M., C. M. Bensimon, and R. E. G. Upshur. 2009. "Your Liberty or Your Life: Reciprocity in the Use of Restrictive Measures in Contexts of Contagion." *Journal of Bioethical Inquiry* 6(2): 207–217.

Viens, A. M., John Coggon, and Anthony S. Kessel, eds. 2013. *Criminal Law, Philosophy and Public Health Practice.* Cambridge University Press.

Weisman, Jonathan. 2012. "Senate Democrats Propose Letting All Tax Cuts Expire." *The New York Times*, July 17, sec. U.S. / Politics. www.nytimes.com/2012/07/18/us/politics/senate-democrats-propose-letting-all-tax-cuts-expire.html.

Wynia, Matthew K. 2007. "Mandating Vaccination: What Counts as a 'Mandate' in Public Health and When Should They Be Used?" *The American Journal of Bioethics* 7(12): 2–6.

6   Vaccine exemptions

"The ethical principle of informed consent to medical risk-taking is protected in vaccine laws when there are flexible medical, religious and conscientious belief exemptions to ensure that human, civil and parental rights are not violated."

(Fisher 2014, 39)

In the previous chapter I defended coercive vaccination policies. I argued that people have reasons to accept coercive vaccination policies that protect children's interests, prevent serious harms to others, and fairly distribute the costs of valuable public goods. In this chapter I discuss whether and how a state may *exempt* people from coercive vaccination laws. For example, I consider whether the state should allow some unvaccinated children to attend school, even if the law requires schoolchildren to be vaccinated.

There are three reasons for offering vaccine exemptions (which are sometimes called vaccine *waivers*). First, it may be *unjust* to subject some people to coercive vaccination, at least on some accounts of public reason liberalism. This is because some people may not have a reason to accept coercive vaccination laws. Second, a commitment to protect *conscience* may tell in favor of exempting people even if it is not unjust to coerce them. This is because some people may falsely believe they have a reason to object to coercive vaccination laws, and the state may give these people waivers to protect them from the moral, psychological, or existential harms they would experience if they were not exempted. Third, a commitment to broader *social and political goals* may count in favor of waiver policies, even if it is not unjust to coerce people to vaccinate, and even if vaccine refusers are not conscientious objectors. For example, the state may decide to offer waivers to prevent parents from becoming vocal anti-vaccine activists.

In the early sections of this chapter, I argue that these three reasons count in favor of waiver policies, but are not decisive. In particular, I argue that the case for vaccine waivers is not as strong as it may initially appear to be. In the later sections of this chapter, I take for granted that vaccine exemption policies are firmly entrenched in many communities and are unlikely to be eliminated in the near future. So, even though I do not think that the case for vaccine waivers is very strong, I argue that there are better and worse ways for exemption programs to be run.

Let's begin with current practice: All fifty states in the United States offer *medical* exemptions. Unvaccinated children may be allowed to attend school if their physicians determine that they are too immunocompromised to be safely vaccinated. I think that at least some medical exemptions should be uncontroversial. If a child is at heightened risk of vaccine complications, you won't protect her interests by coercively vaccinating her. Also, it is unreasonable to vaccinate immunocompromised children to prevent them from infecting others or to get them to contribute to herd immunity, since the risks to the vaccinated child may be too high. I often disagree with Barbara Loe Fisher, but I agree that "[i]t is not humane or just to compel everyone to use a pharmaceutical product that carries a greater risk of injury or death for those more vulnerable to suffering harm from use of that product" (Fisher 2014, 40).

Medical exemptions should be relatively non-controversial. The interesting questions are about *nonmedical* exemptions. These waivers go to people who object to vaccination for religious, moral, or philosophical reasons. Exemption policies often distinguish between exemptions for people who object for religious reasons and exemptions for people who object for secular reasons. The former are called 'religious' exemptions, while the latter are usually called 'personal belief' or 'philosophical' exemptions. Many communities make it easier to receive religious exemptions. Either they offer *only* religious exemptions or they make the process for receiving a philosophical exemption more burdensome. For example, in the United States, forty-eight states offer religious waivers, but a far smaller number offer philosophical waivers (seventeen or nineteen depending on the demarcation criteria) (Fisher 2014; National Conference of State Legislatures (NCSL) 2012).[1] Even states that offer philosophical exemptions often make it easier to receive religious exemptions. For example, as of May 2014, California grants religious exemptions to anyone who makes a religious objection, but it requires people who want personal belief exemptions to meet with a physician to discuss vaccines (California Department of Public Health 2013b).

Nonmedical exemption rates are increasing in many communities (Butz 2014; California Department of Public Health 2013a; Centers for Disease Control and Prevention 2013; Rockoff 2010). And disease outbreaks are more likely in communities with higher rates of nonmedical exemptions (Imdad et al. 2013; Omer et al. 2012). Furthermore, the communities that make nonmedical exemptions easier to receive tend to have higher rates of nonmedical exemptions (Blank, Caplan, and Constable 2013).[2] When exemptions are easier to get, more people get them. Therefore, communities with more permissive exemption policies are at greater risk of disease outbreaks. Finally, there is evidence that communities can lower their rates of higher-incidence diseases by making nonmedical exemption policies more restrictive (Szabo 2012; Yang and Debold 2014).

The evidence I discuss in the previous paragraph indicates that one way to protect communities from disease outbreaks is to make nonmedical exemption policies more restrictive. One strategy is to eliminate nonmedical exemptions entirely. For example, California Governor Jerry Brown announced in 2015 that he was open to legislative efforts to eliminate all nonmedical exemptions in his state (McGreevy and Lin II 2015). Another strategy is to eliminate one of the categories of nonmedical exemptions; in most all cases, people want to eliminate philosophical exemptions. For example, in 2014 the editorial board of USA *Today* – the widest circulated print newspaper in the United States – called for an end to personal belief waivers (USA Today Editorial Board 2014). A further strategy is to make (some kinds of) nonmedical exemptions more difficult to receive. For one example, as of 2014 children throughout Australia may be enrolled in a childcare facility only if their parents provide documentation that the children are fully vaccinated (Hansen 2014). An exemption is made for parents who document that they are 'conscientious objectors' to vaccination, and who get a physician to sign a form attesting to the fact that the parents have been informed about vaccine safety and efficacy. Even though this new law makes vaccine refusal more burdensome, some in Australia worry that it does not yet make it burdensome enough, and they support eliminating personal belief exemptions entirely (Ngo 2014). For another example, my home state of Michigan now requires all parents who want their children exempted from mandatory vaccination laws to attend education sessions run by county health departments (Michigan Department of Public Health 2015). Other states in the United States – including Oregon, California, Vermont, and Washington – have recently passed similar laws (Moody 2014; Warner 2014), while legislators are pushing for more restrictive nonmedical exemption laws in many other states, including Colorado (Fowler 2014; WAMC Editor 2014).

My goal in this chapter is to engage with contemporary debates about nonmedical exemptions in the following way. First, I clarify the ways in which liberal justice, concern for conscience, and pragmatic considerations may tell in favor of offering vaccine waivers. However, I conclude that it is unlikely that these kinds of considerations justify nonmedical exemption policies. In particular, I argue that nonmedical vaccine exemptions may undermine the goals of coercive vaccination laws: individual and herd immunity. Furthermore, I argue that it is both difficult and unjustifiable to prioritize exemptions for people who make religious objections. And I conclude by arguing that policies that make it more difficult to receive vaccine waivers may be proxy policies. They may help to distribute exemptions to people for whom reasons of liberal justice, concern for conscience, and pragmatic consideration count in favor of receiving waivers.

Rules and exemptions

How should a society respond to the fact that reasons of liberal justice, considerations of conscience, or pragmatic concerns count against a coercive law?

First, a state could eliminate a law if considerations of liberal justice, conscience, or political pragmatism counted against subjecting people to it. In this case, there would be no exemptions, because there would not be a law to exempt people from. A second possibility is universal enforcement. In this case, the state would conclude that the goals served by the law were sufficiently important to justify the (potentially) unjust coercion of some members of society, the violation of some people's conscience, or potentially harmful consequences for other valuable social and political projects. This is a suboptimal outcome, but it may sometimes be the best that the state can do. A third option is to enforce the law, but to exempt some people from it. This is what Brian Barry calls a 'rule-plus-exemption' strategy (Barry 2001).[3] In this case, the state concludes that some combination of liberal justice, concern for conscience, and pragmatic considerations lead to the conclusion that the 'objectionable' law should be selectively enforced.

Exemption policies to general laws may seem to occupy an unstable middle ground, because the considerations that count in favor of a general law also count in favor of universal compliance with the law (Barry 2001, 39).[4] At the same time, considerations that tell in favor of exempting people from a law also tell in favor of abolishing the law (and exempting everyone).

Some laws have such weighty reasons in favor of them, that the state ought to insist on universal compliance, even if some people have reasons to object conscientiously, or even if they would make trouble if they were not exempted. For example, consider a law that outlaws Female Genital Cutting (FGC).[5] This rule aims to protect young girls from procedures that cause pain, diminish future sexual pleasure, and increase the risks of childbirth complications. But some parents (and children) may believe that a law prohibiting FGC forces them to violate their religious and cultural values. They may have a reason to reject this law, or at least their conscience may tell them not to follow it. And parents who object to laws prohibiting FGC may also make trouble for politicians and public authorities, if they are not given waivers. Even though these are significant considerations, I think it is clear that the state's responsibility to protect the current and future interests of children is sufficient to rule out exemptions to laws that prohibit FGC. This may mean that anti-FGC laws are imperfectly just or unavoidably indifferent to the demands of conscience. But in some circumstances, these imperfections may be the price a society pays for a law that promotes especially important political goals.

Other laws to which people object seem like they should not be laws at all. For example, many societies prohibit people from wearing head coverings in photographs for official identification cards. However, states often provide waivers for people who have religious reasons for covering the head, as long as the headwear does not obstruct the face (Foreign & Commonwealth Office of the United Kingdom 2014; U.S. Department of State 2014).[6] I assume (for the sake of this example) that the state's interest in using identification cards to *identify* people is not much compromised by allowing headwear in official photos, under the restrictions included in current exemptions (e.g. that religious head coverings not block the face). But if this is the case, then it is unclear why anyone should be prohibited from wearing unobtrusive head coverings in their official photographs. From the point of view of liberal justice, the fact that someone loves his sports team, or is ashamed of his bald spot, or participates in popular forms of contemporary masculinity (which require the wearing of baseball caps or fedoras) seems to be as good a reason for him to wear a head covering as is the fact that his religion or culture tells him not to leave his head bare. And from the point of view of the state, the public purpose of the official photograph would still be served if everyone wore a hat when they had their pictures taken. In this case, a general interest in liberty counts in favor of a more permissive law, rather than the (current) combination of a general prohibition on headwear with selective exemptions.

Advocates of a particular rule-plus-exemption scheme must defend against the charge that the law ought to be universally applied or eliminated. They must show that their rule-plus-exemption scheme occupies a middle ground between laws such as those prohibiting FGC and laws such as those requiring head coverings in official photographs.

A paradigm example of a justified rule-plus-exemption scheme is the case of exemptions for conscientious objectors to combat military service.

On one hand, I take for granted that states have a right to use coercion to compel people to participate in military service, if doing so is necessary for national security. A fundamental purpose (perhaps *the* fundamental purpose) of the state is to defend its members from external attack. Therefore, constraints that are necessary for national defense are paradigm cases of justified state coercion. These are laws that political communities may sometimes be unable to do without.

On the other hand, I take for granted that there are very good reasons not to compel at least some people to participate in combat military service. Indeed, there is a broad international consensus that conscientious objectors to combat military service ought generally to be exempted from laws that compel such service.[7] For example, the United States has a long history of granting exemptions to some general conscientious objectors.[8] The same is true of most other countries, and of the international community, where there is an emerging consensus that conscientious objectors are entitled to exemptions as a matter of human rights (Lippman 1990; Lubell 2002; Major 2001; Marcus 1997). In particular, the 1948 Universal

Declaration of Human Rights (UDHR) affirms that all people are entitled to freedom of thought and conscience, which includes a right to manifest their beliefs in their lives (United Nations General Assembly 1948). The United Nations Commission on Human Rights has argued that Article 18 of the UDHR grounds exemption rights for conscientious objectors to military service (Takemura 2009, chap. 2).

But the fact that there may be good reasons to offer exemptions does not mean that the state *should* offer exemptions. Recall that some parents and children may object to laws prohibiting FGC, but universal compliance is called for in that case. What makes the case of military conscientious objection different? I think the relevant difference is that offering exemptions to people who conscientiously object to military service is almost always consistent with protecting national defense – the fundamental goal of laws that coerce military service. Most societies will be able to meet their national security needs with only a small percentage of their members serving in combat roles. And very few citizens are likely to request exemptions. Consider that only about 60,000 Britons applied for conscientious objector status during World War II, when millions of Britons served in uniform (Kramer 2013). So, even during wartime and full mobilization, conscientious objector policies are unlikely to undermine national defense. Also, coercing sincere conscientious objectors into combat service may be *counterproductive* to the goals of military readiness, since placing conscientious objectors alongside willing soldiers may undermine morale. Indeed, military commanders have often supported permissive exemption policies, since generals have not wanted pacifist soldiers in the ranks.

There is also a consensus international view that military conscientious objector exemptions may be rescinded if they undermine military readiness. For example, in *Gillette v. United States*, the US Supreme Court decided that the government may deny exemptions when doing so is required for national security (Gillette v. United States 1971). The international community has recognized a similar conditionality for conscientious objector policies. For example, the United Nations Human Rights Committee has determined that the freedom of religion and conscience does not include an absolute right to act in accordance with one's beliefs, but may be constrained for national security purposes.[9]

Another goal of military conscription is to fairly distribute the human costs of providing for national defense. So, we might object to conscientious objector exemption policies if they allowed someone to avoid contributing to public efforts to promote national defense. However, many people who have been exempted from combat military service have provided alternative service, either in noncombatant military roles or elsewhere. For example, during World War II some conscientious objectors defused bombs, and during the US war in Vietnam some conscientious objectors served as medics. It counts in favor of a rule-plus-exemption policy if exempted individuals do not unfairly increase the burdens borne by others (Leiter 2013, 101).

Exemptions and the goals of vaccination policy

Do vaccine waiver laws occupy a middle ground between universal compliance and universal legal permissiveness?

On one hand, there are weighty reasons for the state to use coercion if it is necessary to ensure mass vaccination. This was the thesis of chapter five, where I argued that coercive vaccination may be justified when it is necessary to protect children's interests, prevent people from harming each other, and fairly distribute the burdens of creating herd immunity. The reasons in favor of using coercion to promote vaccination (when voluntary methods are unlikely to succeed) seem as strong as the reasons for using coercion to ensure military readiness (when voluntary military service will not suffice). Millions have died in wars, but millions more have died from diseases. Diseases are responsible for most wartime deaths, too. If mass vaccination were feasible in the 17th century, I think it's likely that Hobbes and Locke would have declared that the generation and maintenance of herd immunity is one of the core purposes of the state. The case for coercive vaccination is about as strong as a case for state coercion could be.

On the other hand, there are weighty reasons for the state not to compel parents to vaccinate their children (see e.g. Asveld 2008; Sutton and Upshur 2010). For example, a parent who believes that God prohibits vaccination may have a reason to object to vaccination laws. At the very least, she likely faces a huge moral or psychological burden if the state compels her to violate the dictates of her conscience. Therefore, reasons of liberal justice or considerations of conscience may tell in favor of offering parents exemptions to mandatory vaccination laws.

I do not think that liberal justice or concern for conscience suffices to justify exemption policies for vaccine refusers. This is because vaccine exemption policies undermine the goals coercive vaccination laws promote.

First, vaccine exemption policies may compromise herd immunity (Atwell et al. 2013; Blank, Caplan, and Constable 2013; Constable, Blank, and Caplan 2014; Lee, Rosenthal, and Scheffler 2013; Omer et al. 2012; Salmon et al. 1999; Yang and Debold 2014). The numbers matter. As I have mentioned at various points in this book, herd immunity may require vaccination rates between 80% (e.g. for rubella and mumps) and 95% (e.g. for measles). In the 2013–2014 school year, CDC found that most states failed to reach the target of having 95% of children entering kindergarten complete the two-dose MMR vaccine sequence (Centers for Disease Control and Prevention 2014). This target must be met to preserve the herd against measles. Some states were far below this level. For example, in Colorado, less than 85% of children entering kindergarten had received both doses of MMR.

Some states already offer too many nonmedical exemptions, and others cannot allow any more. Some states are fine for now, but would do well to try to prevent increases in their nonmedical exemption rates. Furthermore, the fact that nonmedical exemptions are geographically clustered means that even relatively low national or state exemption rates may result in local breakdowns in herd immunity (Gahr et al. 2014; Gaudino and Robison 2012; May and Silverman 2003; Omer et al. 2008). Douglas Diekema says:

> The state of Washington, for example, reported a statewide exemption rate of 5.6% for students enrolled in kindergarten through twelfth grade during the 2011–2012 school year. Exemption rates by county, however, ranged between 1% (Garfield) and 30% (Ferry), with exemption rates exceeding 10% in 7 of 37 counties reporting data.
>
> (Diekema 2014, 284)

Nonmedical exemptions may have weakened or destroyed herd immunity in Ferry County, Washington. And herd immunity is also at risk in the many Washington counties with exemption rates greater than 10%, even though the state's overall exemption rate is not nearly so high. The same can be said about county-specific vulnerabilities in many other states (see e.g. Omer et al. 2008).

The fact that herd immunity requires such high vaccination rates means that coercive vaccination laws are unable to promote their goals with even moderate exemption rates. Notice the contrast with exemptions for military conscientious objectors. Relatively few members of society are needed for combat military service and there are unlikely to be very many conscientious objectors, especially during just wars. Or consider a contemporary policy question: whether the state should permit business owners to refuse to provide goods and services for same-sex weddings, when business owners have heartfelt religious objections to participating in these events (Kaplan 2015; Muskal 2015). Some people defend exemption rights in this sort of case, on the grounds that business owners who object are usually able to refer people to other businesses (bakers, florists, etc.) who will work with them.

A second way that vaccine exemptions undermine the goals of coercive vaccination laws is by compromising individual immunity. One of the main purposes of coercive vaccination laws is to give individual children immunity against diseases, and to prevent them from infecting others, even in the absence of herd immunity. But vaccine exemptions allow parents to withhold vital preventative medical care from their children and to negligently make their children potential vectors of disease. Avoiding these outcomes is among the goals at which coercive vaccination policies aim. The fact that vaccine exemptions directly undermine these goals is an especially weighty reason not to allow vaccine exemptions.

Someone might respond that individual immunity is superfluous when herd immunity exists. So, if a nonmedical exemption policy did not undermine herd immunity, then it would not matter that exempted people did not develop individual immunity. In response, individual immunity offers protection even when herd immunity exists, since people from outside the community may infect someone who lacks individual immunity, even when herd immunity exists. Therefore, the fact that nonmedical exemptions prevent children from developing individual immunity *does* count against exemption policies, even when herd immunity exists.

I have shown that vaccine exemptions are not likely to be a requirement of liberal justice or of giving due consideration to the demands of conscience. Of course, requiring universal compliance with vaccination laws may not protect conscience (and may not be fully just). But this may be the least bad option available. Liberal justice and conscience do not exhaust the reasons for vaccine exemptions. In the next section I discuss pragmatic reasons to offer vaccine waivers.

Pragmatic reasons for exemptions

Exempting people from coercive vaccine laws may serve broader social and political purposes.

First, people tend to mobilize when they believe a law is unjustly coercing them.[10] We generally do more to resist laws to which we object than to defend laws that we support, especially if our objection is forceful or our approval is not animated by powerful emotions. Therefore, groups who object to a particular law are likely to have a disproportionate voice in public debates about that law. Politicians who want to satisfy the demands of their most engaged constituents have pragmatic reasons to offer exemptions.

Second, offering exemptions to the most committed vaccine refusers may prevent criticism of coercive vaccination programs. The history of early compulsory vaccination shows how unhelpful it can be to coerce people who are willing to face great sacrifices to avoid vaccination. Some people went to prison, or had their homes seized and sold by the state, because they refused to pay fines for refusing vaccines. And many people who were otherwise sympathetic with vaccination programs were aghast at the coercive tactics the state used to promote public health (Colgrove 2006; Durbach 2005; Porter and Porter 1988). Of course, contemporary vaccination programs are usually not as coercive as 19th-century programs were. (As I discussed in chapter five, vaccine programs used to be more *compulsory*, but are now usually only *mandatory*.) However we may still worry that coercive public health efforts are counterproductive. For example, we have reason to offer exemptions if doing so will avoid creating a class of popular 'martyrs'. It does not help the cause of mass vaccination if television programs and websites are full of stories about how the government prevented innocent children from attending school, just because their mothers were (perhaps overzealously) protective of their health. Even when public health officials are on the side of both truth and morality, parents (and others) may sympathize with the plight of children who have been banished from schools or daycare. Offering exemptions may limit the number of these sorts of stories.

Finally, vaccine waivers keep kids in school and keep parents engaged with broader social programs. Some parents respond to mandatory vaccination policies by withdrawing their children from school and daycare. This is a problem, because school and daycare offer important educational and developmental benefits to children. Among other things, formal schooling often offers the only opportunities some children have for developing the skills they will need to access higher education and professional careers. And we should not underestimate the potential of formal education to develop the habits of good citizenship. In particular, participation in public institutions (such as public schools) helps to build the shared culture of a society, and society suffers when more families pull their children out of the public sphere and choose to retreat to within the home.[11] (I assume that students at many private schools also realize these benefits.) We may also hope that vaccine exemption policies may cause vaccine refusers to place greater trust in public health authorities than they otherwise would. At the very least, if they can be exempted from vaccination laws, vaccine refusers may be less adversarial when they respond to other public health initiatives or to other government programs.

I do not know if these pragmatic considerations are sufficient to require states to adopt vaccine exemption policies. This conclusion requires empirical knowledge that I do not have. But at the very least, these pragmatic considerations identify reasons to support exemption policies, beyond considerations of liberal justice and conscience.

Prioritizing religion?

I have so far discussed ways in which liberal justice, concern for conscience, and pragmatic considerations could count in favor of vaccine exemptions. Ultimately, I do not think these considerations suffice to justify vaccine exemptions, or at least I don't have sufficient evidence to conclude that they do. However, if we take for granted that some vaccine exemptions scheme is going to exist, we can focus on how best to restrict exemptions, so as to minimize the harms to individuals and to herd immunity. I begin this part of the chapter – which takes the existence of some form of vaccine waiver scheme for granted – by considering whether exemptions ought to be prioritized for people who object for religious reasons.

Parents in twenty-nine (or thirty-one) of the states in the United States may receive exemptions only if they object for religious reasons.[12] Even communities that grant philosophical exemptions have sometimes made it easier for people with religious objections to get waivers. For example, California Governor Jerry Brown uttered the following when he signed a recent law tightening access to nonmedical vaccine exemptions:

> I will direct the Department [of Public Health] to allow for a separate religious exemption on the form … in this way, people whose religious beliefs preclude vaccinations will not be required to seek a health practitioner's signature.
>
> (Shute 2013)

The California *statute* treats all nonmedical exemptions equally. It requires everyone who wants an exemption to complete a form signed by a physician attesting to the fact that they have been informed about the science of vaccines. However, Brown's *signing statement* created a more permissive standard for religious waivers (California Department of Public Health 2013b).[13]

If the state prioritizes exemptions for people who make religious objections, then the state has to decide what counts as a religion (Barry 2001, 52). There are both conceptual and epistemological problems with the state getting into the business of defining religions and determining whether people have religious reasons for their objections.

There is a conceptual problem: There are no obvious criteria for the state to use to distinguish between religious and non-religious objections. The mere fact that someone says that their objection is 'religious' should not be enough. But at the same time, we should not limit religious exemptions to people who espouse popular (and easily recognizable) religious beliefs. That would be unjustifiably discriminatory against members of minority religious groups. But objective criteria that would include all clear cases of religion are also likely to be more expansive than they first appear to be. For example, consider the distinguishing features of religion proposed by Brian Leiter. On Leiter's view, religions offer "existential consolation" and make "categorical demands that are insulated from evidence" (Leiter 2013, 52, 63). Leiter's account of the distinctive features of religion includes clear cases of religion, but also seems to place both Kantianism and the 'ethics of purity' within the sphere of the religious. The followers of Ayn Rand may count as religious acolytes, too; I have met people who have received 'existential consolation' from her work, and they often seem unresponsive to evidence. Recall that one reason to prioritize religious exemptions is to limit the number of exemptions the state hands out, e.g. by making it harder or impossible for people to receive philosophical waivers. But it's not clear that conceptions of 'religion' that are expansive enough to admit clear cases will be restrictive enough to justify many restrictions on exemptions. However, conceptions of religion that would result in significantly lower exemption rates (i.e. in communities that offered only religious waivers) may not include clear cases of religion. For example, if we supposed that a 'religion' must include a deity, then some forms of Buddhism would be out.[14]

There is also an epistemological problem: Even if we could solve the conceptual problem, it is not clear how the state would distinguish between cases in which people are motivated by sincere religious beliefs and cases in which people insincerely invoke religion to receive special treatment. Current practice in most communities with vaccine exemption policies has been to take people at their word when they claim to have religious objections. But this practice encourages people to invent new 'religions' in order to take advantage of the priority that the law grants to religious objectors. Consider the lighthearted attempt by some atheists to claim religious exemptions on the grounds of their adherence to 'Pastafarianism', a faith that involves devotion to the 'Flying Spaghetti Monster' and the wearing of pasta strainers (colanders) on the head. (A Pastafarian in Austria was permitted to wear a colander on his head in his driver's license photograph (Peralta 2011).) To be clear, Pastafarians' requests for religious exemptions are usually intended as humorous criticism of the priority that states often grant to religious believers. All the same, the success of Pastafarians in receiving exemptions points to deficiencies in the state's capacity (or willingness) to distinguish religious from non-religious sources of objection.[15]

More worrisome, at least from the point of view of vaccine policy, are efforts by some Australian vaccine refusers to identify vaccine refusal *as a religion*. They have formed the 'Church of Conscious Living', which teaches that "the human body is a sacred space and ... should not be contaminated by external toxic forces ... [which include] orthodox vaccination" (Cusack 2013). The Australian government has so far been hesitant to declare that this church does not practice a 'real' religion. And given the conceptual problem I discuss above, it is not obvious what standard the government would use if it wanted to make such a declaration. Accordingly, Australians who claim membership in the Church of Conscious Living have received religious exemptions to mandatory vaccination policies (Hansen 2013).

More common than the opportunistic *creation* of new anti-vaccine religions has been the opportunistic *invocation* of religious objections that are not actually based in religious teachings (Associated Press 2007). Some parents may be confused when they claim that their religions prohibit vaccination, since most parents who claim religious objections do not practice religions that prohibit vaccination (Grabenstein 2013). But Dorit Reiss argues persuasively that most people who claim to object to vaccines for religious reasons are lying (Reiss 2014). They know that their religions (if they are religious at all) do not prohibit vaccination, but they are willing to do whatever is necessary to get a waiver for their children.

I think the conceptual and epistemological problems with prioritizing religious waivers are sufficiently powerful to warrant the conclusion that we ought not to (try to) prioritize exemptions for religious objectors. But another problem with prioritizing religion is that it's not clear why people who make religious objections ought to receive priority treatment. So, even if we *could* prioritize religious waivers, it is not clear that we *should*.

First, liberal justice should not treat religion as a privileged source of reasonable objections to (potential) laws. I agree that public reason liberals ought to be willing to treat religious belief as a possible source of reasons for rejecting laws. (Public justification need not occur only in secular language.) But I see no basis for a principled priority for religious objections, since secular beliefs and values may also be the source of reasons to object to laws.

Second, the fact that a belief is religious is not a reason for thinking that it is more central to conscience. So, a commitment to protect conscience cannot justify prioritizing exemptions for religious objectors. Compelling a person to violate his religious beliefs need not do any more to constrain his liberty or compromise his moral autonomy than compelling a person to violate his secular convictions. A secular commitment to protect human rights, to fulfill one's obligations as a parent, or to act with integrity may be just as conscientious as religious convictions may be. Also, religious beliefs are not in principle more connected to people's emotional and psychological well-being than secular beliefs. Compelling a person to violate his religious convictions need not cause greater emotional or psychological harm than compelling a person to violate secular convictions. I agree that it may be burdensome for a religious believer to worry about spending an eternity in hell. But being forced to act against one's secular convictions could cause comparable emotional and psychological trauma. Of course, a person who believes that she will receive a post-mortem punishment for her wrongdoing may *anticipate* a longer duration for her emotional and psychological pain. But there is no reason to think that the emotional and psychological disturbances religious believers experience in their earthly lives are worse than the disturbances secular people experience.

Finally, I do not think pragmatic considerations tell in favor of prioritizing exemptions for religious objectors. People may be willing to protest vaccine policies or to pull their kids out of school if they have religious reasons to object to vaccines. But people who object to vaccines for secular reasons – perhaps they believe vaccines are very harmful – also seem likely to protest or to pull their children from school.

We might try to avoid the charge that prioritizing religious objections is morally unjustified if we embraced an especially expansive conception of religion. One option is for the state to claim that an objection is 'religious' if it emerges from sincere and deeply held (moral) convictions. The United States has pursued something like this strategy to manage its program for offering exemptions to military conscientious objectors. In *United States v. Seeger*, 380 U.S. 163 (1965), the US Supreme Court determined that a belief qualifies as sufficiently 'religious' (for the purpose of a religious objection to military service) when it is "sincere and meaningful [and] occupies a place in the life of its possessor parallel to that filled by the orthodox belief in God" (United States v. Seeger 1965, 166). Courts and legislatures in the United States have often adopted similar standards for determining whether vaccine objections are 'religious' (Salmon, Sapsin, et al. 2005; Salmon and Siegel 2001). For example, Douglas Diekema observes that "[i]n Oregon ... a religion is defined as 'any system of beliefs, practices, or ethical values'" (Diekema 2014, 285).[16]

Conceptions of 'religion' that assimilate the distinction between religious and non-religious reasons to a distinction between moral and merely prudential reasons make a distinction worth making in exemption policies. But if prioritizing 'religious' over 'secular' objections reduces to prioritizing moral over prudential objections, then it would be best to address this distinction directly, rather than under the confused labels of the 'religious' and the 'secular'.

Moral and prudential objections

One way to limit exemptions is to give them only to people who object for moral reasons (or to make it easier for people who object for moral reasons to get waivers), and not to give waivers to people who object for merely prudential reasons.

Prioritizing exemptions for people who object for moral reasons may be morally defensible. First, considerations of liberal justice may tell in favor of prioritizing exemptions for people who object for moral reasons. This is because moral convictions seem more likely to ground reasons to reject otherwise reasonable laws than do considerations about what might merely promote a person's interests. Second, considerations of conscience tell in favor of prioritizing exemptions for people who have moral reasons for objecting. This is because someone who objects for a moral reason is more likely to be motivated by conscience than someone who objects for reasons of prudence. Finally, pragmatic considerations also tell in favor of prioritizing exemptions for people who object for moral reasons. This is because someone who objects for moral reasons may be more likely to protest vaccine policies or withdraw her children from school than someone who objects for merely prudential reasons. While people sometimes resist state actions that compromise their interests, they seem more likely to resist state actions that compel them to act immorally.

I think there are good reasons to prioritize exemptions for people who object for moral reasons over people who object for merely prudential reasons. However, familiar conceptual and epistemological questions assert themselves when we reflect on how the state ought to distinguish between moral and merely prudential objections.

On one hand, it may not be clear how to distinguish between a parent who objects to vaccination for moral reasons and a parent who objects to vaccination for merely prudential reasons. One of a parent's chief moral duties is to promote her child's interests. Does this mean that a parent has a moral obligation to perform all acts that are in the interests of the child? I think that some vaccine refusers are committed to something like this expansive conception of parental obligations. But this cannot be a correct view. Parents are not morally obligated to do everything they can to promote the interests of their children since they do not even have a moral *right* to do everything they can to promote their children's interests. For example, I argued in chapter four that parents are not morally permitted to promote their children's interests by placing other people at significant risk of serious harm or by free-riding on public goods.

Some critics of vaccine refusal have argued that vaccine refusers usually offer merely prudential objections (Offit 2010, 144–146). I agree that vaccine refusers are sometimes immoral free-riders. But I do not think that vaccine refusers are usually motivated primarily by a desire to promote their children's interests by free-riding. Instead, many vaccine refusers (falsely) believe that vaccines are *so harmful* for their children that allowing their children to be vaccinated would violate their obligation to protect their children from serious avoidable harms. In contrast, some parents may have (roughly) true beliefs about the safety and efficacy of vaccines, but may refuse vaccines in order to *maximize* their children's interests.[17] Hence, in the case of vaccine refusal, the conceptual distinction between moral and merely prudential objections may have more traction than it may first appear to have.

However, even if we can solve the conceptual problem about what *is* a moral objection, we still have a pressing epistemological problem. How can the state tell when someone is making a moral objection to vaccination? Parents will lie to get waivers, and it is unclear whether the state is willing or able to try to distinguish sincere from insincere claims of moral objections.

In the next section, I will argue that making it *burdensome* to receive an exemption may serve as a useful proxy for distinguishing between moral and (merely) prudential objections. People who object because they believe that a law compels them to act immorally are likely driven to object by a greater intensity of feeling than someone who objects because they believe the law does not adequately promote their children's interests. I agree with Philip Kitcher that "the intensity with which an outcome is valued can often be assessed (roughly, to be sure) by considering the ways in which individuals are prepared to sacrifice time and comfort for their causes" (Kitcher 2011, 65). Of course, if we had an easy way to tell whether someone was making a moral objection to vaccination, then it would be fairer to offer them a waiver without making them withstand a burdensome exemption process (Swaine 2008). For example, if we knew that objectors from particular cultural or religious groups were almost certain to be conscientious, then we might forgo burdensome waiver application processes for members of those groups. But, we are generally unable to make these sorts of *ex ante* decisions in the case of vaccine refusal. So, we may have to make the waiver application process burdensome if we want to lower exemption rates while ensuring that people with serious moral objections to vaccination may continue to receive waivers.

Making exemptions burdensome

Some communities have recently decided to make it more difficult for parents to receive exemptions to mandatory vaccination laws. In many cases, communities have continued to grant exemptions for the same reasons as they have in the past, but they have made the application process more difficult to complete. For example, until recently, my county health office (in Oakland, Michigan) granted exemptions to anyone who documented an objection (short personal letters often sufficed). As of January 1, 2015, parents in Oakland County who want to receive a waiver must bring their child to the county health division's offices, and they must participate in a vaccination education session with a public health nurse. Parents will be able to receive a waiver only after they complete the education session.

There is evidence that more burdensome exemption policies – such as the one that Oakland County has introduced – are likely to lower the rates of nonmedical vaccine exemptions (Constable, Blank, and Caplan 2014; Rota et al. 2001; Salmon, Omer, et al. 2005; Yang and Debold 2014). Fewer people will receive exemptions because some people are unwilling to complete burdensome application processes (May and Silverman 2005). At the same time, none of these burdens places insurmountable (or even unreasonable) barriers in the way of parents who want exemptions.

Prioritizing exemptions for people who are willing to bear additional burdens may be a useful proxy for other criteria. First, someone who does not have a reason to accept coercive vaccination laws is likely to complete a more burdensome waiver application process. Second, parents who believe that vaccination violates the dictates of their conscience are also likely to be willing to face moderate burdens to receive an exemption. Finally, people who are willing to become political activists to protest vaccine mandates are likely to put up with minor inconveniences to be exempted from policies they would otherwise be willing to protest.

The people who are going to be discouraged by more burdensome waiver application processes are likely to be people who have the least claim to receive exemptions in the first place. When vaccine exemptions are easy to receive, some parents apply for exemptions because that is easier than getting their children vaccinated, which can involve setting up doctor's appointments, taking kids out of school, and missing work to attend appointments (Omer et al. 2012; Rota et al. 2001). Making it more burdensome to receive vaccine exemptions than to become vaccinated will incentivize some parents to get their children vaccinated, while leaving exemptions available for those who *really* want them.

We may hope that requiring people who want exemptions to complete vaccination education sessions will lead some parents to endorse more accurate views about the safety and efficacy of vaccines, or to place greater trust in mainstream medical authorities. In Oakland County, the new vaccine education sessions are run by trained public health nurses. These nurses are experts at talking to people about communicable diseases. Perhaps they will be able to undermine some parents' confidence in their non-expert intuitive judgments, and perhaps the public health nurses will bolster some parents' willingness to defer to expert consensus views about childhood vaccination. After all, people tend to become less confident in their views when they are exposed to multiple perspectives (Brenner, Koehler, and Tversky 1996; Kahneman 2011, 87, 133). And deviating from a widespread practice – such as routine childhood vaccination – requires someone to sustain a great deal of confidence in their views (Thaler and Sunstein 2009, 6, 27).

It is not unreasonable to be optimistic about the potential for vaccine education sessions to change people's minds, but there are also reasons to be pessimistic. Brendan Nyhan et al. have found that various interventions – providing people with scientific information about vaccines, or telling stories and showing pictures about vaccine-preventable diseases – sometimes lead people to endorse more accurate beliefs about vaccines (Nyhan et al. 2014). But Nyhan et al. found that these interventions did not make people more likely to vaccinate and, in some cases, they made people *less* likely to vaccinate. It may matter that Nyhan et al.'s experiments consisted of automated responses over the Internet. We may hope that in-person interactions would be more effective. Indeed, Opel et al. have shown that pediatricians can affect the rates at which parents vaccinate their children depending on how pediatricians handle discussions with parents about vaccines (Opel et al. 2013). Hendrix et al. reach a similar conclusion about the potential for in-person interactions with pediatricians to increase vaccination rates (Hendrix et al. 2014).[18]

Someone might object that it is unfair to socially disadvantaged people to make it more burdensome to receive vaccine waivers (Sutton and Upshur 2010; Wynia 2006).[19] For example, parents who work multiple jobs or have limited access to transportation may be unable to bring their children to the health department's offices for mandatory education sessions. Also, parents who lack Internet access or computer literacy will face greater burdens when they attempt to complete vaccine webinars. Therefore, vaccine laws that require parents seeking exemptions to complete bur-densome tasks may shift the burden of creating and maintaining herd immunity further onto the backs of the worst-off members of society.[20] This is a real problem, but it may be unavoidable if we are going to reduce vaccine waiver rates.

Conclusion

Vaccine exemption policies are unlikely to go away any time soon. So, even if nonmedical exemptions are not required by liberal justice, concern for conscience, or pragmatic considerations, we ought to reflect on how to best run nonmedical exemption programs. I have argued that it is unjustified to prioritize waivers for people who make religious objections. And I have defended efforts to lower exemption rates that make the application process for waivers more burdensome.

Notes

1 The National Vaccine Information Center (for whom Fisher is writing) does not count either Missouri or New Mexico as offering personal belief exemptions, though the National Council of State Legislatures (NCSL) does. Missouri offers personal belief exemptions only for daycare, preschool, and nursery school (State of Missouri 2014). New Mexico offers only religious exemptions, but one might interpret the statute's authorization of religious objections so as to include a right to personal belief exemptions (Fisher 2014; State of New Mexico 2014).

2 This study concludes that rates of nonmedical exemptions are twice as high in states with permissive nonmedical exemption policies as they are in states with more restrictive policies.

3 I use Barry's term for exemption policies, but I do not rely on his justification for exemption policies.

4 Another way in which rule-plus-exemption policies occupy an unsteady middle ground is raised by Wynia (2007). He argues that *permissive* exemption policies effectively destroy the mandates from which they offer exemptions.

5 I use the term 'Female Genital Cutting' rather than either of the other two common terms ('Female Genital Mutilation' and 'Female Circumcision'). This way, I avoid reading a moral evaluation of the practice into its name. For example 'mutilation' is something bad, and male circumcision is an uncontroversial practice in some communities. Also, by FGC I mean procedures that cause significant harms, including both current pain and future dysfunction. Merely symbolic forms of FGC – that cause very little pain and do not cause future dysfunction – may not be as objectionable.

6 The US State Department says the following about head coverings in photos for US passports: "You may only wear a hat or head covering if you wear it daily for religious purposes. Your full face must be visible and your head covering cannot obscure your hairline or cast shadows on your face" (U.S. Department of State 2014).

7 Here I am discussing only pacifist or *general* objectors.

8 While there have been conscientious objectors in the United States since colonial times, objectors first received statutory exemption rights during World War I. However, conscientious objectors have been able to legally avoid military service in previous American conflicts. For example, during the

Civil War conscripts from the northern states could pay $300 to obtain a replacement conscript (Capozzola 2008, chap. 2; Chambers II 1993).

9 For discussion of these issues, see Lubell (2002, especially 415). By endorsing the conditionality of the freedom of conscience (identified in the UDHR), I reject Sutton and Upshur's claim that freedom of conscience in medical choices may not be jeopardized, even to avoid negative public health consequences (Sutton and Upshur 2010, 342).

10 For discussion of how difficult it would be to eliminate vaccine exemption policies see Offit (2010, 192f).

11 Homeschooling may sometimes be a reasonable (even commendable) choice, such as when public schools are unsafe. My focus here is on the way that coercive vaccination policies may contribute to otherwise avoidable (and unjustified) instances of homeschooling.

12 See note 1 for an explanation of the different ways of counting the number of states that offer only religious exemptions.

13 This more permissive standard for religious objectors is reflected in California's new vaccine waiver form. The new form (which incorporates the direction from Governor Brown's signing statement) may be successfully completed in one of two ways. First, Part A may be completed by an "authorized healthcare practitioner licensed in California," who must attest that she has provided the parent with accurate information about the benefits and risks of immunization to both the individual and the community. Then, the parent must attest, in Part B, that the health care practitioner did what she said she did in Part A. The second way to successfully complete the form is much easier. It requires only that a parent attest that she is a member of a religion that prohibits her from "seeking medical advice or treatment from authorized healthcare practitioners" (California Department of Public Health 2013b).

14 Of course, this is not a criticism of Leiter's view, but only of the idea that prioritizing religious objections would sufficiently limit waivers if religion were defined broadly.

15 An Austrian man who was allowed to wear a spaghetti strainer on his head for his official identification photograph said, "something is going wrong here that there is a part of the population that can exert certain special rights that people like me, that atheist people or non-believers cannot have" (Peralta 2011).

16 For example, in *Sherr and Levy v. Northport East-Northport Union Free School District* (672 F. Supp. 81, 89), the court found that parents who had objected to childhood vaccination for the following reason were entitled to a religious exemption under New York state's vaccine laws: "We feel that any introduction into that process of a foreign element outside the normal processes of the body, is going to affect the body adversely and, therefore, we feel it is a violation in a sense of our nature, physical, spiritual religious nature." Note the similarity of these views and the 'ethics of purity' I discussed in chapter three.

17 Importantly, one need not use the language of free-riding to be motivated by a desire to free-ride. For example, a parent who objects to vaccination because she thinks it best promotes her child's interests to receive the protection of herd immunity without facing a low risk of serious vaccine complications is motivated by a desire to free-ride.

18 It is notable that Hendrix et al. found that pediatricians can increase vaccination rates by emphasizing the direct benefits to the child, but that mentioning the social benefits of vaccination does not lead to increases (or decreases) in vaccination rates.

19 I thank Karl Martin Adam for encouraging me to address questions of fairness that are raised by burdensome exemption programs.
20 The fact that coercive vaccination policies have historically shifted burdens onto the less well-off gives us further reason to worry about the fairness of burdensome exemption policies (Colgrove 2004, 364).

Bibliography

Associated Press. 2007. "Parents Claim Religion to Avoid Vaccines for Kids," October 18. www.nbcnews.com/id/21347434/ns/health-childrens_health/t/parents-claim-religion-avoid-vaccines-kids/.

Asveld, Lotte. 2008. "Mass-Vaccination Programmes and the Respect for Autonomy." *Bioethics* 22(5): 245–257.

Atwell, Jessica E., Josh Van Otterloo, Jennifer Zipprich, Kathleen Winter, Kathleen Harriman, Daniel A. Salmon, Neal A. Halsey, and Saad B. Omer. 2013. "Non-medical Vaccine Exemptions and Pertussis in California, 2010." *Pediatrics* 132(4): 624–630. doi:10.1542/peds.2013–0878.

Barry, Brian. 2001. *Culture and Equality: An Egalitarian Critique of Multiculturalism.* Harvard University Press.

Blank, Nina R., Arthur L. Caplan, and Catherine Constable. 2013. "Exempting Schoolchildren from Immunizations: States with Few Barriers Had Highest Rates of Nonmedical Exemptions." *Health Affairs* 32(7): 1282–1290.

Brenner, Lyle A., Derek J. Koehler, and Amos Tversky. 1996. "On the Evaluation of One-Sided Evidence." *Journal of Behavioral Decision Making* 9(1): 59–70.

Butz, Dolly. 2014. "Vaccination Exemptions on the Rise in Woodbury County." *Sioux City Journal*, January 4. http://siouxcityjournal.com/news/local/a1/vaccination-exemptions-on-the-rise-in-woodbury-county/article_9c92f125-6ce9-55bf-b4a6-d0ba937a7b9e.html.

California Department of Public Health. 2013a. *2012–2013 Kindergarten Immunization Assessment Results.* Accessed June 23, 2015. www.cdph.ca.gov/programs/immunize/Documents/2012-2013%20CA%20Kindergarten%20Immunization%20Assessment.pdf.

California Department of Public Health. 2013b. "Personal Beliefs Exemption to Required Immunizations." Accessed June 23, 2015. http://eziz.org/assets/docs/CDPH-8262.pdf.

Capozzola, Christopher. 2008. *Uncle Sam Wants You: World War I and the Making of the Modern American Citizen.* Oxford University Press.

Centers for Disease Control and Prevention. 2013. "Vaccination Coverage among Children in Kindergarten – United States, 2012–13 School Year." 62(30). *Morbidity and Mortality Weekly Report (MMWR)*, August 2. www.cdc.gov/mmwr/preview/mmwrhtml/mm6230a3.htm.

Centers for Disease Control and Prevention. 2014. "Vaccination Coverage among Children in Kindergarten – United States, 2013–14 School Year." 63(41). *Morbidity and Mortality Weekly Report (MMWR)*, October 17. www.cdc.gov/mmwr/preview/mmwrhtml/mm6341a1.htm.

Chambers II, John Whiteclay. 1993. "Conscientious Objectors and the American State from Colonial Times to the Present." In *The New Conscientious Objection: From Sacred to Secular Resistance*, edited by Charles C. Moskos and John Whiteclay Chambers II, 23–46. Oxford University Press.

Colgrove, James Keith. 2004. "Between Persuasion and Compulsion: Smallpox Control in Brooklyn and New York, 1894–1902." *Bulletin of the History of Medicine* 78(2): 349–378.

Colgrove, James Keith. 2006. *State of Immunity: The Politics of Vaccination in Twentieth-Century America*. University of California Press.

Constable, Catherine, Nina R. Blank, and Arthur L. Caplan. 2014. "Rising Rates of Vaccine Exemptions: Problems with Current Policy and More Promising Remedies." *Vaccine* 32(16): 1793–1797.

Cusack, Catherine. 2013. "Religious Exemption Bid Is Last Sting in Anti-Vaccine Bag of Tricks." *Daily Telegraph*. May 26. www.dailytelegraph.com.au/news/opinion/religious-exemption-bid-is-last-sting-in-anti-vaccine-bag-of-tricks/story-fni0cwl5-1226650426023.

Diekema, Douglas S. 2014. "Personal Belief Exemptions from School Vaccination Requirements." *Annual Review of Public Health* 35(1): 275–292.

Durbach, Nadja. 2005. *Bodily Matters: The Anti-Vaccination Movement in England, 1853–1907*. Duke University Press.

Fisher, Barbara Loe. 2014. *Reforming Vaccine Policy & Law – A Guide*. National Vaccine Information Center. Accessed June 23, 2015. www.nvic.org/CMSTemplates/NVIC/pdf/NVIC_Referenced_Vaccine_Law_Reform_Guide.pdf.

Foreign & Commonwealth Office of the United Kingdom. 2014. "Passport Photo Requirements – GOV.UK." GOV.UK. June 2. www.gov.uk/photos-for-passports.

Fowler, Kelsey. 2014. "Colorado Health Organizations Recommend Making It Harder to Opt-out of Vaccinations." *The Summit Daily*, January 12. www.summitdaily.com/entertainment/9720851-113/colorado-district-exemptions-personal.

Gahr, Pamala, Aaron S. DeVries, Gregory Wallace, Claudia Miller, Cynthia Kenyon, Kristin Sweet, Karen Martin, et al. 2014. "An Outbreak of Measles in an Undervaccinated Community." *Pediatrics* 134(1): e220–228. doi:10.1542/peds.2013-4260.

Gaudino, James A., and Steve Robison. 2012. "Risk Factors Associated with Parents Claiming Personal-Belief Exemptions to School Immunization Requirements: Community and Other Influences on More Skeptical Parents in Oregon, 2006." *Vaccine* 30(6): 1132–1142. doi:10.1016/j.vaccine.2011.12.006.

Gillette v. United States. 1971. 401 U.S. 437.

Grabenstein, John D. 2013. "What the World's Religions Teach, Applied to Vaccines and Immune Globulins." *Vaccine* 31(16): 2011–2023.

Hansen, Jane. 2013. "Real Churches Denounce Cult of Anti-Vaccine." *Daily Telegraph*, June 9. www.dailytelegraph.com.au/news/nsw/real-churches-denounce-cult-of-anti-vaccine/story-fni0cx12-1226660589245.

Hansen, Jane. 2014. "No Jab, No Play Policy Is Now a Reality across NSW." *Daily Telegraph*, January 2. www.dailytelegraph.com.au/news/nsw/no-jab-no-play-policy-is-now-a-reality-across-nsw/story-fni0cx12-1226793383449.

Hendrix, Kristin S., S. Maria E. Finnell, Gregory D. Zimet, Lynne A. Sturm, Kathleen A. Lane, and Stephen M. Downs. 2014. "Vaccine Message Framing and Parents' Intent to Immunize Their Infants for MMR." *Pediatrics* 134(3): e675–683. doi:10.1542/peds.2013-4077.

Imdad, Aamer, Boldtsetseg Tserenpuntsag, Debra S. Blog, Neal A. Halsey, Delia E. Easton, and Jana Shaw. 2013. "Religious Exemptions for Immunization and

Risk of Pertussis in New York State, 2000–2011." *Pediatrics* 132(1): 37–43. doi:10.1542/peds.2013-3449.

Kahneman, D. 2011. *Thinking, Fast and Slow*. Farrar, Straus and Giroux.

Kaplan, Sarah. 2015. "'Relationship with Jesus' Doesn't Justify Florist's Refusal to Serve Gay Couple, Judge Rules." *The Washington Post*, February 19. www.washingtonpost.com/news/morning-mix/wp/2015/02/19/relationship-with-jesus-doesnt-justify-florists-refusal-to-serve-gay-couple-judge-rules/.

Kitcher, Philip. 2011. *Science in a Democratic Society*. Prometheus Books.

Kramer, Ann. 2013. *Conscientious Objectors of the Second World War: Refusing to Fight*. Pen and Sword.

Lee, Emily Oshima, Lindsay Rosenthal, and Gabriel Scheffler. 2013. *The Effect of Childhood Vaccine Exemptions on Disease Outbreaks*. Center for American Progress, November 14. http://americanprogress.org/issues/healthcare/report/2013/11/14/76471/the-effect-of-childhood-vaccine-exemptions-on-disease-outbreaks/.

Leiter, Brian. 2013. *Why Tolerate Religion?* Princeton University Press.

Lippman, M. 1990. "The Recognition of Conscientious Objection to Military Service as an International Human Right." *California Western International Law Journal* 21(1): 31–66.

Lubell, N. 2002. "Selective Conscientious Objection in International Law: Refusing to Participate in a Specific Armed Conflict." *Netherlands Quarterly of Human Rights* 20(4): 407–422.

Major, M. F. 2001. "Conscientious Objection to Military Service: The European Commission on Human Rights and the Human Rights Committee." *California Western International Law Journal* 32(1): 1–38.

Marcus, E. N. 1997. "Conscientious Objection as an Emerging Human Right." *Virginia Journal of International Law* 38: 507.

May, T., and R. D. Silverman. 2003. "'Clustering of Exemptions' as a Collective Action Threat to Herd Immunity." *Vaccine* 21(11–12): 1048–1051.

May, T., and R. D. Silverman. 2005. "Free-Riding, Fairness and the Rights of Minority Groups in Exemption from Mandatory Childhood Vaccination." *Human Vaccines* 1(1): 12–15.

McGreevy, Patrick, and Rong-Gong Lin II. 2015. "California Gov. Jerry Brown Appears Open to Restricting Vaccine Waivers." *Los Angeles Times*, February 4. www.latimes.com/local/politics/la-me-pol-measles-vaccination-20150205-story.html.

Michigan Department of Public Health. 2015. "Immunization Waiver Information." Accessed March 23. www.michigan.gov/mdch/0,4612,7-132-2942_4911_4914_68361-344843-,00.html.

Moody, Jennifer. 2014. "Exclusion Day Coming up Feb. 19." *Albany Democrat Herald*, January 28. http://democratherald.com/news/local/exclusion-day-coming-up-feb/article_7a038050-87ea-11e3-9062-0019bb2963f4.html.

Muskal, Michael. 2015. "Should Religion Give Businesses an Excuse to Not Serve Gay Couples?" *Los Angeles Times*, February 5. www.latimes.com/nation/la-na-gay-marriage-poll-20150205-story.html.

National Conference of State Legislatures (NCSL). 2012. *States with Religious and Philosophical Exemptions from Immunization Requirements, December 2012*. NCSL. www.ncsl.org/research/health/school-immunization-exemption-state-laws.aspx.

Ngo, Cindy. 2014. "Vaccine Objectors Rise as Parents Skirt 'No Jab, No Play' Law." *The Sydney Morning Herald*, January 11. www.smh.com.au/national/hea

lth/vaccine-objectors-rise-as-parents-skirt-no-jab-no-play-law-20140110-30mil. html.

Nyhan, Brendan, Jason Reifler, Sean Richey, and Gary L. Freed. 2014. "Effective Messages in Vaccine Promotion: A Randomized Trial." *Pediatrics* 133(4): e835– e842. doi:10.1542/peds.2013-2365.

Offit, Paul A. 2010. *Deadly Choices: How the Anti-Vaccine Movement Threatens Us All*. Basic Books.

Omer, S. B., K. S. Enger, L. H. Moulton, N. A. Halsey, S. Stokley, and D. A. Salmon. 2008. "Geographic Clustering of Nonmedical Exemptions to School Immunization Requirements and Associations with Geographic Clustering of Pertussis." *American Journal of Epidemiology* 168(12): 1389–1396.

Omer, S. B., Jennifer Richards, Michelle Ward, and Robert Bednarczyk. 2012. "Vaccination Policies and Rates of Exemption from Immunization, 2005– 2011." *New England Journal of Medicine* 367(12): 1170–1171.

Opel, Douglas J., John Heritage, James A. Taylor, Rita Mangione-Smith, Halle Showalter Salas, Victoria DeVere, Chuan Zhou, and Jeffrey D. Robinson. 2013. "The Architecture of Provider-Parent Vaccine Discussions at Health Supervision Visits." *Pediatrics* 132(6): 1–10. doi:10.1542/peds.2013-2037.

Peralta, Eyder. 2011. "Austrian 'Pastafarian': License Photo Was a Win for Freedom from Religion." *NPR.org*, July 15. www.npr.org/blogs/thetwo-way/ 2011/07/15/138162835/austrian-pastafarian-picture-was-a-win-for-freedom-from-religion.

Porter, D., and R. Porter. 1988. "The Politics of Prevention: Anti-Vaccinationism and Public Health in Nineteenth-Century England." *Medical History* 32(3): 231–252.

Reiss, Dorit Rubinstein. 2014. "Thou Shalt Not Take the Name of the Lord Thy God in Vain: Use and Abuse of Religious Exemptions from School Immunization Requirements." *Hastings Law Journal* 65(6): 1551–1602.

Rockoff, Jonathan D. 2010. "More Parents Seek Vaccine Exemption." *Wall Street Journal*, July 6, sec. New York. http://online.wsj.com/news/articles/ SB10001424052748703322204575226460746977850.

Rota, J. S., D. A. Salmon, L. E. Rodewald, R. T. Chen, B. F. Hibbs, and E. J. Gangarosa. 2001. "Processes for Obtaining Nonmedical Exemptions to State Immunization Laws." *American Journal of Public Health* 91(4): 645–648.

Salmon, Daniel A., M. Haber, E. J. Gangarosa, L. Phillips, N. J. Smith, and R. T. Chen. 1999. "Health Consequences of Religious and Philosophical Exemptions from Immunization Laws." *JAMA: The Journal of the American Medical Association* 282(1): 47–53.

Salmon, Daniel A., Saad B. Omer, Lawrence H. Moulton, Shannon Stokley, M. Patricia Dehart, Susan Lett, Bryan Norman, Stephen Teret, and Neal A. Halsey. 2005. "Exemptions to School Immunization Requirements: The Role of School-Level Requirements, Policies, and Procedures." *American Journal of Public Health* 95(3): 436–440. doi:10.2105/AJPH.2004.046201.

Salmon, Daniel A., Jason W. Sapsin, Stephen Teret, Richard F. Jacobs, Joseph W. Thompson, Kevin Ryan, and Neal A. Halsey. 2005. "Public Health and the Politics of School Immunization Requirements." *American Journal of Public Health* 95(5): 778–783.

Salmon, Daniel A., and Andrew W. Siegel. 2001. "Religious and Philosophical Exemptions from Vaccination Requirements and Lessons Learned from Conscientious Objectors from Conscription." *Public Health Reports* 116(4): 289.

Shute, Nancy. 2013. "How a California Law to Encourage Vaccination Could Backfire." *NPR.org*. November 9. www.npr.org/blogs/health/2013/11/09/243937869/how-a-california-law-to-encourage-vaccination-could-backfire.

State of Missouri. 2014. *Mo. Rev. Stat.* § *167.181, 210.003.* Accessed June 30. www.moga.mo.gov/statutes/C100-199/1670000181.HTM.

State of New Mexico. 2014. *N.M. Stat. Ann.* § *24–5-1, 3.* Accessed June 30. www.nmcpr.state.nm.us/nmac/parts/title07/07.005.0003.htm.

Sutton, Erica J., and Ross E. G. Upshur. 2010. "Are There Different Spheres of Conscience?" *Journal of Evaluation in Clinical Practice* 16(2): 338–343.

Swaine, Lucas. 2008. *The Liberal Conscience: Politics and Principle in a World of Religious Pluralism.* Columbia University Press.

Szabo, Liz. 2012. "Lawmakers Weigh Boosting School-Age Vaccines." *USA Today*, August 19. www.usatoday.com/news/health/story/2012-08-19/school children-vaccinations/57146910/1.

Takemura, H. 2009. *International Human Right to Conscientious Objection to Military Service and Individual Duties to Disobey Manifestly Illegal Orders.* Springer Verlag.

Thaler, Richard H., and Cass R. Sunstein. 2009. *Nudge: Improving Decisions about Health, Wealth, and Happiness.* Penguin Books.

United Nations General Assembly. 1948. *Universal Declaration of Human Rights.*

United States v. Seeger. 1965. 380 U.S. 176.

USA Today Editorial Board. 2014. "Vaccine Opt-Outs Put Public Health at Risk: Our View." *USA Today*, April 13. www.usatoday.com/story/opinion/2014/04/13/vaccines-measles-misinformation-risks-editorials-debates/7682093/.

U.S. Department of State. 2014. "Frequently Asked Questions – Photo Requirements." *U.S. Passports & International Travel.* Accessed June 24. http://travel.state.gov/content/passports/english/passports/photos/frequently-asked-questions.html#Photo.

WAMC Editor. 2014. "Debate in Colorado Grows Over Child Vaccinations." *WAMC Northeast Public Radio*, January 20. http://wamc.org/post/debate-colorado-grows-over-child-vaccinations.

Warner, Trevor. 2014. "New Law Changes Immunization Rules for Children." *Paradise Post*, January 24. www.paradisepost.com/breaking-news/ci_24988268/new-law-changes-immunization-rules-children.

Wynia, Matthew K. 2006. "Ethics and Public Health Emergencies: Rationing Vaccines." *The American Journal of Bioethics* 6(6): 4–7.

Wynia, Matthew K. 2007. "Mandating Vaccination: What Counts as a 'Mandate' in Public Health and When Should They Be Used?" *The American Journal of Bioethics* 7(12): 2–6.

Yang, Y. Tony, and Vicky Debold. 2014. "A Longitudinal Analysis of the Effect of Nonmedical Exemption Law and Vaccine Uptake on Vaccine-Targeted Disease Rates." *American Journal of Public Health* 104(2): 371–377.

Conclusion

I think vaccine refusal is usually immoral and that it is often based on false beliefs or unreasonable values. But vaccine refusers are neither irrational nor evil, and they often have good epistemic and moral reasons to refuse vaccines. Their failure to make the right choice is often an understandable consequence of a commendable commitment to make informed decisions about their children's health care. Time and again, I have argued that we can best understand and evaluate vaccine refusal by focusing on the ways in which parental decisions about vaccination are influenced by contested values and by unfortunate social and political circumstances, rather than by the moral and epistemic failures of individuals.

In an ideal world, parents would defer to the recommendations of their children's pediatricians. But parents may have good reasons to be less deferential. Indeed, the more parents learn about the historical and contemporary shortcomings of mainstream medicine – including its frequent cooptation by business interests – the more reasonable it may be for parents to rely on their own judgments (or on the judgments of their resistant epistemic communities). And vaccine refusers often live in do-it-yourself cultures that value epistemic individualism. Unfortunately, epistemic self-reliance is a cardinal cognitive bias. In the absence of adequate practices of accountability and adversariality, self-confidence frequently leads people towards false beliefs when they are considering complicated phenomena outside their expertise, and especially when they are motivated by fear.

Vaccine refusers often live in societies where public institutions are failing and where hyper-individualistic moral and political ideologies are ascendant. For example, citizens of the United States place record low levels of trust in their public institutions (Gallup 2014). And the societies that have the highest rates of vaccine refusal (especially the United States) also do the least to support parents and families (Pew Research Center 2013; UNICEF Innocenti Research Centre 2012). Neoliberal attacks on the welfare state further undermine trust in public institutions, and give parents another reason to prioritize their children's interests. If the public is not going to protect their children, why should parents risk harming their children to protect the public?

I conclude this book by identifying ways in which my arguments could inform public policy debates about vaccine refusal. I tread carefully. Decisions about public policy ought to be enlightened by forms of knowledge and expertise that I lack. However, I think this book supports three broad theses about vaccination policy.

First, making things better is likely to be difficult. Values often contribute to vaccine refusal, but value-based disagreement is often intractable. For example, if someone is a vaccine refuser because she is committed to an 'ethics of purity', then better education about the low risks of vaccine complications is unlikely to change her mind. And it is not clear how or whether public health authorities should try to convince parents that an 'ethics of purity' (or any other value system) is unreasonable or unrealizable. For another example, some people seem committed to vaccine refusal because of their libertarian social and political ideals, but representatives from government institutions are extremely unlikely to convince people to abandon libertarianism.

It will also be difficult to change the social and political conditions that contribute to vaccine denialism and refusal. I have argued that parental distrust of mainstream medical authorities – and parental rejection of paternalistic styles of medicine – may sometimes contribute to vaccine denialism. (Furthermore, paternalistic styles of medicine may be informed by broader forms of gender inequality.) But reforming the practices of mainstream medicine and promoting greater gender equality are enormous tasks, and are far beyond the abilities of public health officials acting in isolation.

Second, making things worse is likely to be easy. We are very fortunate that vaccine denialism and refusal are not yet strongly correlated with a particular political ideology. This is unlike many other areas of popular science contestation, including debates surrounding climate change (Kahan et al. 2012). But things can change quickly. For example, as late as the mid-1990s, beliefs about climate change were not yet strongly correlated with political ideology among the general public, but now this correlation is dramatic (McCright and Dunlap 2011). I am worried that beliefs about coercive vaccination policy (though not yet vaccine science) have become increasingly correlated with political ideology. For example, in 2012 the Texas Republican party added the following to its platform: "All adult citizens should have the legal right to conscientiously choose which vaccines are administered to themselves, or their minor children, without penalty for refusing a vaccine" (Republican Party of Texas 2012). In contrast, the Center for American Progress, one of the most prominent left-leaning think tanks in the United States, released a 2013 report that called for greater restrictions on nonmedical vaccine exemptions, and that proposed an outline for model national vaccine exemption legislation (Lee, Rosenthal, and Scheffler 2013). It is disheartening that the race for the 2016 Republican presidential nomination began with a critical discussion of vaccine policy, led by Senator Paul Ryan and Governor Chris Christie. Of course, it's fine to debate vaccine policy. But I worry that criticizing vaccine policy in the context of a presidential campaign is likely to pollute the science communication environment and cause otherwise avoidable political polarization surrounding vaccine science and vaccination policy (Kahan 2013).

Finally, there are reasons to be hopeful. Mainstream medical institutions are now much less likely to lend legitimacy to vaccine denialism than they were in the past. The most famous example was the 1998 Wakefield et al. paper from *The Lancet*, but papers (believed to be) sympathetic to vaccine denialism were also published by other mainstream journals. And organizations such as CDC and AAP lent legitimacy to vaccine fears when they pushed to have thimerosal removed from vaccines, absent any evidence that this ingredient was harmful (Centers for Disease Control and Prevention 1999; Centers for Disease Control and Prevention 2001). Those days are gone. This is not only because questions about the supposed link between vaccines and autism have been definitively answered by research scientists, but also because mainstream medical institutions are on greater alert to avoid inadvertently granting legitimacy to vaccine denialist views.

Another reason to be hopeful about the future of vaccination policy is that current and future outbreaks of communicable diseases may be sufficiently frightening to encourage parents to vaccinate, and to encourage communities to make it more difficult for parents to receive vaccine exemptions. This is a sad occasion for hope, and it is regrettable that people may have to get sick and die for rates of vaccine refusal to decline. Unfortunately, small outbreaks – such as the 2011–2012 pertussis outbreak in Washington state – may be insufficient to increase vaccination rates (Wolf et al. 2014). But we may hope that we will not have to witness the complete collapse of herd immunity before parents change their minds.

Bibliography

Centers for Disease Control and Prevention. 1999. "Thimerosal in Vaccines: A Joint Statement of the American Academy of Pediatrics and the Public Health Service." July 9. www.cdc.gov/mmwr/preview/mmwrhtml/mm4826a3.htm.

Centers for Disease Control and Prevention. 2001. "Impact of the 1999 AAP/USPHS Joint Statement on Thimerosal in Vaccines on Infant Hepatitis B Vaccination Practices." *Morbidity and Mortality Weekly Report (MMWR)* 50(6): 94.

Gallup. 2014. *Americans Losing Confidence in All Branches of U.S. Gov't.* Gallup, June 30. www.gallup.com/poll/171992/americans-losing-confidence-branches-gov.aspx.

Kahan, Dan M. 2013. "A Risky Science Communication Environment for Vaccines." *Science* 342(6154): 53–54.

Kahan, Dan M., Ellen Peters, Maggie Wittlin, Paul Slovic, Lisa Larrimore Ouellette, Donald Braman, and Gregory Mandel. 2012. "The Polarizing Impact of

Science Literacy and Numeracy on Perceived Climate Change Risks." *Nature Climate Change* 2(10): 732–735.

Lee, Emily Oshima, Lindsay Rosenthal, and Gabriel Scheffler. 2013. *The Effect of Childhood Vaccine Exemptions on Disease Outbreaks.* Center for American Progress, November 14. http://americanprogress.org/issues/healthcare/report/2013/11/14/76471/the-effect-of-childhood-vaccine-exemptions-on-disease-outbreaks/.

McCright, Aaron M., and Riley E. Dunlap. 2011. "The Politicization of Climate Change and Polarization in the American Public's Views of Global Warming, 2001–2010." *The Sociological Quarterly* 52(2): 155–194.

Pew Research Center. 2013. *Among 38 Nations, U.S. Is the Outlier When It Comes to Paid Parental Leave,* December 12. www.pewresearch.org/fact-tank/2013/12/12/among-38-nations-u-s-is-the-holdout-when-it-comes-to-offering-paid-parental-leave/.

Republican Party of Texas. 2012. *Report of Platform Committee.* Republican Party of Texas. www.texasgop.org/wp-content/themes/rpt/images/2012Platform_Final.pdf.

UNICEF Innocenti Research Centre. 2012. *Measuring Child Poverty: New League Tables of Child Poverty in the World's Richest Countries.* Innocenti Report Card 10. UNICEF International Research Centre, May. www.unicef-irc.org/publications/pdf/rc10_eng.pdf.

Wolf, Elizabeth R., Douglas Opel, M. Patricia DeHart, Jodi Warren, and Ali Rowhani-Rahbar. 2014. "Impact of a Pertussis Epidemic on Infant Vaccination in Washington State." *Pediatrics* 134(3): 456–464. doi:10.1542/peds.2013-3637.

Index